Medical Terminology

MASTERING THE BASICS

Second Edition

By

Cindy Destafano, BS, RT(R)
Instructor
Radiologic Technologist
Conestoga, Pennsylvania

Fran Federman, MSEd
Instructor/Educational Consultant
York, Pennsylvania

Publisher
The Goodheart-Willcox Company, Inc.
Tinley Park, IL
www.g-w.com

The Goodheart-Willcox Company, Inc. Brand Disclaimer: Brand names, company names, and illustrations for products and services included in this text are provided for educational purposes only and do not represent or imply endorsement or recommendation by the author or the publisher.

The Goodheart-Willcox Company, Inc. Safety Notice: The reader is expressly advised to carefully read, understand, and apply all safety precautions and warnings described in this book or that might also be indicated in undertaking the activities and exercises described herein to minimize risk of personal injury or injury to others. Common sense and good judgment should also be exercised and applied to help avoid all potential hazards. The reader should always refer to the appropriate manufacturer's technical information, directions, and recommendations; then proceed with care to follow specific equipment operating instructions. The reader should understand these notices and cautions are not exhaustive.

The publisher makes no warranty or representation whatsoever, either expressed or implied, including but not limited to equipment, procedures, and applications described or referred to herein, their quality, performance, merchantability, or fitness for a particular purpose. The publisher assumes no responsibility for any changes, errors, or omissions in this book. The publisher specifically disclaims any liability whatsoever, including any direct, indirect, incidental, consequential, special, or exemplary damages resulting, in whole or in part, from the reader's use or reliance upon the information, instructions, procedures, warnings, cautions, applications, or other matter contained in this book. The publisher assumes no responsibility for the activities of the reader.

The Goodheart-Willcox Company, Inc. Internet Disclaimer: The Internet resources and listings in this Goodheart-Willcox Publisher product are provided solely as a convenience to you. These resources and listings were reviewed at the time of publication to provide you with accurate, safe, and appropriate information. Goodheart-Willcox Publisher has no control over the referenced websites and, due to the dynamic nature of the Internet, is not responsible or liable for the content, products, or performance of links to other websites or resources. Goodheart-Willcox Publisher makes no representation, either expressed or implied, regarding the content of these websites, and such references do not constitute an endorsement or recommendation of the information or content presented. It is your responsibility to take all protective measures to guard against inappropriate content, viruses, or other destructive elements.

Cover Image Credit: kurhan/Shutterstock.com

Names: Destafano, Cindy, author. | Federman, Fran M., author.
Title: Medical terminology : mastering the basics / by Cindy Destafano, Fran Federman.
Description: Second edition. | Tinley Park, IL : Goodheart-Willcox Company, Inc., [2020] | Includes index.
Identifiers: LCCN 2018032042 | ISBN 9781635636062
Subjects: | MESH: Terminology as Topic | Problems and Exercises
Classification: LCC R123 | NLM W 18.2 | DDC 610.1/4--dc23 LC record available at https://lccn.loc.gov/2018032042

Brief Contents

Chapter 1   Introduction to Medical Terminology 2

Chapter 2   The Integumentary System 44

Chapter 3   The Digestive System 88

Chapter 4   The Musculoskeletal System 132

Cumulative Review: Chapters 2–4 190

Chapter 5   The Lymphatic and Immune Systems 194

Chapter 6   Special Sensory Organs: Eye and Ear 236

Chapter 7   The Nervous System 278

Cumulative Review: Chapters 5–7 318

Chapter 8   The Male and Female Reproductive Systems 322

Chapter 9   The Respiratory System 364

Chapter 10   The Cardiovascular System 402

Cumulative Review: Chapters 8–10 440

Chapter 11   The Endocrine System 444

Chapter 12   The Urinary System 482

Cumulative Review: Chapters 11–12 525

Appendix A   Medical Word Elements 528

Appendix B   Medical Abbreviations and Acronyms 535

Index 536

About the Authors

Cindy Destafano, as an instructor at the Consolidated School of Business in Lancaster, Pennsylvania, has taught courses in a variety of allied health subjects, including medical terminology, anatomy and physiology, law and ethics for medical careers, medical coding, and medical transcription. She was also the program coordinator for the Medical Administrative Assistant degree program, for which she developed and wrote the curriculum. Before joining the Consolidated School of Business, she served as the program director for the Radiologic Technology degree program at Lancaster Regional Medical Center and taught courses in medical imaging. Destafano is the coauthor of *Essentials of Medical Transcription*, *Advanced Medical Transcription*, and *The Mentor Program Workbook*. She is a member of the American Society of Radiologic Technology and the American Registry of Radiologic Technology. She is a graduate of Elizabethtown College with a bachelor of science in business administration. Destafano is also a registered radiologic technologist and graduated from the Lancaster General Hospital School of Radiologic Technology.

Fran Federman served for many years as a business instructor and educational consultant in York, Pennsylvania. She taught courses in the Microsoft Office software suite, business principles, entrepreneurship, accounting, and medical billing and reimbursement. She has also developed curricula for a variety of subjects, including business management, personal finance, and sports marketing. After earning a bachelor of science degree in business education from the City University of New York (CUNY), Federman obtained a teaching certificate and launched her career as a business education instructor. She was a curriculum director for the Consolidated School of Business, where she assisted in the development and coordination of internship and cooperative programs. She holds a master of science degree in education from Virginia Tech and completed additional postgraduate coursework at Gratz College. Federman is the author or coauthor of several books and journal articles, including *Essentials of Medical Transcription*, *Advanced Medical Transcription*, *The Mentor Program Workbook*, and *The Role of the Business Teacher in Guidance*. Federman continues to provide consulting services.

New to This Edition

The second edition of *Medical Terminology: Mastering the Basics* has been updated with new, improved digital offerings; clear, detailed images; and updated content:

- **EduHub:** This edition includes a subscription to the new EduHub platform. EduHub enables students and instructors to access premium digital content, such as autograded activities, audio pronunciations of medical terms, and print and digital flash cards, all in one place. EduHub also includes the interactive eBook for this text with note-taking, magnification, and highlighting features.
- **Photography Program:** The photography program for *Medical Terminology: Mastering the Basics* was enhanced for this edition. New photographs of diseases, including acromegaly, psoriasis, and osteomyelitis, were added to improve student understanding of symptoms and pathology.
- **Illustration Program:** New, professionally rendered illustrations were created to help students visualize medical terms. Some of these new illustrations include those showing anatomical terms of position, direction, and location and diseases such as bursitis and joint effusion.
- **Updated Content:** Updates were made to ensure the medical language in this text is current and in line with today's healthcare field. For example, this edition refers to *sexually transmitted infections (STIs)* in place of *sexually transmitted diseases (STDs)*.

Guided Tour

Teach and test the meanings of medical word parts

Knowing the meanings of word parts is the first, foundational step toward mastering medical terminology. In *Medical Terminology: Mastering the Basics*, prefixes, combining forms, and suffixes are introduced in clear, easy-to-read charts organized by body system. This organization helps students relate medical word parts to anatomy concepts and understand and memorize the pieces that make up a medical term. Review opportunities include matching exercises in the book, cumulative reviews, and e-flash cards available on EduHub.

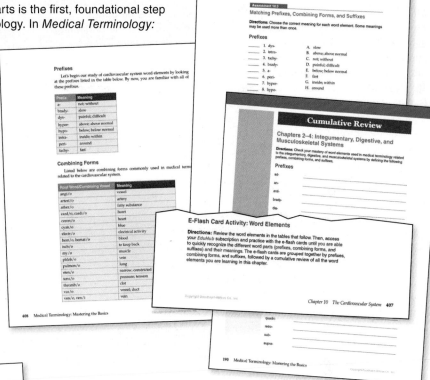

Expand students' medical vocabularies

Interactive, hands-on activities challenge students to recall and apply their knowledge of medical word parts. Activities can be completed both in the text and online. In each chapter, common medical terms related to anatomy and physiology, diagnostic tests and procedures, and therapeutic treatments are introduced. A phonetic spelling for each term is provided, and audio pronunciations of terms are available on EduHub. *Break It Down* and *Build It* activities provide the opportunity to dissect and form medical terms. These activities reinforce understanding of common medical terms and demonstrate how knowing word parts improves the comprehension of unfamiliar terms.

Guided Tour

Prepare students for the field of healthcare

Medical Terminology: Mastering the Basics teaches the language needed to enter the field of healthcare with confidence. At the beginning of each chapter, *Intern Experience* scenarios are presented. These scenarios feature diverse types of healthcare professionals and conditions, illustrating how medical terminology is used to handle healthcare situations and communicate with patients and coworkers. Near the end of each chapter, students will revisit the *Intern Experience* scenario and use their knowledge of medical terminology to interpret a medical record related to the scenario. An audio recording of this medical record is available on EduHub to provide practice listening to and interpreting medical language.

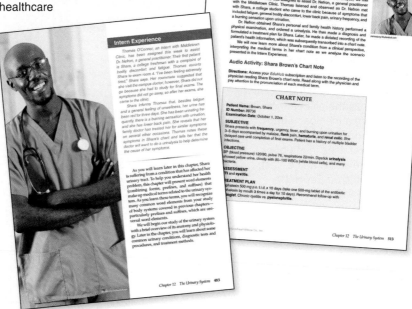

Provide practice interpreting medical records

Like any language, medical terminology is both written and spoken. *Medical Terminology: Mastering the Basics*'s write-in format provides many opportunities to write and read medical terms. At the end of each chapter, written and audio medical records can be interpreted using the medical terms learned. The EduHub subscription accompanying this text offers the opportunity to listen to medical records and identify and define medical terms. Practice with interpreting medical records will prepare students to enter the healthcare field.

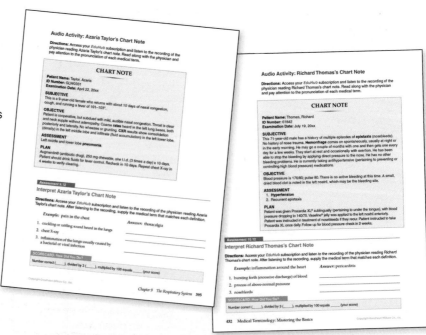

Guided Tour

Show how medical terminology relates to anatomy

Medical Terminology: Mastering the Basics is organized by body system, relating new word parts to the structures of the human body. Learning about the 11 body systems will help students visualize and apply medical terms, and each chapter begins with a brief anatomy overview to introduce medical terms related to that body system. Detailed, professional illustrations bring the structures of the human body to life and demonstrate the locations of body parts and anatomical terms related to position and direction.

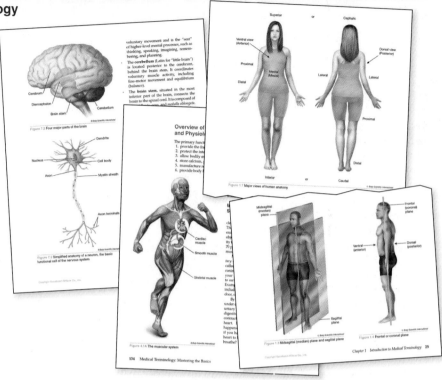

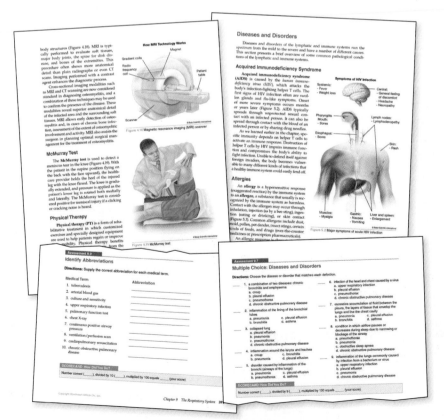

Introduce common diseases and disorders, procedures, and treatments

Each chapter in *Medical Terminology: Mastering the Basics* includes medical terms related to common diseases and disorders, diagnostic tests and procedures, and therapeutic treatments. Easy-to-follow explanations introduce conditions and treatments, and detailed illustrations provide visuals of the words presented. Multiple choice and fill-in-the-blank activities challenge students to recall and use these terms and their abbreviations, strengthening understanding.

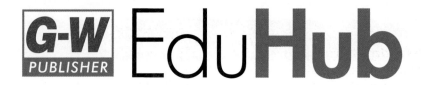

Be Digital Ready on Day One with EduHub

EduHub provides a solid base of knowledge and instruction for digital and blended classrooms. This easy-to-use learning hub delivers the foundation and tools that improve student retention and facilitate instructor efficiency. For the student, EduHub offers an online collection of eBook content, interactive practice, and test preparation. Additionally, students have the ability to view and submit assessments, track personal performance, and view feedback via the Student Report option. For instructors, EduHub provides a turnkey, fully integrated solution with course management tools to deliver content, assessments, and feedback to students quickly and efficiently. The integrated approach results in improved student outcomes and instructor flexibility.

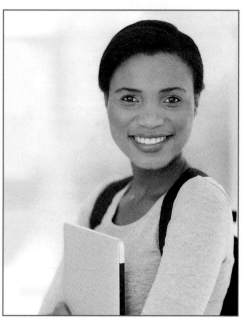

Michael Jung/Shutterstock.com

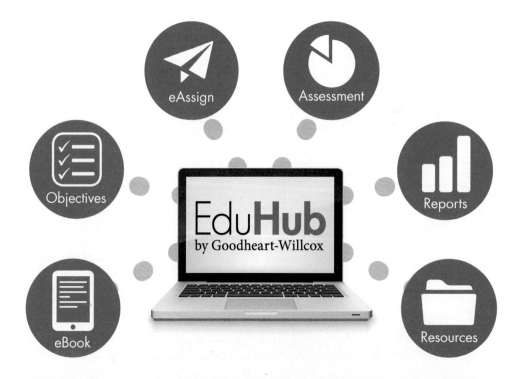

eBook

The EduHub eBook engages students by providing the ability to take notes to improve comprehension and highlight key concepts to remember. The fixed layout maintains the look and feel of a printed textbook, while links to vocabulary practice activities, e-flash cards, and audio pronunciations and recordings provide reinforcement and enrich understanding.

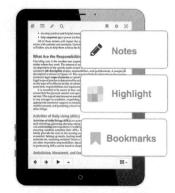

Objectives

Course objectives at the beginning of each eBook chapter help students stay focused and provide benchmarks for instructors to evaluate student progress.

eAssign

eAssign makes it easy for instructors to assign, deliver, and assess student engagement. Coursework can be administered to individual students or the entire class.

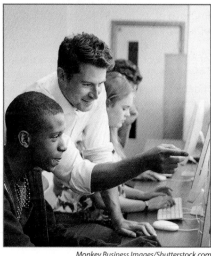

Monkey Business Images/Shutterstock.com

Assessment

Self-assessment opportunities enable students to gauge their understanding as they progress through the course. In addition, formative assessment tools for instructor use provide efficient evaluation of student mastery of content.

	🖨 Print	⬇ Export
Score	**Items**	
100%	⦿	⦿
80%	⦿	●
100%	⦿	⦿
80%	⦿	●
100%	⦿	⦿
100%	⦿	⦿

Reports

Reports, for both students and instructors, provide performance results in an instant. Analytics reveal individual student and class achievements for easy monitoring of success.

Instructor Resources

Instructors will find all the support they need to make preparation and classroom instruction more efficient and easier than ever. Lesson plans, answer keys, and PowerPoint® presentations provide an organized, proven approach to classroom management.

Learn more about EduHub at www.g-w.com/eduhub

EduHub

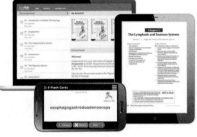

EduHub provides a solid base of knowledge and instruction for digital and blended classrooms. This easy-to-use learning hub provides the foundation and tools that improve student retention and facilitate instructor efficiency.

For the student, EduHub offers an online collection of eBook content, interactive practice, and test preparation. Additionally, students have the ability to manage class activity and assignments, track personal performance, and view feedback via the Student Report option. For instructors, EduHub provides a turnkey, fully integrated solution with course management tools to deliver content, assessments, and feedback to students quickly and efficiently. The integrated approach results in improved student outcomes and instructor flexibility. Be digital ready on day one with EduHub!

- *eBook Content*: EduHub includes the text in an online format. The eBook is interactive, with highlighting, magnification, and note-taking features.
- *Vocabulary Practice*: E-flash cards are available for the word parts and vocabulary terms introduced in each chapter. Flash cards can be printed or reviewed online with accompanying audio pronunciations. Additional vocabulary practice games help students review word parts and terminology.
- *Audio Pronunciations*: A complete audio glossary includes audio pronunciations of the medical terms in each chapter, giving students the tools they need to interpret and communicate. Audio recordings of medical records in the text also provide practice listening to the language of medicine and comprehending important terms and abbreviations.
- *Assignments*: In EduHub, students can complete the text activities online. Instructors can assign activities and chapter tests that challenge students to define word parts, break down and build medical terms, use medical dictionaries to answer questions, and interpret medical records. Many activities are autograded for easy class assessment and management.

Student Tools

Student Text

Medical Terminology: Mastering the Basics is an interactive, online and print work text that leverages a printed book and interactive digital activities to help students learn the language of medicine (introduce and reinforce). Through numerous activities, students will learn the meanings of word parts and spell, pronounce, break down, and build medical terms integral to the field of health sciences. Organized by body system, this work text covers essential root words, prefixes, suffixes, and abbreviations and also summarizes common diseases and disorders, diagnostic tests and procedures, and therapeutic treatments. Students will not only learn, but will also practice, using these terms as they interpret written and audio examples of medical records and become comfortable with the word parts they need to master medical terminology.

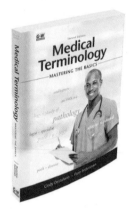

Instructor Tools

Annotated Instructor's Edition

The Instructor's Edition for *Medical Terminology: Mastering the Basics* includes the full student text and instructional resources and pacing charts for course planning. This edition also includes in-line answers for all of the activities in the text, making it easy to plan, review, and grade assignments.

LMS Integration

Integrate Goodheart-Willcox content in your Learning Management System for a seamless user experience for both you and your students. Contact your G-W Educational Consultant for ordering information or visit www.g-w.com/lms-integration.

Instructor Resources

The Instructor Resources provide all the support needed to make preparation and classroom instruction easier than ever. Included are the annotated Instructor's Edition for *Medical Terminology: Mastering the Basics* and time-saving preparation tools such as answer keys, editable lesson plans, chapter outlines and handouts, and other teaching aids. In addition, presentations for PowerPoint® and assessment software with question banks are provided for your convenience. These resources can be accessed at school, at home, or on the go.

Instructor's Presentations for PowerPoint®

Instructor's Presentations for PowerPoint® provide a useful teaching tool when presenting the concepts introduced in the text. These fully customizable, richly illustrated slides help you teach and visually reinforce the key concepts from each chapter. Slides include the list of Chapter Objectives; reviews of word parts and abbreviations; and illustrations of common diseases and disorders, diagnostic procedures, and therapeutic treatments.

Assessment Software with Question Banks

Administer and manage assessments to meet your classroom needs. The following options are available through the Respondus Test Bank Network.

- A Respondus 4.0 license can be purchased directly from Respondus, which enables you to easily create tests that can be printed on paper or published directly to a variety of Learning Management Systems. Once the question files are published to an LMS, exams can be distributed to students with results reported directly to the LMS gradebook.

- Respondus LE is a limited version of Respondus 4.0 and is free with purchase of the Instructor Resources. It allows you to download test banks and create assessments that can be printed or saved as a paper test.

G-W Integrated Learning Solution

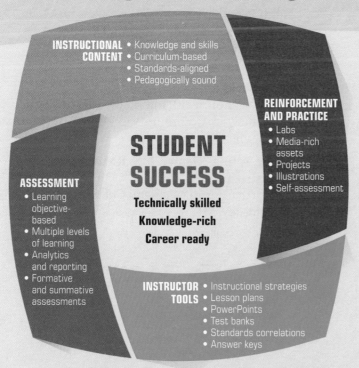

INSTRUCTIONAL CONTENT
- Knowledge and skills
- Curriculum-based
- Standards-aligned
- Pedagogically sound

REINFORCEMENT AND PRACTICE
- Labs
- Media-rich assets
- Projects
- Illustrations
- Self-assessment

STUDENT SUCCESS

Technically skilled
Knowledge-rich
Career ready

ASSESSMENT
- Learning objective-based
- Multiple levels of learning
- Analytics and reporting
- Formative and summative assessments

INSTRUCTOR TOOLS
- Instructional strategies
- Lesson plans
- PowerPoints
- Test banks
- Standards correlations
- Answer keys

The G-W Integrated Learning Solution offers easy-to-use resources that help students and instructors achieve success.

▶ **EXPERT AUTHORS**
▶ **TRUSTED REVIEWERS**
▶ **100 YEARS OF EXPERIENCE**

EMPLOYABILITY SKILLS · TECHNICAL SKILLS · ACADEMIC KNOWLEDGE · INDUSTRY RECOGNIZED STANDARDS

Reviewers

Goodheart-Willcox Publisher would also like to thank the following instructors who reviewed selected manuscript chapters and provided valuable input into the development of this textbook program.

Muriel Adams
Instructor
Prince George's Community College
Largo, MD

Emily Bedsted
Instructor
Anoka-Hennepin School District
Anoka, MN

Jane Best
Instructor
Chesapeake Public Schools
Chesapeake, VA

Amy Bledsoe
Instructor
Spokane Community College
Spokane, WA

Deborah Clarke
Instructor
Littleton Public Schools
Littleton, CO

Molly Day, RRT, RCP, BS Ed
Allied Health Instructor
Bainbridge State College
Bainbridge, GA

Tina Evans, PhD
Associate Professor of Health Sciences
Pennsylvania College of Technology
Williamsport, PA

Coleen Kumar, RN, MS
Professor of Nursing
Kingsborough Community College
Brooklyn, NY

Dr. Amy Lemkuil
Health and Safety Instructor
Madison Area Technical College
Madison, WI

Joan Lynch, RN, MS, MA
Medical Terminology Instructor
Academy of Allied Health and Science
Neptune, NJ

Veronique Parker
Health Professions Program Director
Phoenix College
Phoenix, AZ

Maryanna Perry
Instructor
Franklin Technology Center
Joplin, MO

Laura Sargent, MA, RN
Medical Terminology Instructor
Academy of Allied Health and Science
Neptune, NJ

Leslie Watson, BBA, RT
Associate Instructor
Virginia Western Community College
Roanoke, VA

Heidi Weingart
Medical Assisting Program Director
Santa Fe Community College
Santa Fe, NM

Zada Wicker
Director of Health Information Technology
Brunswick Community College
Bolivia, NC

Sonya Young-Riemer, MS, RMA, LCMT
Instructor
North Central Michigan College
Petoskey, MI

Contents

Chapter 1 Introduction to Medical Terminology 2

  Brief Overview of Medical Terminology 4

  Analyzing and Defining Medical Terms 6

  Medical Word Parts 9

    Prefixes 9

    Root Words and Combining Forms 10

    Suffixes 11

  Breaking Down and Building Medical Terms 14

    Breaking Down Medical Terms: Summary of Steps 14

    Building Medical Terms: Summary of Steps 17

  Building Plural Forms 21

  Pronouncing Medical Terms 22

  Spelling Medical Terms 24

  Overview of Anatomical Positions, Planes,
    Directions, and Locations 24

  Body Cavities 32

  Common Medical Abbreviations for Anatomical Terms
    of Position, Direction, and Location 34

  Body Systems 35

  Mastering Medical Terminology 38

  Chapter Review 39

Chapter 2 The Integumentary System 44

  Intern Experience 45

  Overview of Integumentary System Anatomy and Physiology 46

  Word Elements 50

  Breaking Down and Building Integumentary System Terms 54

  Diseases and Disorders 69

  Procedures and Treatments 73

  Analyzing the Intern Experience 77

  Working with Medical Records 78

  Chapter Review 81

Chapter 3   **The Digestive System** 88

Intern Experience. 89

Overview of Digestive System Anatomy and Physiology. 90

Word Elements. 94

Breaking Down and Building Digestive System Terms 100

Diseases and Disorders 110

Procedures and Treatments 114

Analyzing the Intern Experience 120

Working with Medical Records 121

Chapter Review 124

Chapter 4   **The Musculoskeletal System**. 132

Intern Experience. 133

Overview of Musculoskeletal System Anatomy and Physiology. 134

Word Elements. 140

Breaking Down and Building Musculoskeletal System Terms 146

Diseases and Disorders 162

Procedures and Treatments 168

Analyzing the Intern Experience 175

Working with Medical Records 176

Chapter Review 179

Cumulative Review: Chapters 2–4 190

Chapter 5   **The Lymphatic and Immune Systems**. .194

Intern Experience. 195

Overview of Lymphatic and Immune System
Anatomy and Physiology 196

Word Elements. 202

Breaking Down and Building Terms Related to the
Lymphatic and Immune Systems 205

Diseases and Disorders 215

Procedures and Treatments 219

Analyzing the Intern Experience 224

Working with Medical Records 225

Chapter Review 228

Chapter 6   **Special Sensory Organs: Eye and Ear** 236

    Intern Experience. 237

    Overview of Anatomy and Physiology of the Eye and Ear 238

    Word Elements. 243

    Breaking Down and Building Terms Related
      to the Eye and Ear. 248

    Diseases and Disorders 259

    Procedures and Treatments 263

    Analyzing the Intern Experience 270

    Working with Medical Records 271

    Chapter Review 273

Chapter 7   **The Nervous System** 278

    Intern Experience. 279

    Overview of Nervous System Anatomy and Physiology 280

    Word Elements. 285

    Breaking Down and Building Nervous System Terms 289

    Diseases and Disorders 296

    Procedures and Treatments 300

    Analyzing the Intern Experience 307

    Working with Medical Records 308

    Chapter Review 312

Cumulative Review: Chapters 5–7 318

Chapter 8   **The Male and Female Reproductive Systems**. 322

    Intern Experience. 323

    Overview of Reproductive System Anatomy and Physiology 324

    Word Elements. 328

    Breaking Down and Building Reproductive System Terms 332

    Diseases and Disorders 342

    Procedures and Treatments 347

    Analyzing the Intern Experience 354

    Working with Medical Records 355

    Chapter Review 358

Chapter 9   The Respiratory System 364

Intern Experience. 365

Overview of Respiratory System Anatomy and Physiology. 366

Word Elements. 369

Breaking Down and Building Respiratory System Terms 373

Diseases and Disorders 382

Procedures and Treatments 386

Analyzing the Intern Experience 392

Working with Medical Records 393

Chapter Review 396

Chapter 10   The Cardiovascular System 402

Intern Experience. 403

Overview of Cardiovascular System Anatomy and Physiology. 404

Word Elements. 407

Breaking Down and Building Cardiovascular System Terms 412

Diseases and Disorders 420

Procedures and Treatments 423

Analyzing the Intern Experience 429

Working with Medical Records 430

Chapter Review 433

Cumulative Review: Chapters 8–10 440

Chapter 11   The Endocrine System 444

Intern Experience. 445

Overview of Endocrine System Anatomy and Physiology. 446

Word Elements. 450

Breaking Down and Building Endocrine System Terms. 453

Diseases and Disorders 462

Tests and Procedures 466

Analyzing the Intern Experience 472

Working with Medical Records 473

Chapter Review 477

Chapter 12   The Urinary System 482

    Intern Experience. 483

    Overview of Urinary System Anatomy and Physiology 484

    Word Elements. 488

    Breaking Down and Building Urinary System Terms 493

    Diseases and Disorders 504

    Procedures and Treatments 507

    Analyzing the Intern Experience 513

    Working with Medical Records 514

    Chapter Review 518

Cumulative Review: Chapters 11–12 525

Appendix A   Medical Word Elements 528

Appendix B   Medical Abbreviations and Acronyms 535

Index 536

Chapter 1

Introduction to Medical Terminology

Chapter Organization

- Brief Overview of Medical Terminology
- Analyzing and Defining Medical Terms
- Medical Word Parts
- Breaking Down and Building Medical Terms
- Building Plural Forms
- Pronouncing Medical Terms
- Spelling Medical Terms
- Overview of Anatomical Positions, Planes, Directions, and Locations
- Body Cavities
- Common Medical Abbreviations for Anatomical Terms of Position, Direction, and Location
- Body Systems
- Mastering Medical Terminology
- Chapter Review

Chapter Objectives

After completing this chapter, you will be able to

1. describe the origins of medical language;
2. identify the four basic word parts that form many medical terms;
3. describe characteristics of prefixes, combining forms, and suffixes;
4. explain the differences between prefixes, suffixes, root words, and combining vowels;
5. understand that the process of building and dissecting a medical term based on its prefix, root word, and suffix enables you to analyze an extremely large number of medical terms beyond those presented in this chapter;
6. pronounce and spell medical terms introduced in this chapter;
7. recognize common Latin and Greek singular nouns and form their plurals;
8. identify the anatomical planes of the human body;
9. identify major anatomical positions, locations, and directions; and
10. identify the eleven body systems and cite their primary functions.

Your *EduHub* subscription that accompanies this text provides access to online assessments, assignments, activities, and resources. Throughout this chapter, access *EduHub* to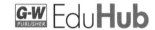

- use e-flash cards to review the medical terminology and word parts you learn;
- listen to the correct pronunciations of medical terms; and
- complete medical terminology activities and assignments.

Before you begin this chapter...

Welcome to medical terminology! Why are you taking this class? Perhaps your school catalog states that you must take this course if you want to pursue a career in the healthcare profession. But why is it necessary to begin with medical terminology? Why not just start with coursework in anatomy and physiology or dive right into the study of diseases and disorders?

Whether your goal is a career in nursing, medical assisting, physical therapy, pharmacology, or any other medical profession, all of these careers begin with an understanding of medical terminology, the language of medicine. When you are at work, the medical community—your coworkers and other healthcare professionals with whom you will have daily contact—will expect you to "speak the language." Being able to speak this language means that you can read and interpret medical documents and correctly write, spell, and pronounce medical terms.

The ability to understand and correctly use medical terminology is essential to your success in the healthcare field. Besides having an outstanding GPA and an excellent attendance record, you need to "walk the talk." This is why you are taking a medical terminology class. Now, let's get started!

Good Luck!

Cindy Destafano and Fran Federman

Brief Overview of Medical Terminology

Learning medical terminology is similar to learning a foreign language. To succeed in any allied health or medical profession, you must understand the language upon which it is founded. Just as a person unfamiliar with Spanish would have difficulty pursuing a career in a country where Spanish is the primary language, so, too, will the healthcare employee who doesn't understand the language of medicine.

Medical Terminology: Mastering the Basics will give you a solid foundation in the language of the healthcare profession and will help you learn this language in a straightforward, engaging, and fun manner.

To master the basics of medical terminology, you will

- memorize word parts: prefixes, root words, and suffixes;
- analyze, dissect, and build medical terms using word parts;
- understand word parts as they relate to diseases and disorders of the different body systems, as well as common diagnostic procedures and therapeutic treatments; and
- reinforce your knowledge, skills, and self-confidence by completing the exercises in this textbook and practicing with the flash cards and vocabulary games included in your *EduHub* subscription.

The language of medicine is derived primarily from Latin and Greek words, and some terms come directly from modern languages such as French and German (Figure 1.1). Many terms can be represented as abbreviations or acronyms, providing valuable shortcuts to communication among healthcare professionals. Some medical terms take the form of eponyms. (An *eponym* is a person after whom a discovery, invention, or other notable achievement has been named.) Furthermore, some medical terms are not built from word parts—that is, they cannot be divided into a prefix, root word, and suffix. For these words, you will need to use a medical dictionary to learn the correct spelling and definition.

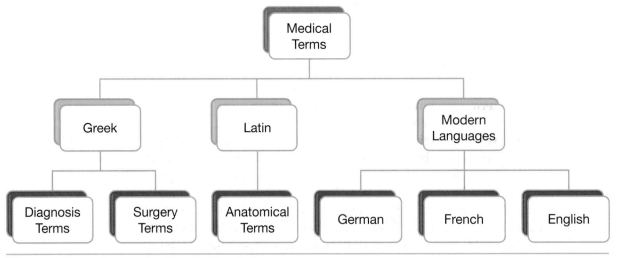

Figure 1.1 Linguistic sources of medical terminology

Medical terminology is a dynamic, fluid, and ever-evolving discipline in which terms are created to describe pioneering surgical procedures, cutting-edge technological innovations, and newly discovered pathological conditions. As a result, new medical terms are constantly being absorbed into the vast body of knowledge that is medical terminology.

A large number of medical terms are built from word parts. There are four types of word parts in medical terminology:

Word Part	Definition
Prefix	A single letter or a group of letters placed before a root word (or series of root words). The prefix shows a particular relationship, such as prepositional or adverbial. In general, most prefixes in medical terminology are used in everyday speech.
Root Word	The word part (or parts) that provides the main meaning of a medical term.
Suffix	A single letter or a group of letters added to the end of a root word (or series of root words). The suffix indicates the grammatical function of the medical term (noun, adjective, verb, or adverb).
Combining Vowel	A vowel that links together word parts for ease of pronunciation. Usually, the combining vowel is **o**, but occasionally it will be **a**, **e**, **i**, or **u**.

Together, a root word and combining vowel are called a **combining form**. For simplicity, each root word introduced in this textbook is presented with its combining vowel.

Word parts may be combined in any of several different ways to build a medical term:

- Prefix, root word, and suffix
- Prefix, root word, combining vowel, and suffix
- Prefix and root word
- Prefix and suffix
- Root word, combining vowel, and suffix
- Root word and suffix

Some medical terms contain more than one prefix, root word, and suffix.

Learning medical terminology requires the memorization of root words, prefixes, and suffixes. Although this process may seem challenging, this textbook provides plenty of skill-building exercises and digital resources to help you learn the material. Using your *EduHub* subscription, you can access print and e-flash cards using any Internet-enabled device. You can also play additional vocabulary practice games and complete the assessment and review activities your instructor assigns. Audio recordings of medical term pronunciations and chart notes can help you practice hearing, interpreting, and using the language of medical terminology.

Follow the processes described in this textbook. Read the material, practice using the e-flash cards (or make your own flash cards), and do some of the digital exercises on a daily basis. Don't wait until the day before a test to study. It doesn't work. Mastering the basics of medical terminology requires a commitment of time and effort. Repetition is a key factor in memorizing medical word parts and their meanings.

To simplify the learning process, we will look at a medical term and then break it down into its word parts. Once you understand how to dissect the term into its word parts, we will put it back together and discuss its meaning and correct pronunciation.

Analyzing and Defining Medical Terms

Let's analyze a medical term and its word parts by following a basic process that will help you develop important skills in mastering the basics of medical terminology. You will learn how to dissect a medical term into its individual word parts and then reconstruct those word parts to determine the meaning of the term as a whole.

At this point, don't worry that you don't know the meanings of the word parts; just pay attention to the *process* of analyzing the term. You will be able to use this process (breaking down a word into its prefix, root word, and suffix) to understand a medical term that you have never seen before. We will illustrate the process using the four medical terms below:

- *gastrology*
- *gastroenterology*
- *intragastric*
- *gastrectomy*

EXAMPLE 1

The medical term *gastrology* is defined as "the study of the stomach." This term contains a combining form (root word plus combining vowel) and a suffix.

Follow these steps to analyze the medical term *gastrology*:

1. Divide the term into its word parts. Note that a slash is used to separate each word part.

Medical Term	Dissection
gastrology	gastr/o/logy

2. Define each word part.

Word Part	Type of Word Part	Meaning of Word Part
gastr/o	root word + combining vowel = combining form	gastr = stomach o = combining vowel
logy	suffix	logy = study of

3. Arrange the word parts in the correct order. To figure out the meaning of a medical term, begin with the suffix. Then go back to the beginning of the term and work your way across.

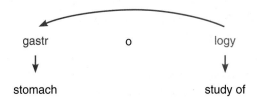

gastr o logy

stomach study of

gastrology = the study of the stomach

EXAMPLE 2

The medical term *gastroenterology* means "the study of the stomach and the intestines." (Typically, the combining form **enter/o** is used to refer to the small intestine.) This term contains two root words, two combining vowels, and a suffix.

Follow these steps to analyze the medical term *gastroenterology*:

1. Divide the term into its word parts by placing a slash between each word part.

Medical Term	Dissection
gastroenterology	gastr/o/enter/o/logy

2. Define each word part.

Word Part	Type of Word Part	Meaning of Word Part
gastr/o	root word + combining vowel = combining form	gastr = stomach o = combining vowel
enter/o	root word + combining vowel = combining form	enter = intestines o = combining vowel
logy	suffix	logy = study of

3. Arrange the word parts in the correct order. Begin with the suffix; then go back to the beginning of the term and work your way across.

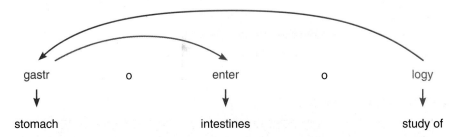

gastr o enter o logy

stomach intestines study of

gastroenterology = the study of the stomach and intestines

EXAMPLE 3

The medical term *intragastric* means "pertaining to within the stomach." This term contains a prefix, a root word, and a suffix. It does not require any combining vowels.

Follow these steps to analyze the medical term *intragastric*:

1. Divide the term into its word parts by placing a slash between each word part.

Medical Term	Dissection
intragastric	intra/gastr/ic

2. Define each word part.

Word Part	Type of Word Part	Meaning of Word Part
intra	prefix	intra = within
gastr	root word	gastr = stomach
ic	suffix	ic = pertaining to

3. Arrange the word parts in the correct order.

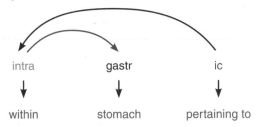

intragastric = pertaining to within the stomach

EXAMPLE 4

Gastrectomy is defined as "the excision (surgical removal) of the stomach." This term contains a root word and a suffix. It does not require a combining vowel.

Follow these steps to analyze the medical term *gastrectomy*:

1. Divide the term into its word parts by placing a slash between each word part.

Medical Term	Dissection
gastrectomy	gastr/ectomy

2. Define each word part.

Word Part	Type of Word Part	Meaning of Word Part
gastr	root word	gastr = stomach
ectomy	suffix	ectomy = excision or surgical removal

3. Arrange the word parts in the correct order.

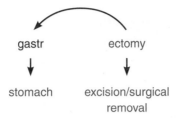

gastrectomy = the excision or surgical removal of the stomach

Medical Word Parts

Now that you understand how a medical term is built from prefixes, root words, and suffixes, we will discuss each of these word parts in more detail.

Prefixes

A **prefix** is a single letter or group of letters that appears at the beginning of a medical term before the root word(s). When written by itself, a prefix is usually followed by a hyphen.

Medical prefixes often express information about diseases or abnormal conditions; anatomical position, location, or direction; measurement; time; number; and color. Adding or changing a prefix changes the meaning of the medical term.

As you progress through this textbook, you will see that many of the same prefixes are used in medical terms relating to multiple body systems. You will also find that a large number of medical terms do not contain a prefix.

Following are some common prefixes that denote number, quantity, position, location, and direction in medical terminology.

Prefixes that Indicate Number

Prefix	Meaning
bi-	two
di-	two; double
quad-	four
tri-	three
uni-	one

Prefixes that Indicate Quantity, Size, or Magnitude

Prefix	Meaning
hemi-	half
hyper-	above normal
hypo-	below normal
poly-	many; much

Prefixes that Indicate Position, Direction, or Location

Prefix	Meaning
ab-	away from
ad-	toward
endo-	within
hypo-	below
inter-	between
intra-	within
para-	near; beside
peri-	around
post-	after
pre-	before
sub-	beneath; below
trans-	through; across

Root Words and Combining Forms

A **root word** is the foundation of most medical terms and gives the essential meaning of the term. Most medical terms are derived from Greek or Latin. These were the languages of the early scholars who discovered many of the concepts that make up the core knowledge base of biology and medicine. The ancient Greeks were the first to study medicine and to formulate a systematized vocabulary. When the Roman Empire began to displace Greek civilization, Roman scholars adopted many of the medical terms that had been developed by the Greeks. The ancient Romans also modified many Greek medical terms to conform to the alphabet and grammar of the Latin language.

Almost all medical terms have one or more root words. The root word often indicates a body part, but it may also denote an anatomical or physiological quality or condition. If a medical term contains more than one root word, those root words are typically joined by a combining vowel. Together, a root word and a combining vowel are called a **combining form**.

In most medical terms, a **combining vowel** is placed between word parts to facilitate pronunciation of the term. Take, for example, the word *gastroenterology*:

gastr/o/enter/o/logy

The combining vowel **o** is inserted after the root words **gastr** and **enter**, both of which end in consonants, to make pronunciation of the term easier. The combining vowels do not change the meanings of the root words.

Some medical terms do not contain a combining vowel. The word *gastrectomy* is an example. It is composed of a root word and a suffix:

gastr/ectomy

General Rules for Use of Combining Vowels

Following are a few general rules concerning the use of combining vowels in medical terms:

1. A combining vowel is not used between a prefix and a root word (trans/derm/al) or a prefix combined with a suffix (quadri/plegic).
2. A combining vowel may be used between two root words (electr/o/cardi/o/gram) or between a root word and a suffix (angi/o/plasty).
3. The combining vowel is usually the letter **o**. In some medical terms, however, the combining vowel is **a**, **e**, **i**, or **u**.

Suffixes

A **suffix** is a single letter or group of letters added to the end of a prefix, root word, or combining form. A suffix modifies the meaning of the word part to which it is added. When written by itself, a suffix is preceded by a hyphen.

Following is an example of a suffix modifying the word part to which it is added. In this example, the suffix is attached to a root word.

Word Part	Type of Word Part	Meaning of Word Part
muscul	root word	muscle
ar	suffix	pertaining to

muscul + ar = muscular

The term *muscular* means "pertaining to muscle."

Suffixes modify medical terms by denoting information about diseases or abnormal conditions, surgical procedures, diagnostic procedures, medical specialties, or healthcare specialists and practitioners. Suffixes are not associated with one particular body system or medical specialty; as you will see, the same suffixes are used in many medical terms. In addition, different suffixes may have the same meaning. For example, the suffixes **-ac**, **-al**, **-ar**, and **-ary** all mean "pertaining to." Not all medical terms have a suffix.

Following are some common suffixes used in medical terminology.

Suffixes Associated with Diseases and Disorders

Suffix	Meaning
-ac	pertaining to
-al	pertaining to
-algia	pain
-cele	hernia; swelling; protrusion
-ectasis	dilatation; dilation; expansion
-edema	swelling
-emia	blood condition
-ia	condition
-iasis	abnormal condition
-itis	inflammation
-malacia	softening
-megaly	large; enlargement
-oma	tumor; mass
-osis	abnormal condition
-pathy	disease
-penia	deficiency; abnormal reduction
-rrhexis	rupture
-trophy	development

Suffixes Associated with Diagnostic Procedures

Suffix	Meaning
-gram	record; image
-graph	instrument used to record an image
-graphy	process of recording an image
-meter	instrument used to measure
-metry	process of measuring
-scope	instrument used to observe
-scopy	process of observing

Suffixes Associated with Surgical Procedures

Suffix	Meaning
-centesis	surgical puncture (to remove fluid)
-ectomy	surgical removal; excision
-lysis	breakdown; loosening; dissolving
-pexy	surgical fixation
-plasty	surgical repair
-rrhaphy	suture
-stomy	new opening (created surgically)
-tomy	incision; cut into
-tripsy	crushing

General Rules for Use of Suffixes

Following are some general rules concerning the use of suffixes in medical terms:

1. **If a suffix begins with a consonant:** Insert a combining vowel between the root word and the suffix.

Examples:

   A. The term *melanocyte* is made up of the root word melan (which means "black") and the suffix -cyte (which means "cell"). The suffix -cyte begins with a consonant; therefore, we insert a combining vowel between the root word and the suffix:

   melan/o/cyte = cell that is black (black cell)

   B. The term *colonoscopy* consists of the root word colon ("large intestine or colon") and the suffix -scopy ("process of observing"). The suffix -scopy begins with a consonant, so we insert a combining vowel between the root word and the suffix:

   colon/o/scopy = process of observing the large intestine or colon

   C. The term *pathologist* consists of the root word path ("disease") and the suffix -logist ("specialist in the study and treatment of"). The suffix -logist begins with a consonant, so a combining vowel is inserted between the root word and the suffix:

   path/o/logist = specialist in the study and treatment of disease

2. **If a suffix begins with a vowel:** Attach the suffix directly to the root word. A combining vowel is not needed.

Examples:

   A. The term *onychosis* is made up of the root word onych (which means "nail") and the suffix -osis (which means "abnormal condition").

The suffix -osis begins with a vowel; therefore, a combining vowel does not need to be added. The suffix is attached directly to the root word:

onych/osis = abnormal condition of a nail

B. The term *melanoma* consists of the root word melan ("black") and the suffix -oma ("tumor or mass"). Because the suffix -oma begins with a vowel, we attach it to the suffix without inserting a combining vowel:

melan/oma = tumor that is black (black tumor)

C. The medical term *bronchitis* consists of the root word bronch ("bronchial tube or bronchus") and the suffix -itis ("inflammation"). The suffix -itis begins with a vowel, so it is attached directly to the suffix:

bronch/itis = inflammation of the bronchial tube or bronchus

Breaking Down and Building Medical Terms

You have learned the process of analyzing the parts of a medical term to decode its meaning. You have learned that prefixes, combining forms (root words plus combining vowels), and suffixes are meaningful word parts in medical terminology. Whether you want to understand television shows with medical content, comprehend what your doctor is saying to you, or prepare for a career in the healthcare field, the ability to recognize and understand these word parts is key to mastering medical terminology.

Once you have mastered the meanings of the medical word parts presented throughout this textbook, you will have the ability to understand a vast number of medical terms. Medical terminology is logical and systematic: Simply by analyzing and breaking down a term into the word parts that comprise it, you can decode the meaning of a medical term that you have never seen or heard before.

Breaking Down Medical Terms: Summary of Steps

When you encounter an unfamiliar medical term, don't panic. You can decode the meaning of any medical term by following these simple steps:
1. Divide the medical term into its word parts: prefix, root word(s), combining vowel(s), and suffix.
2. Define each word part.
3. Arrange the word parts in the correct order. Begin with the suffix; then go back to the beginning of the term and work your way across to figure out the term's meaning.

Break It Down

Directions: Study the prefixes, combining forms, and suffixes in the charts that follow until you are familiar with each word part and its meaning. Then do the exercise that appears after the charts.

Prefix	Meaning
brady-	slow
endo-	within
epi-	upon
para-	near; beside
supra-	above
tachy-	fast

Combining Form (Root Word plus Combining Vowel)	Meaning
card/o, cardi/o	heart
dermat/o	skin
gastr/o	stomach
myc/o	fungus
neur/o	nerve
ophthalm/o	eye
pharyng/o	throat

Suffix	Meaning
-al	pertaining to
-ia	condition
-ic	pertaining to
-itis	inflammation
-logist	specialist in the study and treatment of
-logy	study of
-tic	pertaining to

Break It Down

Directions: Dissect each medical term by identifying and filling in its component word parts (prefix, root word, combining vowel, and suffix). If a term does not have a combining vowel, list *None* in the Combining Vowel column. Finally, define each term. You can also complete this activity online using *EduHub*.

Medical Term	Prefix	Root Word	Combining Vowel	Suffix
1. cardiologist		Cardi	o	logist

Definition: _____

_____

2. ophthalmology

Definition: _____

_____

3. paraneural

Definition: _____

_____

4. epigastric

Definition: _____

_____

5. suprapharyngeal

Definition: _____

_____

6. bradycardia

Definition: _____

_____

Medical Term	Prefix	Root Word	Combining Vowel	Suffix
7. endocarditis	_____	_____	_____	_____

Definition: _____

_____

| 8. tachycardia | _____ | _____ | _____ | _____ |

Definition: _____

_____

| 9. dermatology | _____ | _____ | _____ | _____ |

Definition: _____

_____

| 10. mycotic | _____ | _____ | _____ | _____ |

Definition: _____

_____

SCORECARD: How Did You Do?

Number correct (_____), divided by 10 (_____), multiplied by 100 equals _____ (your score)

Building Medical Terms: Summary of Steps

The process of building a medical term is almost the reverse of breaking it down. You can construct any medical term by following these steps:
1. Choose the word parts (prefix, root word(s), combining vowel(s), and suffix) that you need to build the medical term.
2. Place the word parts in the correct order.
3. Remember that the first word in the definition of a medical term usually is its suffix.

Build It

Directions: Study the prefixes, combining forms, and suffixes in the charts that follow until you are familiar with each word part and its meaning. Then do the exercise that appears after the charts.

Prefix	Meaning
intra-	within
peri-	around
poly-	many

Combining Form (Root Word plus Combining Vowel)	Meaning
aden/o	gland
angi/o	vessel
cardi/o	heart
crani/o	skull
dermat/o	skin
enter/o	intestines (usually the small intestine)
gastr/o	stomach
neur/o	nerve
pulmon/o	lung

Suffix	Meaning
-al	pertaining to
-asthenia	weakness
-ectomy	surgical removal; excision
-gram	record; image
-itis	inflammation
-logist	specialist in the study and treatment of
-logy	study of
-oma	tumor; mass
-tomy	incision; cut into

Build It

Directions: Build the medical term that matches each definition by supplying the correct word parts. Follow the color-coded key as a guide for completing this assessment. You can also complete this activity online using *EduHub*.

P (Prefixes) = Green
RW (Root Words) = Red
S (Suffixes) = Blue
CV (Combining Vowel) = Purple

1. surgical removal or excision of a vessel

   _____ _____
          RW   S

2. inflammation of the stomach

   _____ _____
          RW   S

3. pertaining to around the heart

   _____ _____ _____
     P   RW   S

4. record of blood vessels

   _____ _____ _____
          RW   CV   S

5. specialist in the study and treatment of the stomach and intestines

   _____ _____ _____ _____ _____
          RW   CV   RW   CV   S

6. tumor of the gland

   _____ _____
          RW   S

7. inflammation of many nerves

_____ _____ _____
  P   RW   S

8. specialist in the study and treatment of the skin

_____ ____ _____
      RW   CV   S

9. incision to the skull

_____ ____ _____
      RW   CV   S

10. inflammation of the skin

_____ _____
      RW   S

11. pertaining to within the skull

_____ _____ _____
  P   RW   S

12. weakness of the nerve

_____ _____
      RW   S

13. study of the lung

_____ ____ _____
      RW   CV   S

14. specialist in the study and treatment of the heart

_____ ____ _____
      RW   CV   S

Building Plural Forms

As you have learned, most medical terms are composed of Latin or Greek word parts; therefore, some of the rules for building plural nouns in medical terminology differ from those in everyday English. You will, however, notice some similarities because many words in the English language have retained their original Latin and Greek forms. Whenever you are in doubt about how to represent the plural form of a medical term, consult a medical dictionary.

Following are some general rules for changing a singular noun to a plural noun in medical terminology.

General Rules for Building Plurals	Examples	
	Singular	Plural
1. If the noun ends in **s**, add **es**.	sinus virus	sinuses viruses
2. If the noun ends in **a**, add **e**.	pleura vertebra	pleurae vertebrae
3. If the noun ends in **ax**, drop the **x** and add **ces**.	anthrax thorax	anthraces thoraces
4. If the noun ends in **ex**, drop the **ex** and add **ices**.	cortex index	cortices indices
5. If the noun ends in **is**, drop the **is** and add **es**.	diagnosis metastasis	diagnoses metastases
6. If the noun ends in **ix**, drop the **x** and add **ces**.	appendix helix	appendices helices
7. If the noun ends in **ma**, add **ta**.	sarcoma stigma	sarcomata stigmata
8. If the noun ends in **on**, drop the **on** and add **a**.	ganglion spermatozoon	ganglia spermatozoa
9. If the noun ends in **um**, drop the **um** and add **a**.	bacterium ovum	bacteria ova
10. If the noun ends in **us**, drop the **us** and add **i**.	alveolus fungus	alveoli fungi
11. If the noun ends in **x**, drop the **x** and add **ges**.	larynx phalanx	larynges phalanges
12. If the noun ends in **y**, drop the **y** and add **ies**.	biopsy deformity	biopsies deformities

Building Plural Forms

Directions: For each medical term, supply its missing plural or singular form. You can also complete this activity online using *EduHub*.

1. bursa _____
2. diverticulum _____
3. adenoma _____
4. ganglion _____
5. index _____
6. diagnosis _____
7. alveolus _____
8. bacterium _____
9. bronchus _____
10. phalanx _____
11. nucleus _____
12. apex _____

SCORECARD: How Did You Do?

Number correct (_____), divided by 12 (_____), multiplied by 100 equals _____ (your score)

Pronouncing Medical Terms

Throughout this textbook, a phonetic spelling (pronunciation) is provided in parentheses for each new medical term that is introduced. Each pronunciation contains diacritical marks, or accent marks. These diacritical marks appear above vowels and provide guidance in pronouncing the vowel sounds in a term. The **macron** (‾), for example, is used to indicate a long vowel sound (ā, ē, ī, ō, ū). The **breve** (˘) is used to indicate a short vowel sound (ă, ĕ, ĭ, ŏ, ŭ). Nearly all vowel sounds in the medical terms presented in this textbook are shown with diacritical marks. The only exception is terms that contain the **r**-controlled vowel sound "**or**." There is only one way to pronounce this **r**-controlled vowel sound; therefore, a diacritical mark does not appear above the "**o**," as illustrated in the following examples:

anteroposterior	(ĂN-tĕr-ō-pōs-TĒR-ē-or)
oropharynx	(or-ō-phăr-ĭngks)
osteoporosis	(ŎS-tē-ō-por-Ō-sĭs)

In addition to diacritical marks, which indicate the correct way to pronounce the vowel sounds in a medical term, uppercase and lowercase letters are used in phonetic spellings to show syllabic emphasis. A syllable represented in uppercase letters indicates primary emphasis on that syllable. A syllable represented in lowercase letters indicates lack of emphasis on that syllable. For the purposes of this introductory textbook, no distinction is made between primary and secondary syllabic emphasis.

Take, for example, the medical term *osteoporosis*. The pronunciation of this term is as follows:

ŎS   tē   ō   por   Ō   sĭs

Uppercase letter =
Syllable is emphasized
during pronunciation.

Uppercase letter =
Syllable is emphasized
during pronunciation.

Pronunciation of medical terms may seem challenging at first, but with practice, your skill and confidence will grow. When you encounter a new medical term, the acts of reading it, writing it, and pronouncing it correctly will help you form an accurate visual and aural memory for the term.

To hear the correct pronunciations of medical terms throughout this textbook, access your *EduHub* subscription and listen to the audio recordings using the audio glossary, Pronounce It activities, or e-flash cards.

The ability to pronounce medical terms correctly is not only essential to effective communication in the medical profession, but is also crucial to patient safety and care. Medical terms are often difficult to pronounce; however, the rules for pronunciation, like the rules for building plural forms, are fairly systematic.

There are 26 letters in the alphabet that in various combinations produce 60 different sounds. Certain letter combinations and vocal sounds are attributed to letters based on their placement within a medical term, as illustrated below.

General Rules of Medical Terminology Pronunciation	Examples
1. In the letter combinations **ae**, **nd**, and **oe**, the second vowel is pronounced.	bursae roentgen
2. The letter combination **ch** is sometimes pronounced like the letter **k**.	cholera
3. When the letter combination **pn** appears at the beginning of a medical term, the **p** is silent; only the **n** is pronounced.	pneumonia
4. When the letter combination **pn** appears in the middle of a medical term, both letters are pronounced.	dyspnea
5. When the letter combination **ps** appears at the beginning of a medical term, the **p** is silent; only the **s** is pronounced.	psychology
6. When the letter **i** appears at the end of a medical term, it has the "long i" vowel sound as in *eye*. Note: Some terms that end in **i** may also be pronounced with the variant "long e" vowel sound. When in doubt about the correct pronunciation of a term, consult a medical dictionary.	bronchi
7. When **e** and **es** are the final letter(s) of a medical term, the letter(s) are pronounced as separate syllables.	syncope nares

For guidance in pronouncing medical terms, the best resource is a medical dictionary.

Spelling Medical Terms

Correct spelling of medical terms is very important. A spelling error that changes just one or two letters can change the entire meaning of a term. Some medical terms are spelled similarly, but have very different meanings (for example, **arteriosclerosis** and **atherosclerosis**). The first term, *arteriosclerosis*, means "hardening of the arteries." The second term, *atherosclerosis*, means "accumulation of fatty plaques within blood vessels."

As a professional in the medical community, you will enter information into patients' electronic health records on a daily basis. Correctly spelled medical terms are critical to patient care. Furthermore, chart notes, history and physical examination reports, operative reports, and other types of health records are considered legal documents. Therefore, accuracy is essential.

Overview of Anatomical Positions, Planes, Directions, and Locations

Healthcare professionals use specific terms to describe anatomical positions, directions, and locations. These terms are important for a variety of reasons. Before a patient undergoes surgery, for example, the doctor must accurately record the precise location of the part of the body on which the surgical procedure is to be performed.

In this section, we will briefly explore key terms used by medical professionals to communicate information about anatomical positions, planes, directions, and locations.

Anatomical Position

When describing body positions or using directional terms, healthcare professionals visualize the patient in anatomical position, the standard frame of reference for communicating information about positions, planes, directions, and locations in the human body.

In **anatomical position**, a person is standing upright with the legs together, feet pointing forward, arms at the sides, palms facing forward, and head facing forward (Figure 1.2). When you view the patient from the anatomical position, everything that you "see" makes up the **anterior** (**ventral**) or *front surface* of the body. When the patient turns around, what you see is the **posterior** (**dorsal**) or *back surface* of the body.

The terms *anterior* and *ventral* are synonyms that mean "the front of the body." Likewise, the terms *posterior* and *dorsal* are synonyms that mean "the back of the body." *Anterior/ventral* is the opposite of *posterior/dorsal*.

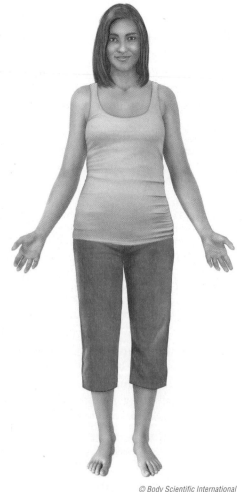

© Body Scientific International

Figure 1.2 Anatomical position

Anatomical position is a reference point that must be remembered. It is the point of origin for understanding anatomical positions, planes, directions, and locations.

Anatomical Planes

In biology and medicine, the human body is divided into imaginary planes or sections that are used as reference points when describing body parts and organs. The human body can be divided into sections along three different planes: the frontal plane (also called the *coronal plane*), the sagittal plane, and the transverse plane.

The **sagittal plane** divides the body into left and right sections. The **midsagittal plane** or *median plane* divides the body into equal right and left halves (Figure 1.3).

The **frontal plane** or *coronal plane* divides the body into front (*anterior/ ventral*) and back (*posterior/dorsal*) sections (Figure 1.4).

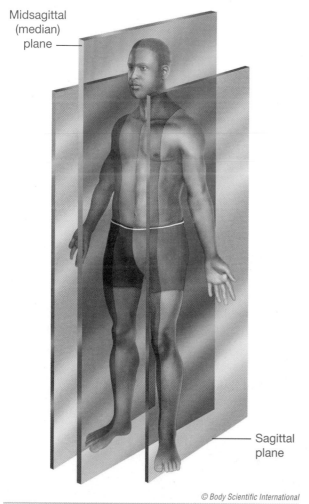

Midsagittal (median) plane

Sagittal plane

© Body Scientific International

Figure 1.3 Midsagittal (median) plane and sagittal plane

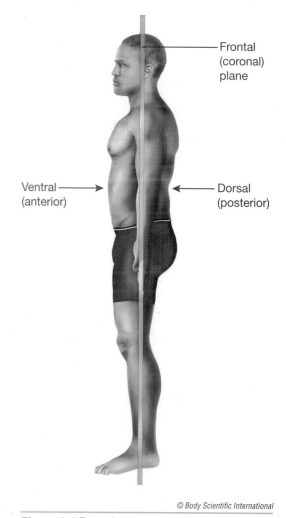

Frontal (coronal) plane

Ventral (anterior)

Dorsal (posterior)

© Body Scientific International

Figure 1.4 Frontal or coronal plane

The **transverse plane** divides the body into upper (*superior*) and lower (*inferior*) sections (Figure 1.5).

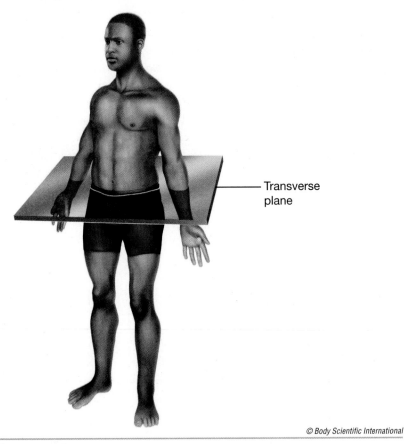

Transverse plane

Figure 1.5 Transverse plane

Assessment 1.4

Anatomical Planes

Directions: Choose the correct term for each definition. You can also complete this activity online using *EduHub*.

_____ 1. divides the body into left and right sections

_____ 2. another term for *frontal plane*

_____ 3. divides the body into front (anterior/ventral) and back (posterior/dorsal) sections

_____ 4. divides the body into equal right and left halves

_____ 5. divides the body into upper (superior) and lower (inferior) sections

_____ 6. another term for *midsagittal plane*

A. frontal plane
B. median plane
C. midsagittal plane
D. transverse plane
E. sagittal plane
F. coronal plane

SCORECARD: How Did You Do?

Number correct (_____), divided by 6 (_____), multiplied by 100 equals _____ (your score)

Terms of Position and Direction

In medical terminology, specific terms are used to describe the relative position of the body or of one body part in relation to another. Terms of position and direction are always based on anatomical position.

Just as road signs indicate the direction of a route (north, south, east, or west), directional terms in anatomy and physiology and in medical terminology often occur in pairs and generally have opposite meanings.

Common terms of position and direction are described in the table below and illustrated in Figures 1.6, 1.7, 1.8, and 1.9 on the pages that follow.

Term of Position or Direction	Definition
anterior	front of the body; ventral
anteroposterior	passing from the anterior (front) of the body to the posterior (rear)
caudal	toward the tailbone
cephalic	toward the head
distal	away from the point of origin
dorsal	back of the body; posterior
external	outer part of the body
inferior	body part located below another part or closer to the feet
internal	deep within the body
lateral	toward the side of the body
medial	toward the midline of the body
posterior	toward the back of the body
posteroanterior	passing from the posterior (rear) of the body to the anterior (front)
prone	lying facedown with the palms facing downward
proximal	closer to the point of origin
superior	body part located above another part or closer to the head
supine	lying on the back with the palms facing upward
ventral	front of the body; anterior

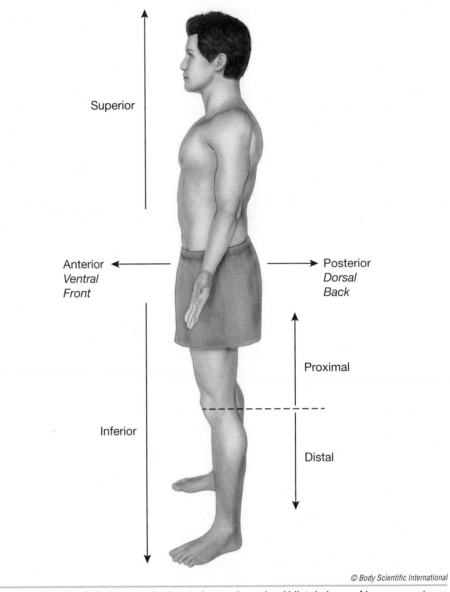

© Body Scientific International

Figure 1.6 Superior/inferior, anterior/posterior, and proximal/distal views of human anatomy

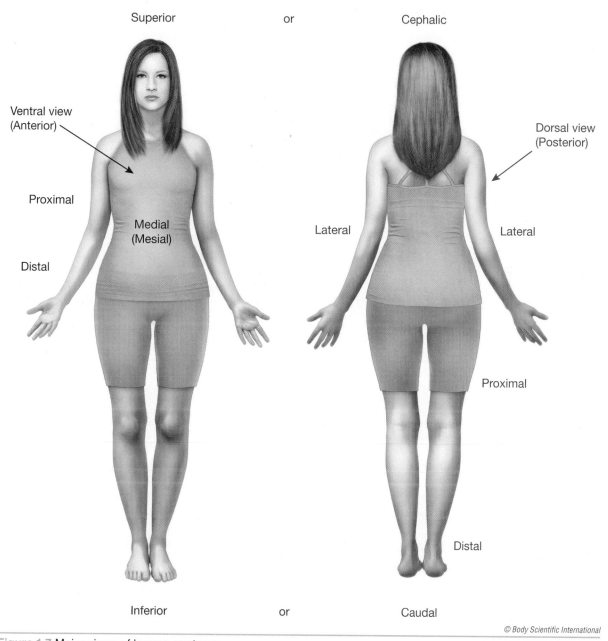

Figure 1.7 Major views of human anatomy

© *Body Scientific International*

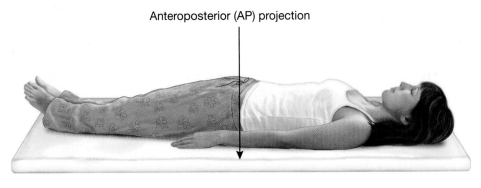

Anteroposterior (AP) projection

Posteroanterior (PA) projection

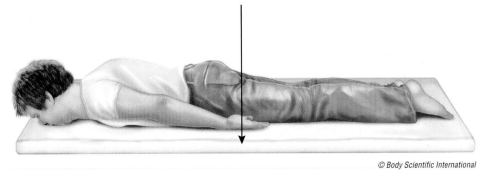

© Body Scientific International

Figure 1.8 Anteroposterior (AP) and posteroanterior (PA) projection

Supine

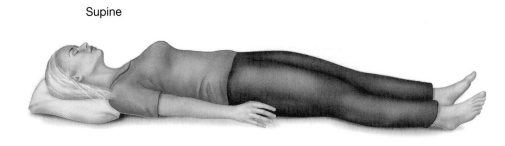

Prone

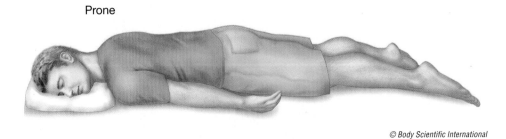

© Body Scientific International

Figure 1.9 Supine and prone positions

Terms of Position and Direction

Directions: Choose the correct term of position or direction for each meaning. You can also complete this activity online using **EduHub**.

_____ 1. passing from the posterior (rear) of the body to the anterior (front)

_____ 2. outer part of the body

_____ 3. toward the head

_____ 4. front of the body; ventral

_____ 5. closer to the point of origin

_____ 6. body part located below another part or closer to the feet

_____ 7. deep within the body

_____ 8. away from the point of origin

_____ 9. lying facedown with the palms facing downward

_____ 10. back of the body; posterior

_____ 11. body part located above another part or closer to the head

_____ 12. front of the body; anterior

_____ 13. toward the tailbone

_____ 14. toward the midline of the body

_____ 15. back of the body; dorsal

_____ 16. lying on the back with the palms facing upward

_____ 17. toward the side of the body

_____ 18. passing from the anterior (front) of the body to the posterior (rear)

A. external
B. prone
C. lateral
D. superior
E. anterior
F. posteroanterior
G. caudal
H. ventral
I. medial
J. distal
K. supine
L. cephalic
M. proximal
N. dorsal
O. anteroposterior
P. internal
Q. posterior
R. inferior

SCORECARD: How Did You Do?

Number correct (_____), divided by 18 (_____), multiplied by 100 equals _____ (your score)

Body Cavities

Body cavities protect and support internal organs (Figure 1.10). The human body contains two major cavities: the **dorsal cavity**, located posteriorly, and the **ventral cavity**, located anteriorly.

The dorsal cavity is subdivided into the **cranial cavity**, which contains the brain, and the **spinal cavity**, which contains the spinal cord. The spinal cavity is also called the *vertebral cavity*.

The ventral cavity is subdivided into the **thoracic** (chest) **cavity** and the **abdominopelvic cavity**. Because the abdominopelvic cavity is large, it is often subdivided into the **abdominal cavity** and the **pelvic cavity**.

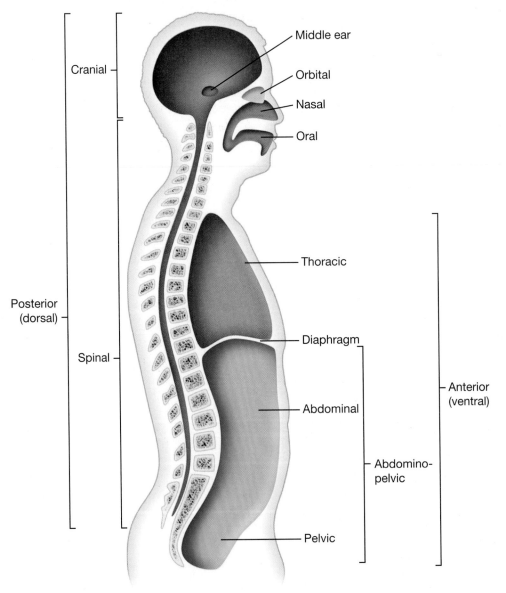

© Body Scientific International

Figure 1.10 Human body cavities

Body Cavities

Directions: Choose the correct body cavity for each description. You can also complete this activity online using *EduHub*.

_____ 1. the part of the dorsal cavity that contains the brain

_____ 2. one of the two major body cavities; located posteriorly

_____ 3. the part of the dorsal cavity that contains the spinal cord

_____ 4. another term for the spinal cavity

_____ 5. chest cavity; part of the ventral cavity

_____ 6. the part of the ventral cavity that contains the abdominal and pelvic cavities

_____ 7. one of the two major body cavities; located anteriorly

A. abdominopelvic cavity

B. ventral cavity

C. thoracic cavity

D. dorsal cavity

E. cranial cavity

F. spinal cavity

G. vertebral cavity

Abdominopelvic Cavity: Quadrants

Because the abdominopelvic cavity is large, it is divided according to one of two systems: quadrants or regions. In the first system, the abdominopelvic cavity is divided into four quadrants (Figure 1.11). These four quadrants consist of the **left upper quadrant (LUQ)**, the **right upper quadrant (RUQ)**, the **left lower quadrant (LLQ)**, and the **right lower quadrant (RLQ)**. The directional terms *right* and *left* refer to the left and right sides of the patient's body, not the perspective of the person viewing it. The quadrant system is used by health-care professionals because the precise locations of internal organs and structures vary from one patient to another.

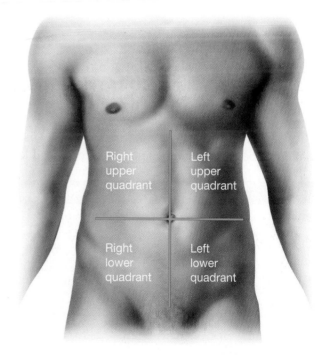

© Body Scientific International

Figure 1.11 Four quadrants of the abdomen

Abdominopelvic Cavity: Regions

In the second, more detailed system of anatomical division, the abdominopelvic cavity is divided into nine regions that resemble the sections of a Tic-Tac-Toe grid (Figure 1.12). The nine regions include the **right and left hypochondriac regions**, the **epigastric region**, the **right and left lumbar regions**, the **umbilical region**, the **right and left inguinal** (or *iliac*) **regions**, and the **hypogastric region**. This method of dividing the abdominopelvic cavity is preferred by anatomists because of its more detailed precision.

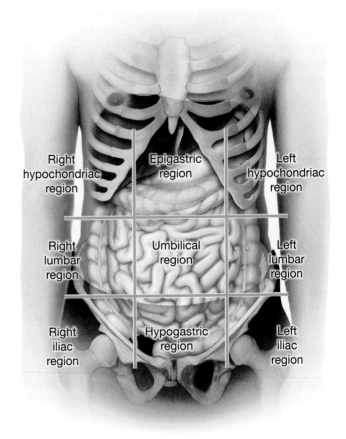

© Body Scientific International

Figure 1.12 Nine regions of the abdomen

Common Medical Abbreviations for Anatomical Terms of Position, Direction, and Location

The following abbreviations are commonly used in place of medical terms that describe anatomical position, direction, and location.

Term	Abbreviation
anterior	Ant
anteroposterior	AP
inferior	Inf
lateral	Lat
left lower quadrant	LLQ
left upper quadrant	LUQ

(Continued)

Term	Abbreviation
medial	Med
posterior	Post
posteroanterior	PA
right lower quadrant	RLQ
right upper quadrant	RUQ
superior	Sup

Abbreviations for Terms of Position, Direction, and Location

Directions: Supply the correct medical term for each abbreviation. You can also complete this activity online using *EduHub*.

1. Ant _____

2. LUQ _____

3. AP _____

4. Inf _____

5. RUQ _____

6. Lat _____

7. Med _____

8. LLQ _____

9. Post _____

10. PA _____

11. RLQ _____

12. Sup _____

SCORECARD: How Did You Do?

Number correct (_____), divided by 12 (_____), multiplied by 100 equals _____ (your score)

Body Systems

From the most basic unit of matter—the microscopic atom—to the intricate architecture of the body systems, human anatomy is wondrously complex. There are 11 major body systems in the human body, each with its own specific function (Figure 1.13 on the next page). Some of these systems function complementarily to maintain homeostasis (a state of internal balance—a concept that will be discussed in more detail later in this book).

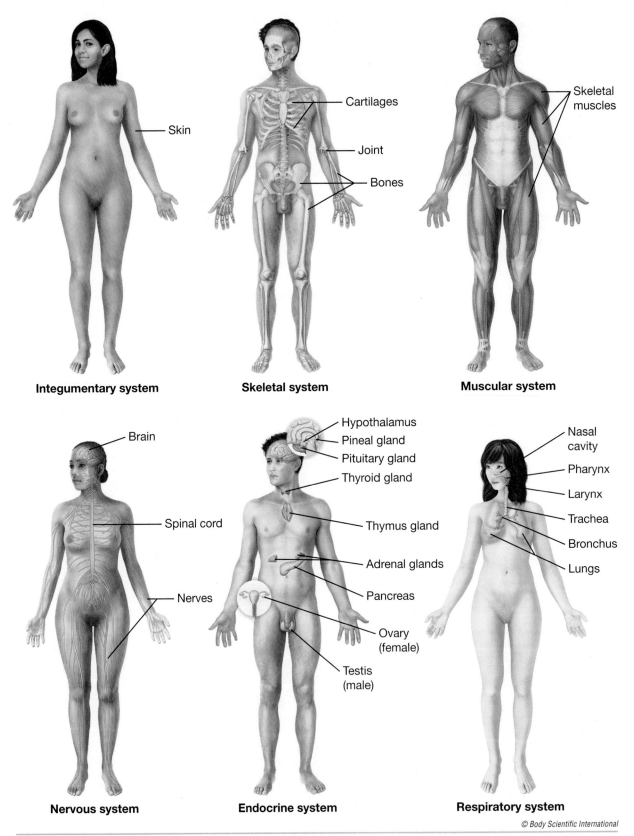

Integumentary system

Skin

Skeletal system

Cartilages

Joint

Bones

Muscular system

Skeletal muscles

Nervous system

Brain

Spinal cord

Nerves

Endocrine system

Hypothalamus
Pineal gland
Pituitary gland
Thyroid gland
Thymus gland
Adrenal glands
Pancreas
Ovary (female)
Testis (male)

Respiratory system

Nasal cavity
Pharynx
Larynx
Trachea
Bronchus
Lungs

© Body Scientific International

Figure 1.13 The 11 body systems

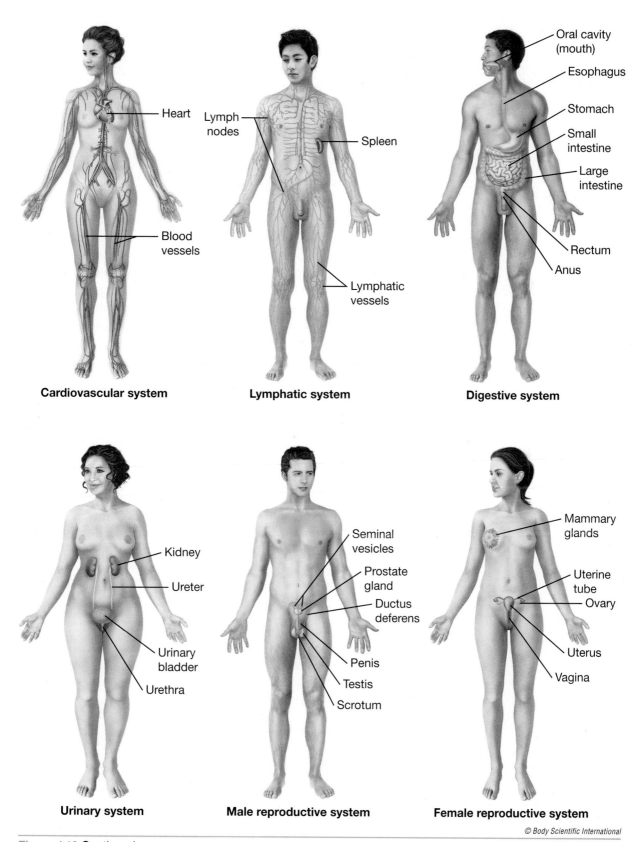

Cardiovascular system

Heart

Blood vessels

Lymphatic system

Lymph nodes

Spleen

Lymphatic vessels

Digestive system

Oral cavity (mouth)

Esophagus

Stomach

Small intestine

Large intestine

Rectum

Anus

Urinary system

Kidney

Ureter

Urinary bladder

Urethra

Male reproductive system

Seminal vesicles

Prostate gland

Ductus deferens

Penis

Testis

Scrotum

Female reproductive system

Mammary glands

Uterine tube

Ovary

Uterus

Vagina

© Body Scientific International

Figure 1.13 Continued

In this textbook, medical terminology pertaining to the muscular and skeletal systems has been combined into one chapter titled *The Musculoskeletal System*. In addition, a separate chapter has been included on the special sensory organs of vision and hearing.

Mastering Medical Terminology

Congratulations! You have completed this chapter and are now ready to learn medical terms relating to the different body systems.

As you are aware, mastery of medical terminology requires memorization of word parts (prefixes, root words, and suffixes) and their meanings. Knowing the meanings of these word parts will enable you to break down and build medical terms that you do not know. As you gain mastery (which comes with practice, time, and patience), you will be able to rely less often on a dictionary to analyze medical terms and interpret their meanings.

Learning a lot of medical terms at once can be overwhelming. Following are some tips to help you study effectively, build mastery, and develop confidence in reading, writing, and speaking the language of medical terminology as you work your way through each chapter of this textbook.

1. Set aside time each day to review the key terms presented in the chapter. To hear the pronunciations of key anatomical and medical terms, access your *EduHub* subscription.
2. Don't wait until the last minute; spend time throughout the week studying the chapter material.
3. Practice with the flash cards provided with your *EduHub* subscription. Flash cards are available digitally and can also be printed. You can also make your own flash cards. Carry the flash cards with you wherever you go, and practice using them whenever you have a few free minutes.
4. Study regularly with a partner from your class, and take turns quizzing each other on the chapter material.

More Practice: Activities and Games

The following activities will help you reinforce your skills and check your mastery of the medical terminology you learned in this chapter. Access your *EduHub* subscription to complete more activities and vocabulary games for mastering the word parts and terms you have learned.

Identifying Anatomical Planes

Directions: Label the diagram of the anatomical planes.

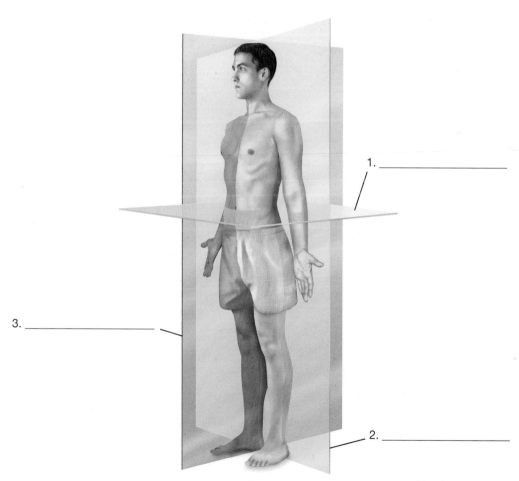

1. _____

3. _____

2. _____

© Body Scientific International

Major Views of Human Anatomy

Directions: Label the diagram showing the major views of human anatomy.

1. _____ or 2. _____

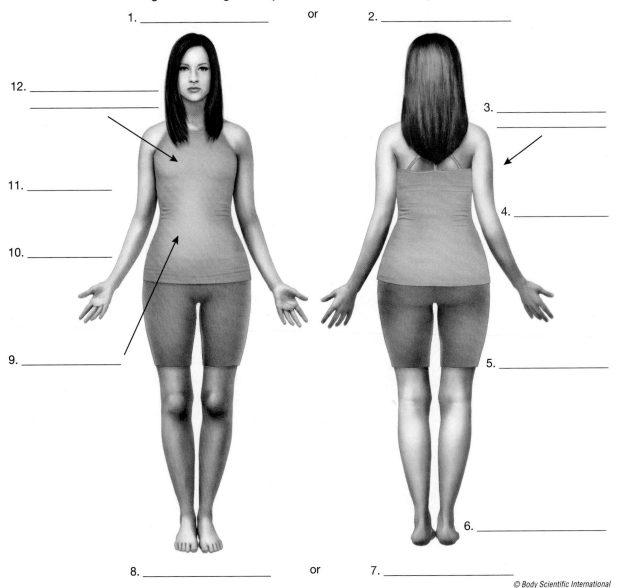

12. _____
_____

11. _____

10. _____

9. _____

3. _____
_____

4. _____

5. _____

6. _____

8. _____ or 7. _____

© *Body Scientific International*

Identifying Prefixes

Directions: Choose the correct meaning for each prefix.

_____ 1. para-

_____ 2. epi-

_____ 3. supra-

_____ 4. brady-

_____ 5. endo-

_____ 6. tachy-

A. fast

B. within

C. upon

D. above

E. near; beside

F. slow

Identifying Suffixes

Directions: Build the correct medical term for each definition. First, choose the correct suffix from the table provided. Add a combining vowel, if one is needed. Then supply the correct medical term.

Suffixes Chart

Suffix	Meaning
-al	pertaining to
-algia	pain
-asthenia	weakness
-eal	pertaining to
-ectomy	surgical removal; excision
-gram	record; image
-itis	inflammation
-logist	specialist in the study and treatment of
-logy	study of
-oma	tumor; mass
-osis	abnormal condition
-pathy	disease
-rrhexis	rupture
-scope	instrument used to observe
-scopy	process of observing
-stomy	new opening (created surgically)

Definition	Root Word	Combining Vowel	Suffix	Build the Medical Term
1. pertaining to the esophagus	esophag	_____	_____	_____
2. the study of the heart	cardi	_____	_____	_____
3. rupture of a vessel	angi	_____	_____	_____
4. cancerous tumor	carcin	_____	_____	_____
5. inflammation of the large intestine	col	_____	_____	_____
6. abnormal condition of the diverticulum	diverticul	_____	_____	_____
7. pain in the stomach	gastr	_____	_____	_____

Definition	Root Word	Combining Vowel	Suffix	Build the Medical Term
8. new surgical opening in the sigmoid colon	sigmoid	_____	_____	_____
9. surgical removal of the thymus gland	thym	_____	_____	_____
10. specialist in the study and treatment of the skin	dermat	_____	_____	_____
11. instrument used to observe the joints	arthr	_____	_____	_____
12. weakness of the muscle	my	_____	_____	_____
13. disease of the bone	oste	_____	_____	_____
14. record or image of the spinal cord	myel	_____	_____	_____
15. new (surgical) opening in the trachea	trache	_____	_____	_____

Forming Plurals

Directions: For each medical term, choose the ending needed to produce the plural form. Then supply the correct plural form for each term.

a   ae   ata   ces   es   ges   i   ices   ies

1. diagnosis   _____
2. vertebra   _____
3. appendix   _____
4. stigma   _____
5. spermatozoon   _____
6. sinus   _____
7. thorax   _____
8. bacterium   _____
9. adenoma   _____
10. ovum   _____
11. phalanx   _____
12. fungus   _____
13. anomaly   _____

True or False

Directions: Indicate whether each statement is true or false.

True or False?

_____ 1. Many medical terms are formed from one or more word parts.

_____ 2. A suffix changes the meaning of a medical term.

_____ 3. Different suffixes may have the same meaning.

_____ 4. Every medical term must have a prefix.

_____ 5. If a suffix begins with a consonant, it must directly follow a root word; a combining vowel should not be inserted.

_____ 6. A prefix always appears at the beginning of a medical term.

_____ 7. All medical terms are formed from word parts such as prefixes, root words, combining forms, and suffixes.

_____ 8. Prefixes are used only in medical terms that pertain to body systems.

_____ 9. All medical terms contain at least two root words.

_____ 10. All medical terms contain a combining vowel.

_____ 11. A spelling error can change the meaning of a medical term.

_____ 12. Diacritical marks are placed above consonants to aid in pronouncing them.

_____ 13. When a patient lies flat on her back with her palms facing upward, she is in the prone position.

_____ 14. The human body can be divided into sections along five different planes.

_____ 15. The coronal plane divides the body into equal right and left halves.

_____ 16. Terms of body position and direction are always based on anatomical position.

_____ 17. For anatomical purposes, the abdomen can be divided into 10 regions.

_____ 18. There are five major cavities in the human body.

_____ 19. When combined, the abdominal cavity and the pelvic cavity are referred to as the *abdominopelvic cavity*.

_____ 20. The skin is part of the integumentary system.

Chapter 2

The Integumentary System

dermat / o / logy: the study of the skin

Chapter Organization

- Intern Experience
- Overview of Integumentary System Anatomy and Physiology
- Word Elements
- Breaking Down and Building Integumentary System Terms
- Diseases and Disorders
- Procedures and Treatments
- Analyzing the Intern Experience
- Working with Medical Records
- Chapter Review

Chapter Objectives

After completing this chapter, you will be able to

1. label an anatomical diagram of the integumentary system;
2. dissect and define common medical terminology related to the integumentary system;
3. build terms used to describe integumentary system diseases and disorders, diagnostic tests and procedures, and therapeutic treatments;
4. pronounce and spell common medical terminology related to the integumentary system;
5. understand that the process of building and dissecting a medical term based on its prefix, root word, and suffix enables you to analyze an extremely large number of medical terms beyond those presented in this chapter;
6. interpret the meaning of abbreviations associated with the integumentary system; and
7. interpret medical records containing terminology and abbreviations related to the integumentary system.

Your *EduHub* subscription that accompanies this text provides access to online assessments, assignments, activities, and resources. Throughout this chapter, access *EduHub* to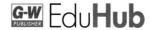

- use e-flash cards to review the medical terminology and word parts you learn;
- listen to the correct pronunciations of medical terms; and
- complete medical terminology activities and assignments.

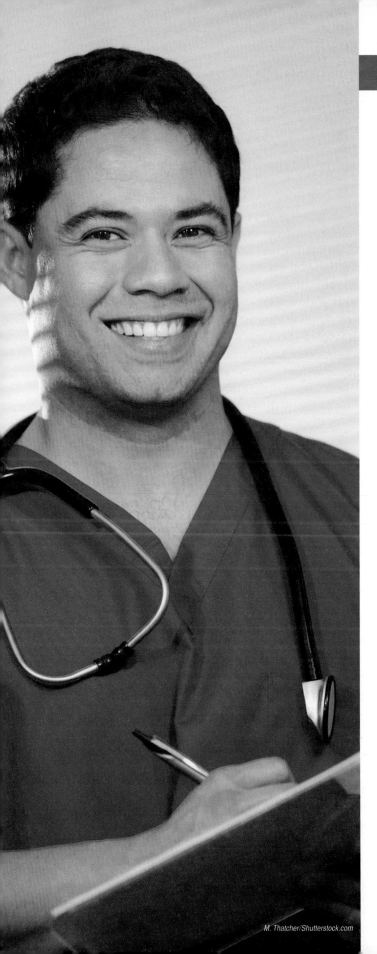

Intern Experience

Adrián Hernandez, an intern with Dr. Gaskins' office, meets Kate and one of her friends in examination room 1. Adrián learns that Kate and several of her friends, all members of the local high school lacrosse team, were watching a movie on TV, eating pizza, and painting their nails when Kate noticed redness and swelling in her right big toe, thickness and discoloration in the toenail, and pus around the nail. Her friends became nervous. With the prom only two weeks away, they persuaded Kate to go to the clinic.

Kate is experiencing a problem with her integumentary system, the body system that consists of the skin and related structures, including the nails, sweat and sebaceous glands, and hair. To help you understand what's happening to Kate, this chapter will present word elements (combining forms, prefixes, and suffixes) that make up medical terminology related to the integumentary system. As you continue to read, you will see many word parts that are also used in medical terms related to other body systems.

Before you begin this chapter, take some time to review the strategies presented in chapter 1 for analyzing medical terms. Reviewing these strategies will help you understand and recall the word elements and terms that you are about to learn.

After you have learned the medical terminology presented in this chapter, you will practice analyzing medical records, commonly known as *patient chart notes*. Accurate interpretation of these chart notes will demonstrate that you have a solid understanding of medical terminology related to the integumentary system.

Let's begin our study with a brief overview of integumentary system anatomy and physiology.

Overview of Integumentary System Anatomy and Physiology

The **integumentary** (ĭn-TĔG-yū-MĔN-tă-rē) system is the body system made up of skin, hair, nails, sweat glands, and oil-secreting glands. The word *integumentary* comes from the Latin word *integumentum*, which means "covering." The skin covers the entire body and is the largest organ of the body. The skin and accessory structures of the integumentary system—hair, nails, sweat glands, and oil-secreting glands—protect us from the external environment by preventing harmful substances from entering our bodies.

The sweat glands, called **sudoriferous** (sū-dō-RĬF-ĕr-ŭs) glands, cool the body by secreting perspiration, or sweat. The oil-secreting **sebaceous** (sĕ-BĀ-shŭs) glands produce an oily substance called **sebum** (SĒ-bŭm), which lubricates the skin, keeping it soft and supple.

The skin is our first line of defense against microorganisms that cause infection or disease, the ultraviolet (UV) rays of the sun, and harmful chemicals. The skin also protects internal body structures from injuries caused by blows, cuts, and burns. The terms **cutaneous** (kyŭ-TĀ-nē-ŭs) and **dermal** (DĔR-măl) are synonyms that both mean "pertaining to the skin." Although the integumentary system performs many different functions, its primary role is that of protection.

Main Functions of the Integumentary System

The primary functions of the integumentary system are to
1. protect the body by serving as a physical barrier between the internal organs and the external environment. The integumentary system protects us from pathogenic (disease-causing) microorganisms, harmful chemicals, the UV rays of the sun, and bodily harm due to physical trauma. It keeps harmful substances out of the body and helps prevent fluid loss by retaining water and electrolytes;
2. produce vitamin D, which is necessary for the absorption of calcium in the intestines;
3. regulate body temperature through blood vessels and sweat glands; and
4. provide sensory information to the brain about pain, pressure, touch, texture, and temperature through nerve receptors in the skin.

Major Structures of the Integumentary System

We mentioned that the skin—which includes the hair, nails, sweat and sebaceous glands, and specialized nerve receptors—is the most extensive organ of the body. Figure 2.1 shows the two layers that make up the skin: the outer layer, or **epidermis** (ĕp-ĭ-DĔR-mĭs), and the inner layer, or dermis.

The epidermis is composed of epithelial (ĕp-ĭ-THĒ-lē-ăl) tissue, or membranous tissue that covers the surface of the body, and does not contain blood vessels. Within the epidermis are **melanocytes** (MĔL-ăn-ō-sīts), specialized cells responsible for the production of a pigment called **melanin** (MĚL-ă-nĭn). Melanin may be black, dark brown, or reddish-brown. Our skin color is determined primarily by the amount of melanin produced by melanocytes. The darker the skin, the greater the concentration of melanin.

Beneath the epidermis is the **dermis**, sometimes referred to as the "true skin," as most of the essential functions of the skin are performed within this layer. The dermis is thicker than the epidermis, is made of connective tissue, and contains blood vessels. Beneath the dermis is the **subcutaneous** (sŭb-kyū-TĀ-nē-ŭs) layer, which contains adipose (fat) tissue that provides insulation to the body (Figure 2.1).

Dermatology (dĕr-mă-TŎL-ō-jē) is the study of the skin and related structures. A **dermatologist** (dĕr-mă-TŎL-ō-jĭst) is a physician who specializes in the study and treatment of the skin and related structures.

Dermatologists commonly **biopsy** (BĪ-ŏp-sē) skin tissue (that is, remove the tissue for microscopic examination) and send the specimen to a **pathologist** (pă-THŎL-ō-jĭst). A pathologist is a physician who specializes in the study, diagnosis, and treatment of disease and examines cells, tissues, and bodily fluids. The pathologist examines the specimen to determine the **etiology** (ē-tē-ŎL-ō-jē), or cause, of a disease. The pathologist's report is correlated with the clinical findings of the dermatologist. Then a diagnosis, treatment plan, and **prognosis** (expected outcome) are determined.

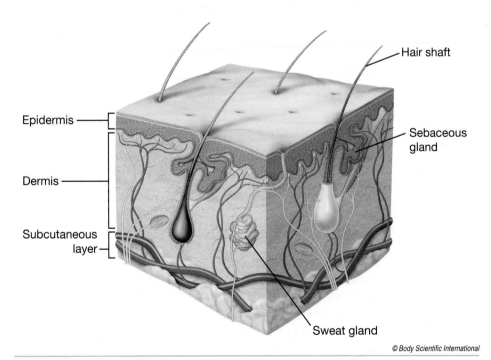

Epidermis

Dermis

Subcutaneous layer

Hair shaft

Sebaceous gland

Sweat gland

© Body Scientific International

Figure 2.1 Structures of the integumentary system

Anatomy and Physiology Vocabulary

Now that you have been introduced to the basic structure and functions of the integumentary system, let's explore in more detail the key terms presented in the introduction.

Key Term	Definition
biopsy	removal of tissue for microscopic examination
cutaneous	pertaining to the skin
dermal	pertaining to the skin, especially the dermis
dermatologist	physician who specializes in the study and treatment of the skin and related structures
dermatology	study of the skin and related structures
dermis	the layer of skin beneath the epidermis; the "true skin"
epidermis	the outer layer of the skin
etiology	cause of a disease or disorder
integumentary	pertaining to the covering of the body
melanin	pigment that is primarily responsible for skin color
melanocytes	specialized cells in the epidermis that produce skin pigment
pathologist	physician who specializes in the study, diagnosis, and treatment of disease
prognosis	expected outcome
sebaceous	pertaining to oil
sebum	oily substance secreted by the sebaceous glands
subcutaneous	beneath the skin (pertaining to the layer of skin that lies below the dermis)
sudoriferous	pertaining to the sweat glands

E-Flash Card Activity: Anatomy and Physiology Vocabulary

Directions: After you have reviewed the anatomy and physiology vocabulary related to the integumentary system, access your *EduHub* subscription and practice with the e-flash cards until you are comfortable with the spelling and definition of each term.

Identifying Major Structures of the Integumentary System

Directions: Label the diagram of the integumentary system. You can also complete this activity online using *EduHub*.

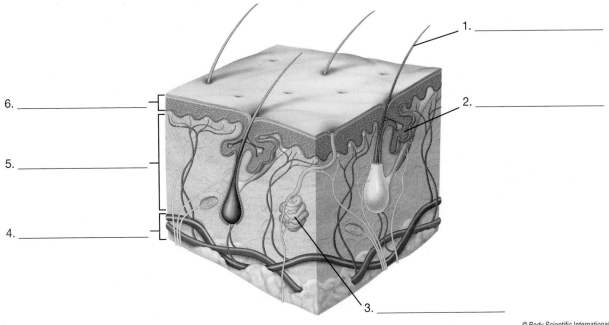

1. _____

2. _____

3. _____

4. _____

5. _____

6. _____

© Body Scientific International

SCORECARD: How Did You Do?

Number correct (_____), divided by 6 (_____), multiplied by 100 equals _____ (your score)

Matching Anatomy and Physiology Vocabulary

Directions: Choose the correct vocabulary term for each meaning. You can also complete this activity online using *EduHub*.

_____ 1. pertaining to the skin

_____ 2. the study of the skin and related structures

_____ 3. the outer layer of the skin

_____ 4. removal of tissue for microscopic examination

_____ 5. the layer of skin beneath the epidermis; the "true skin"

_____ 6. pertaining to the covering of the body

_____ 7. expected outcome

_____ 8. cause of a disease or disorder

_____ 9. pigment primarily responsible for skin color

_____ 10. oily substance secreted by the sebaceous glands

_____ 11. pertaining to oil

_____ 12. pertaining to the sweat glands

_____ 13. beneath the skin (below the dermis)

_____ 14. physician who specializes in the study and treatment of the skin and related structures

_____ 15. physician who specializes in the study, diagnosis, and treatment of disease

_____ 16. specialized cells in the epidermis that produce skin pigment

A. dermatologist

B. melanin

C. dermis

D. prognosis

E. biopsy

F. etiology

G. sebum

H. epidermis

I. sudoriferous

J. cutaneous

K. sebaceous

L. subcutaneous

M. integumentary

N. dermatology

O. pathologist

P. melanocytes

SCORECARD: How Did You Do?

Number correct (_____), divided by 16 (_____), multiplied by 100 equals _____ (your score)

Word Elements

In this section, you will learn word elements—prefixes, combining forms, and suffixes—that are common to the integumentary system. By learning these word parts and understanding how they are combined to build medical terms, you will be able to analyze Kate's skin problem (described in the Intern Experience at the beginning of this chapter) and identify a large number of terms associated with the integumentary system.

E-Flash Card Activity: Word Elements

Directions: Review the word elements in the tables that follow. Then, access your *EduHub* subscription and practice with the e-flash cards until you are able to quickly recognize the different word parts (prefixes, combining forms, and suffixes) and their meanings. The e-flash cards are grouped together by prefixes, combining forms, and suffixes, followed by a cumulative review of all the word elements you are learning in this chapter.

Prefixes

Let's start our study of integumentary system word elements by looking at the prefixes listed in the table below. These prefixes appear not only in medical terms related to the integumentary system, but also in many terms pertaining to other body systems.

Prefix	Meaning
epi-	upon
hypo-	below; below normal
intra-	within
per-	through
sub-	beneath; below
trans-	across

Combining Forms

Listed below are common combining forms used in medical terms related to the integumentary system. As you will discover, some of these combining forms are used in medical terms related to other body systems as well.

Root Word/Combining Vowel	Meaning
carcin/o	cancer
contus/o	bruising
cry/o	cold
cutane/o	skin
cyan/o	blue
cyst/o	sac containing fluid
derm/a, derm/o, dermat/o	skin
ecchym/o	blood in the tissues
erythemat/o	redness
erythr/o	red
hemat/o	blood
lip/o	fat
malign/o	causing harm; cancer
melan/o	black

(Continued)

Root Word/Combining Vowel	Meaning
myc/o	fungus
necr/o	death
onych/o	nail
path/o	disease
prurit/o	itching
py/o	pus
schiz/o	split
seb/o	oil or sebum
squam/o	scale-like
topic/o	place
trich/o	hair
xer/o	dry

Suffixes

Listed below are suffixes used in medical terms pertaining to the integumentary system. You will also encounter these suffixes in your study of terms related to other body systems.

Suffix	Meaning
-al	pertaining to
-ancy	state of
-cyte	cell
-ectomy	surgical removal; excision
-gen	producing; originating; causing
-ia	condition
-ic	pertaining to
-ion	condition
-itis	inflammation
-logist	specialist in the study and treatment of
-logy	study of
-oid	like; resembling
-oma	tumor; mass
-osis	abnormal condition
-ous	pertaining to
-rrhea	flow; discharge
-tic	pertaining to
-tomy	incision; cut into

Matching Prefixes, Combining Forms, and Suffixes

Directions: Choose the correct meaning for each word element. Some meanings may be used more than once. You can also complete this activity online using *EduHub*.

Prefixes

_____ 1. per-

_____ 2. epi-

_____ 3. trans-

_____ 4. sub-

_____ 5. hypo-

_____ 6. intra-

A. across

B. within

C. below; below normal

D. upon

E. beneath; below

F. through

Combining Forms

_____ 1. schiz/o

_____ 2. melan/o

_____ 3. cyan/o

_____ 4. malign/o

_____ 5. xer/o

_____ 6. carcin/o

_____ 7. myc/o

_____ 8. prurit/o

_____ 9. trich/o

_____ 10. topic/o

_____ 11. seb/o

_____ 12. cry/o

_____ 13. derm/a, derm/o, dermat/o

_____ 14. erythemat/o

_____ 15. cutane/o

_____ 16. py/o

_____ 17. lip/o

_____ 18. squam/o

_____ 19. ecchym/o

_____ 20. contus/o

_____ 21. onych/o

A. causing harm; cancer

B. dry

C. split

D. fat

E. nail

F. skin

G. scale-like

H. hair

I. itching

J. black

K. cold

L. place

M. oil or sebum

N. fungus

P. pus

Q. blue

R. death

S. cancer

T. red

U. bruising

V. blood

_____ 22. erythr/o   W. redness

_____ 23. necr/o   X. blood in the tissues

_____ 24. hemat/o   Y. sac containing fluid

_____ 25. cyst/o   Z. disease

_____ 26. path/o

Suffixes

_____ 1. -al   A. pertaining to

_____ 2. -cyte   B. specialist in the study and treatment of

_____ 3. -rrhea   C. surgical removal; excision

_____ 4. -ectomy   D. state of

_____ 5. -tic   E. like; resembling

_____ 6. -ia   F. inflammation

_____ 7. -ic   G. condition

_____ 8. -itis   H. tumor; mass

_____ 9. -logist   I. study of

_____ 10. -logy   J. flow; discharge

_____ 11. -oid   K. cell

_____ 12. -oma   L. producing; originating; causing

_____ 13. -tomy   M. abnormal condition

_____ 14. -ancy   N. incision; cut into

_____ 15. -ion

_____ 16. -ous

_____ 17. -gen

_____ 18. -osis

SCORECARD: How Did You Do?

Number correct (_____), divided by 50 (_____), multiplied by 100 equals _____ (your score)

Breaking Down and Building Integumentary System Terms

You are now able to dissect and build medical terms pertaining to the integumentary system. Whether you merely want to understand TV shows with medical content, interpret what your doctor is saying to you, or prepare for a career in healthcare, the ability to recognize the prefixes, combining forms, and suffixes used in medical terms is essential. In fact, having a solid grasp of these medical word parts gives you the ability to figure out the definitions of an enormous number of medical terms. Simply by breaking down a word into its prefix, combining form(s), and suffix, you can determine the meaning of a medical term that you have never seen before.

Below are some common medical terms related to the integumentary system. For each term, a dissection has been provided, along with the meaning of each word part and the definition of the term as a whole.

Term	Dissection	Word Part/Meaning	Term Definition
Note: *For simplification, combining vowels have been omitted from the Word Part/Meaning column.*			
1. **contusion** (kŏn-TŪ-zhŭn)	contus/ion	**contus** = bruising **ion** = condition	condition of bruising
2. **cyanodermal** (SĪ-ă-nō-DĔR-măl)	cyan/o/derm/al	**cyan** = blue **derma** = skin **al** = pertaining to	pertaining to blue skin
3. **cyanosis** (sī-ă-NŌ-sĭs)	cyan/osis	**cyan** = blue **osis** = abnormal condition	abnormal condition of blue
4. **cystic** (SĬS-tĭk)	cyst/ic	**cyst** = sac containing fluid **ic** = pertaining to	pertaining to a sac containing fluid
5. **dermal** (DĔR-măl)	derm/al	**derm** = skin **al** = pertaining to	pertaining to the skin
6. **dermatitis** (DĔR-mă-TĪ-tĭs)	dermat/itis	**dermat** = skin **itis** = inflammation	inflammation of the skin
7. **dermatologist** (dĕr-mă-TŎL-ō-jĭst)	dermat/o/logist	**dermat** = skin **logist** = specialist in the study and treatment of	specialist in the study and treatment of the skin
8. **dermatology** (dĕr-mă-TŎL-ō-jē)	dermat/o/logy	**dermat** = skin **logy** = study of	study of the skin
9. **ecchymosis** (ĕk-ĭ-MŌ-sĭs)	ecchym/osis	**ecchym** = blood in the tissues **osis** = abnormal condition	abnormal condition of blood in the tissues
10. **epidermal** (ĕp-ĭ-DĔR-măl)	epi/derm/al	**epi** = upon **derm** = skin **al** = pertaining to	pertaining to upon the skin
11. **epidermis*** (ĕp-ĭ-DĔR-mĭs)	epi/dermis	**epi** = upon **dermis** = skin	upon the skin
12. **erythematous** (ĕr-ĭ-THĔM-ă-tŭs)	erythemat/ous	**erythemat** = redness **ous** = pertaining to	pertaining to redness
Prefixes = **Green** Root Words = **Red** Suffixes = **Blue**			

*The term *epidermis* is made up of the prefix *epi-* and an unusual blending of the Greek word *derma*, which means "skin," and the Latin word *cutis*, which means "surface layer of the skin."

Term	Dissection	Word Part/Meaning	Term Definition
13. **erythrodermal** (ĕ-RĬTH-rō-DĔR-măl)	erythr/o/derm/al	**erythr** = red **derm** = skin **al** = pertaining to	pertaining to red skin
14. **hematoma** (hēm-ă-TŌ-mă)	hemat/oma	**hemat** = blood **oma** = tumor; mass	tumor/mass of blood
15. **hypodermic** (hī-pō-DĔR-mĭk)	hypo/derm/ic	**hypo** = below **derm** = skin **ic** = pertaining to	pertaining to below the skin
16. **intradermal** (ĭn-tră-DĔR-măl)	intra/derm/al	**intra** = within **derm** = skin **al** = pertaining to	pertaining to within the skin
17. **lipocyte** (LĬP-ō-sīt)	lip/o/cyte	**lip** = fat **cyte** = cell	fat cell
18. **lipoid** (LĬP-oyd)	lip/oid	**lip** = fat **oid** = like; resembling	like or resembling fat
19. **lipoma** (lĭ-PŌ-mă)	lip/oma	**lip** = fat **oma** = tumor; mass	tumor/mass of fat
20. **malignancy** (mă-LĬG-năn-sē)	malign/ancy	**malign** = causing harm; cancer **ancy** = state of	state of cancer
21. **melanocyte** (MĔL-ăn-ō-sīt)	melan/o/cyte	**melan** = black **cyte** = cell	black cell
22. **melanoma** (mĕl-ă-NŌ-mă)	melan/oma	**melan** = black **oma** = tumor; mass	black tumor
23. **mycotic** (mī-KŎT-ĭk)	myc/o/tic	**myc** = fungus **tic** = pertaining to	pertaining to fungus
24. **necrotic** (nĕ-KRŎT-ĭk)	necr/o/tic	**necr** = death **tic** = pertaining to	pertaining to death
25. **onychectomy** (ŏn-ĭ-KĔK-tō-mē)	onych/ectomy	**onych** = nail **ectomy** = surgical removal; excision	excision of the nail (of a finger or toe)
26. **onychoma** (ŏn-ĭ-KŌ-mă)	onych/oma	**onych** = nail **oma** = tumor; mass	tumor of the nail
27. **onychomycosis** (ŎN-ĭ-kō-mī-KŌ-sĭs)	onych/o/myc/osis	**onych** = nail **myc** = fungus **osis** = abnormal condition	abnormal condition of nail fungus
28. **onychosis** (ŏn-ĭ-KŌ-sĭs)	onych/osis	**onych** = nail **osis** = abnormal condition	abnormal condition of the nail
29. **onychotomy** (ŏn-ĭ-KŎT-ō-mē)	onych/o/tomy	**onych** = nail **tomy** = incision; cut into	incision/cut into the nail

Prefixes = **Green**   Root Words = **Red**   Suffixes = **Blue**

Term	Dissection	Word Part/Meaning	Term Definition
30. **pathologist** (pă-THŎL-ō-jĭst)	path/o/logist	**path** = disease **logist** = specialist in the study and treatment of	specialist in the study and treatment of disease
31. **percutaneous** (pĕr-kyū-TĀ-nē-ŭs)	per/cutane/ous	**per** = through **cutane** = skin **ous** = pertaining to	pertaining to through the skin
32. **pruritic** (prū-RĬT-ĭk)	prurit/ic	**prurit** = itching **ic** = pertaining to	pertaining to itching
33. **pyogenic** (pī-ō-JĔN-ĭk)	py/o/gen/ic	**py** = pus **gen** = producing **ic** = pertaining to	pertaining to producing pus
34. **pyorrhea** (pī-ō-RĒ-ă)	py/o/rrhea	**py** = pus **rrhea** = flow; discharge	flow/discharge of pus
35. **schizotrichia** (skĭt-sō-TRĬK-ē-ă)	schiz/o/trich/ia	**schiz** = split **trich** = hair **ia** = condition	condition of split hair
36. **seborrhea** (sĕb-ō-RĒ-ă)	seb/o/rrhea	**seb** = sebum or oil **rrhea** = flow; discharge	flow/discharge of sebum or oil
37. **squamous** (SKWĀ-mŭs)	squam/ous	**squam** = scale-like **ous** = pertaining to	pertaining to scale-like
38. **subcutaneous** (sŭb-kyū-TĀ-nē-ŭs)	sub/cutane/ous	**sub** = beneath; below **cutane** = skin **ous** = pertaining to	pertaining to beneath the skin
39. **topical** (TŎP-ik-ăl)	topic/al	**topic** = place **al** = pertaining to	pertaining to place
40. **transdermal** (trans-DĔR-măl)	trans/derm/al	**trans** = across **derm** = skin **al** = pertaining to	pertaining to across the skin
41. **trichomycosis** (trĭk-ō-mī-KŌ-sĭs)	trich/o/myc/osis	**trich** = hair **myc** = fungus **osis** = abnormal condition	abnormal condition of fungus in the hair
42. **xeroderma** (zē-rō-DĔR-mă)	xer/o/derma	**xer** = dry **derma** = skin	dry skin

Prefixes = Green   Root Words = Red   Suffixes = Blue

Using the pronunciation guide in the Breaking Down and Building chart, practice saying each medical term aloud. To hear the pronunciation of each term, complete the Pronounce It activity on the next page.

Studying medical terminology is similar to learning a foreign language. At first, pronouncing new medical terms can be challenging. To develop fluency, it is necessary to practice pronouncing the terms until you are comfortable saying them aloud.

Audio Activity: Pronounce It

Directions: Access your *EduHub* subscription and listen to the correct pronunciations of the following medical terms. Practice pronouncing the terms until you are comfortable saying them aloud.

contusion
(kŏn-TŪ-zhŭn)

cyanodermal
(SĪ-ă-nō-DĔR-măl)

cyanosis
(sī-ă-NŌ-sĭs)

cystic
(SĬS-tĭk)

dermal
(DĔR-măl)

dermatitis
(DĔR-mă-TĪ-tĭs)

dermatologist
(dĕr-mă-TŎL-ō-jĭst)

dermatology
(dĕr-mă-TŎL-ō-jē)

ecchymosis
(ĕk-ĭ-MŌ-sĭs)

epidermal
(ĕp-ĭ-DĔR-măl)

epidermis
(ĕp-ĭ-DĔR-mĭs)

erythematous
(ĕr-ĭ-THĔM-ă-tŭs)

erythrodermal
(ĕ-RĬTH-rō-DĔR-măl)

hematoma
(hēm-ă-TŌ-mă)

hypodermic
(hī-pō-DĔR-mĭk)

intradermal
(ĭn-tră-DĔR-măl)

lipocyte
(LĬP-ō-sīt)

lipoid
(LĬP-oyd)

lipoma
(lĭ-PŌ-mă)

malignancy
(mă-LĬG-năn-sē)

melanocyte
(MĔL-ăn-ō-sīt)

melanoma
(mĕl-ă-NŌ-mă)

mycotic
(mī-KŎT-ĭk)

necrotic
(nĕ-KRŎT-ĭk)

onychectomy
(ŏn-ĭ-KĔK-tō-mē)

onychoma
(ŏn-ĭ-KŌ-mă)

onychomycosis
(ŎN-ĭ-kō-mī-KŌ-sĭs)

onychosis
(ŏn-ĭ-KŌ-sĭs)

onychotomy
(ŏn-ĭ-KŎT-ō-mē)

pathologist
(pă-THŎL-ō-jĭst)

percutaneous
(pĕr-kyū-TĀ-nē-ŭs)

pruritic
(prū-RĬT-ĭk)

pyogenic
(pī-ō-JĔN-ĭk)

pyorrhea
(pī-ō-RĒ-ă)

schizotrichia
(skĭt-sō-TRĬK-ē-ă)

seborrhea
(sĕb-ō-RĒ-ă)

squamous
(SKWĀ-mŭs)

subcutaneous
(sŭb-kyū-TĀ-nē-ŭs)

topical
(TŎP-ik-ăl)

transdermal
(trans-DĔR-măl)

trichomycosis
(trĭk-ō-mī-KŌ-sĭs)

xeroderma
(zē-rō-DĔR-mă)

Assessment 2.4

Audio Activity: Spell It

Directions: Access your *EduHub* subscription and listen to the pronunciation for each number. As you hear each term, write its correct spelling.

1. _____
2. _____
3. _____
4. _____
5. _____
6. _____
7. _____
8. _____
9. _____
10. _____

11. _____
12. _____
13. _____
14. _____
15. _____
16. _____
17. _____
18. _____
19. _____
20. _____

21. _____   32. _____

22. _____   33. _____

23. _____   34. _____

24. _____   35. _____

25. _____   36. _____

26. _____   37. _____

27. _____   38. _____

28. _____   39. _____

29. _____   40. _____

30. _____   41. _____

31. _____   42. _____

Assessment 2.5

Break It Down

Directions: Dissect each medical term into its word parts (prefix, root word, combining vowel, and suffix) using one or more slashes. Then define each term. You can also complete this activity online using *EduHub*.

Example:

Medical Term: schizotrichia

Dissection: schiz/o/trich/ia

Definition: condition of split hair (ends)

Medical Term	Dissection
1. cyanodermal	c y a n o d e r m a l

Definition: _____

_____

| 2. onychosis | o n y c h o s i s |

Definition: _____

_____

Medical Term	Dissection
3. schizotrichia	s c h i z o t r i c h i a

Definition: _____

_____

4. ecchymosis   e c c h y m o s i s

Definition: _____

_____

5. lipocyte   l i p o c y t e

Definition: _____

_____

6. contusion   c o n t u s i o n

Definition: _____

_____

7. erythematous   e r y t h e m a t o u s

Definition: _____

_____

8. pyogenic   p y o g e n i c

Definition: _____

_____

9. cyanosis   c y a n o s i s

Definition: _____

_____

10. melanocyte   m e l a n o c y t e

Definition: _____

_____

Medical Term	Dissection
11. percutaneous	p e r c u t a n e o u s

Definition: _____

_____

| 12. onychectomy | o n y c h e c t o m y |

Definition: _____

_____

| 13. subcutaneous | s u b c u t a n e o u s |

Definition: _____

_____

| 14. cystic | c y s t i c |

Definition: _____

_____

| 15. erythrodermal | e r y t h r o d e r m a l |

Definition: _____

_____

| 16. pathologist | p a t h o l o g i s t |

Definition: _____

_____

| 17. lipoma | l i p o m a |

Definition: _____

_____

| 18. onychomycosis | o n y c h o m y c o s i s |

Definition: _____

_____

Medical Term	Dissection
19. dermal	d e r m a l

Definition: _____

_____

20. xeroderma   x e r o d e r m a

Definition: _____

_____

21. topical   t o p i c a l

Definition: _____

_____

22. dermatology   d e r m a t o l o g y

Definition: _____

_____

23. transdermal   t r a n s d e r m a l

Definition: _____

_____

24. hypodermic   h y p o d e r m i c

Definition: _____

_____

25. epidermis   e p i d e r m i s

Definition: _____

_____

26. squamous   s q u a m o u s

Definition: _____

_____

Medical Term	Dissection
27. malignancy	m a l i g n a n c y

Definition: _____

_____

| 28. mycotic | m y c o t i c |

Definition: _____

_____

| 29. dermatitis | d e r m a t i t i s |

Definition: _____

_____

| 30. onychotomy | o n y c h o t o m y |

Definition: _____

_____

| 31. onychoma | o n y c h o m a |

Definition: _____

_____

| 32. pruritic | p r u r i t i c |

Definition: _____

_____

| 33. dermatologist | d e r m a t o l o g i s t |

Definition: _____

_____

| 34. intradermal | i n t r a d e r m a l |

Definition: _____

_____

Medical Term	Dissection
35. necrotic	n e c r o t i c

Definition: _____

_____

36. hematoma   h e m a t o m a

Definition: _____

_____

37. epidermal   e p i d e r m a l

Definition: _____

_____

38. melanoma   m e l a n o m a

Definition: _____

_____

39. seborrhea   s e b o r r h e a

Definition: _____

_____

40. lipoid   l i p o i d

Definition: _____

_____

41. pyorrhea   p y o r r h e a

Definition: _____

_____

42. trichomycosis   t r i c h o m y c o s i s

Definition: _____

_____

SCORECARD: How Did You Do?

Number correct (_____), divided by 42 (_____), multiplied by 100 equals _____ (your score)

Build It

Directions: Build the medical term that matches each definition by supplying the correct word parts. You can also complete this activity online using *EduHub*.

P (Prefixes) = Green
RW (Root Words) = Red
S (Suffixes) = Blue
CV (Combining Vowel) = Purple

1. pertaining to blue skin

    _____   _____ _____   _____
    RW   CV   RW   S

2. specialist in the study and treatment of disease

    _____   _____ _____
    RW   CV   S

3. fat cell

    _____   _____ _____
    RW   CV   S

4. pertaining to red skin

    _____   _____ _____   _____
    RW   CV   RW   S

5. pertaining to through the skin

    _____ _____   _____
    P   RW   S

6. tumor of blood

    _____   _____
    RW   S

7. pertaining to a sac containing fluid

    _____   _____
    RW   S

8. condition of bruising

    _____   _____
    RW   S

9. pertaining to producing pus

    _____   _____ _____ _____
    RW   CV   S   S

10. condition of split hair

_____ ____ _____ ____
RW   CV   RW   S

11. inflammation of the skin

_____ _____
RW   S

12. abnormal condition of nail fungus

_____ ____ _____ ____
RW   CV   RW   S

13. pertaining to scale-like

_____ _____
RW   S

14. pertaining to below the skin (two possible answers)

_____ _____ _____
P   RW   S

_____ _____ _____
P   RW   S

15. flow or discharge of pus

_____ ____ ____
RW   CV   S

16. pertaining to the skin

_____ _____
RW   S

17. black cell

_____ ____ ____
RW   CV   S

18. pertaining to upon the skin

_____ _____ _____
P   RW   S

19. flow or discharge of sebum or oil

_____ ____ ____
RW   CV   S

20. incision/cut into the nail

——————————— ——— ———
         RW   CV   S

21. specialist in the study and treatment of the skin

——————————— ——— ———
         RW   CV   S

22. pertaining to death

——————————— ——— ———
         RW   CV   S

23. abnormal condition of blood in the tissues

——————————— ————————
         RW   S

24. abnormal condition of fungus in the hair

——————————— ——— ——————————— ———
         RW   CV   RW   S

25. upon the skin

——— ———————————
   P   RW

26. tumor of fat

——————————— ————————
         RW   S

27. pertaining to across the skin

——— ——————————— ————————
   P   RW   S

28. abnormal condition of blue

——————————— ————————
         RW   S

29. the study of the skin

——————————— ——— ———
         RW   CV   S

30. tumor of the nail

——————————— ————————
         RW   S

31. pertaining to within the skin

_____ _____ _____
    P   RW   S

32. state of cancer

_____ _____
       RW   S

33. like or resembling fat

_____ _____
       RW   S

34. pertaining to itching

_____ _____
       RW   S

35. pertaining to fungus

_____ _____ _____
       RW   CV   S

36. abnormal condition of the nail

_____ _____
       RW   S

37. surgical removal/excision of the nail

_____ _____
       RW   S

38. black tumor

_____ _____
       RW   S

39. pertaining to place

_____ _____
       RW   S

40. dry skin

_____ _____ _____
       RW   CV   RW

SCORECARD: How Did You Do?

Number correct (_____), divided by 40 (_____), multiplied by 100 equals _____ (your score)

Diseases and Disorders

Diseases and disorders of the integumentary system range from the mild to the severe, and they have a wide variety of causes. We will now take a look at some problems that commonly affect this body system.

Acne

Acne is a disorder that affects the sebaceous glands. It is most common during puberty when the sebaceous glands secrete large amounts of sebum, predominantly on the face, shoulders, and back.

Acne develops when excess sebum accumulates around the hair shaft and then hardens, blocking the hair follicle. Oily sebum traps dirt, enlarges the skin pore, and then turns black when exposed to air. The result is a *comedo*, or blackhead. A hardened white bump, or *whitehead,* appears when the pore becomes clogged with sebum that cannot reach the skin's surface. Bacteria may also invade the clogged pore, causing the formation of a small, infected skin elevation called a *pustule*. When the pustule becomes red and inflamed, it is called a *pimple* (Figure 2.3).

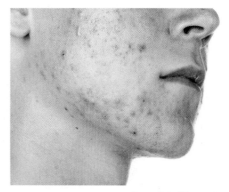

Suzanne Tucker/Shutterstock.com

Figure 2.3 Acne

Alopecia

Alopecia is an acute or chronic loss of scalp hair. Acute hair loss is usually a side effect of radiation or chemotherapy treatment in cancer patients. It can also be caused by a fungal infection or damage to the hair shaft or follicles.

There are two main forms of chronic hair loss. Chronic alopecia, also called *androgenetic alopecia,* is an inherited condition that typically begins during middle age and gradually worsens as a person gets older. Androgenetic alopecia is characterized by thinning of the hair on the top of the scalp; eventually, the hair disappears (Figure 2.4 on the next page). Hormonal changes in susceptible men and women may also lead to alopecia, known as *male-pattern baldness* and *female-pattern baldness.* In some cases, a genetic predisposition may cause hair loss in men and women beginning in their twenties.

The second main form of chronic hair loss, *alopecia areata*, is caused by an autoimmune disorder. An autoimmune disorder is one in which the immune system of the body attacks its own tissues because it does not recognize and distinguish between a normal part of the body (self) and a substance that is foreign to the body (non-self). In alopecia areata, the body's immune system attacks its own hair follicles, causing hair to fall out all over the body. (You will learn more about autoimmune disorders in Chapter 5: The Lymphatic and Immune Systems.) Young children can be affected by alopecia areata.

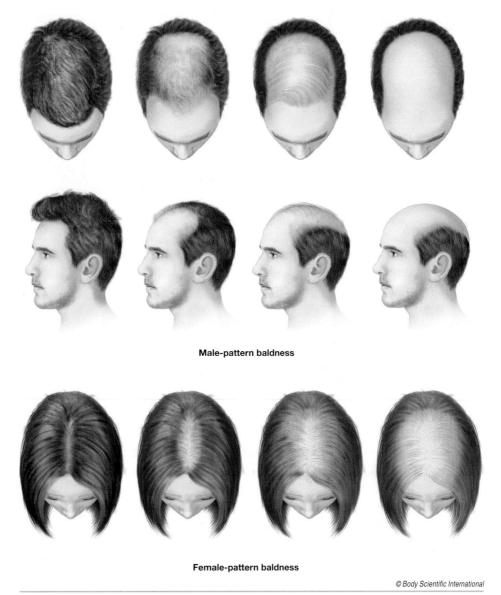

Male-pattern baldness

Female-pattern baldness

© Body Scientific International

Figure 2.4 Androgenetic alopecia

Burns

Heat, electricity, chemicals, or radiation can cause burns to the skin. The severity of a burn is classified based on two factors: depth and extent of injury.

First-degree burns (Figure 2.5A) are mild burns that involve only the epidermis. They result in edema (swelling), pain, and **erythema** (ĕr-ĭ-THĒ-mă), or redness. Generally, however, first-degree burns do not produce scarring.

Second-degree burns (Figure 2.5B) extend through the epidermis and into the dermis, causing blisters, erythema, pain, edema, and sometimes scarring. A second-degree burn is also known as a *partial-thickness burn*.

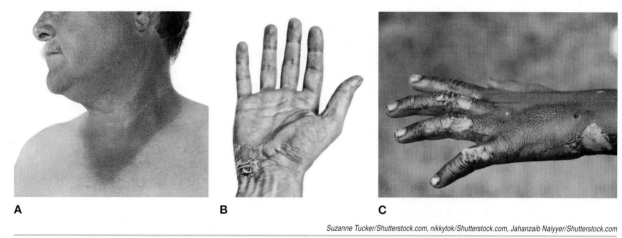

A **B** **C**

Figure 2.5 Different types of burns. A—First-degree burn. B—Second-degree burn. C—Third-degree burn.

Third-degree burns (Figure 2.5C) affect the epidermis, dermis, and sometimes the subcutaneous tissue and muscle. Third-degree burns, also called *full-thickness burns*, cause charred (black) skin and formation of a thick, crusty scar of necrotic tissue. Third-degree burns can become infected and delay healing, so they must be surgically removed.

Cancer of the Skin

Cancer is divided into two categories: **benign** (noncancerous) and **malignant** (causing cancer). **Malignant melanoma** is an aggressive form of skin cancer that originates in the melanocytes of the epidermis and quickly **metastasizes** (grows and spreads) to other parts of the body (Figure 2.6). Skin cancer can arise in areas that have been chronically exposed to the damaging ultraviolet light (UVA and UVB rays) of the sun.

People susceptible to UV damage include those with fair skin, which contains less melanin to absorb radiation, and older adults, who have endured a lifetime of sunlight exposure. Regular self-examination of the skin, along with the use of sunscreen and avoidance of prolonged exposure to the sun, not only reduces damage to the skin, but also helps prevent the development of skin cancer. Irregular changes in the color, shape, or size of skin moles or lesions should be examined by a dermatologist.

Contact Dermatitis

Contact dermatitis occurs when the skin comes in contact with an allergen or irritant, causing edema and pruritic (itchy) skin (Figure 2.7). Chemicals contained in deodorants,

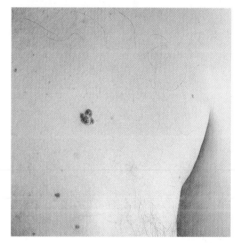

Figure 2.6 Skin cancer

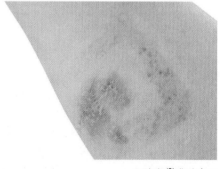

Figure 2.7 Contact dermatitis caused by exposure to poison ivy

soaps, perfumes, or makeup may cause the skin to become inflamed, red, and irritated. Small vesicles (fluid-filled sacs) may appear on the skin. Contact dermatitis may also be caused by exposure to animal dander, poison ivy, or synthetic products containing latex.

Edema

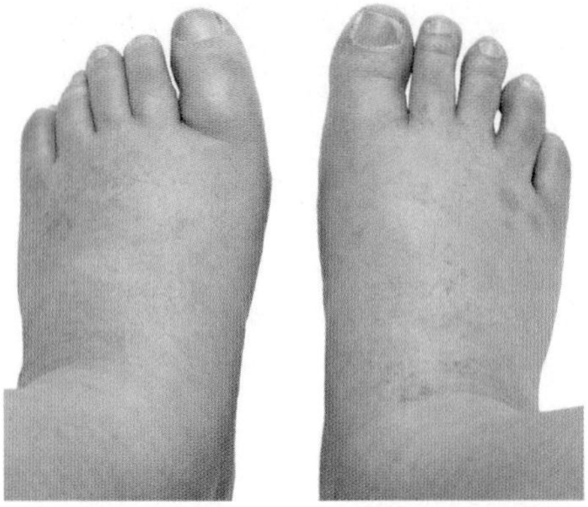

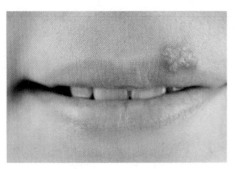

tugolukof/Shutterstock.com

Figure 2.8 Edema

Edema comes from the Greek word *oidēma*, which means "swelling." This disorder is characterized by the buildup of excessive fluid in the body tissues, causing them to swell (Figure 2.8). Edema may result from large amounts of fluid moving from the blood into the dermis or subcutaneous tissues. Localized infections, allergic reactions, and some cardiovascular and urinary system diseases produce edema.

Herpes

Herpes comes from a Greek word meaning "to creep," an appropriate derivation given that this inflammatory disease is characterized by vesicles that appear to "creep" across the skin. Other symptoms include erythema, edema, and pain. Itching and soreness are usually present before the development of erythematous (ĕr-ĭ-THĔM-ă-tŭs) (red) patches. When the vesicles rupture, they release fluid that forms a crust.

The two most common types of herpes are herpes simplex and herpes zoster. **Herpes simplex** is caused by *herpes simplex virus 1* (HSV-1), which produces painful blisters on or around the lips (Figure 2.9). These blisters, commonly called *cold sores* or *fever blisters,* tend to recur during illness or stress. Topical or oral antiviral drugs are typically prescribed for herpes simplex.

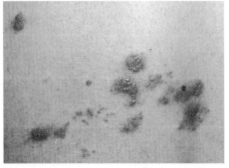

Levent Konuk/Shutterstock.com

Figure 2.9 Herpes simplex viral infection

Herpes zoster is an acute viral disease marked by inflammation of a nerve root, causing the appearance of painful blisters along the path of the nerve (Figure 2.10). Herpes zoster is more commonly called *shingles*. The herpes zoster virus is the same virus that causes chickenpox. The virus remains dormant in the nerves long after recovery from chickenpox, and it can become active due to stress or an immune system weakened with age.

Psoriasis

Psoriasis is a chronic skin disorder characterized by scaly, silvery-white patches and erythematous skin. The excessive production of epidermal cells associated with psoriasis is thought to be the result of an autoimmune disorder.

Stephen VanHorn/Shutterstock.com

Figure 2.10 Herpes zoster infection

The pruritic, erythematous, silvery scales and plaques (small, abnormal patches) caused by psoriasis usually appear on the scalp, elbows, hands, and knees (Figure 2.11). Psoriasis has a hereditary component, and the condition seems to worsen during physical, mental, or emotional stress. Because its etiology is unknown, there is no cure for psoriasis. Treatment consists of topical coal tar drugs, corticosteroid drugs, vitamin A and D supplements, and ultraviolet light therapy.

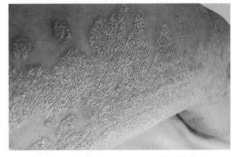

Figure 2.11 Psoriasis is characterized by pruritic, erythematous, silvery patches.

Procedures and Treatments

In this section, we will briefly describe some common diagnostic procedures used to help identify disorders and diseases of the integumentary system, as well as common therapeutic procedures used to treat certain conditions.

Biopsy

A **biopsy (Bx)** is a surgical procedure performed to remove all or part of a skin lesion for pathological evaluation (Figure 2.12). It may be performed using a knife, needle, brush, or punch (a sharp, round instrument). The biopsy specimen is sent to a laboratory, where a pathologist examines it under a microscope. The pathologist's findings are used to help make a diagnosis.

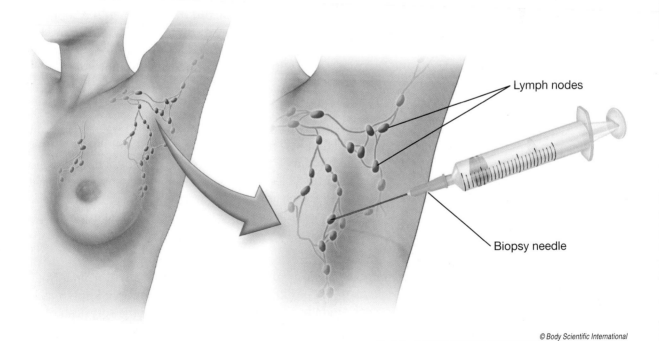

Lymph nodes

Biopsy needle

Figure 2.12 Needle biopsy

Cryosurgery

Cryosurgery is a technique in which liquid nitrogen, an extremely low-temperature fluid, is used to freeze and destroy abnormal skin cells or lesions (Figure 2.13). The nitrogen gas is applied directly to the tissue using an applicator, probe, or spray. This quick, simple, low-risk procedure can be performed in a doctor's office to freeze and destroy warts, moles, other benign lesions, or some small, malignant lesions.

Debridement

Debridement is a medical procedure in which damaged and necrotic tissue or foreign material is removed from a skin wound. Debridement of a wound prevents an infection from developing and helps the physician determine the depth and extent of the wound. Debridement is also used to remove thick, crusty, necrotic tissue that forms on a third-degree burn.

Incision and Drainage

Incision and drainage (I&D) is a dermatologic procedure commonly performed to treat a cyst or abscess. A scalpel or needle is used to puncture or cut the skin lesion above the cyst or abscess, which is then drained of fluid or pus.

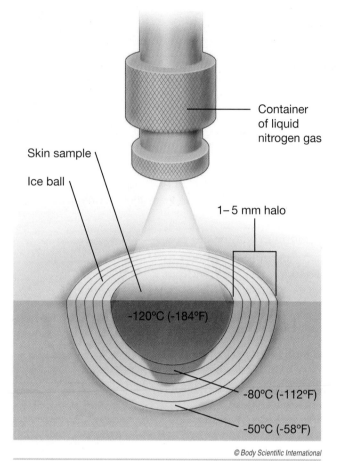

Container of liquid nitrogen gas

Skin sample

Ice ball

1–5 mm halo

-120°C (-184°F)

-80°C (-112°F)

-50°C (-58°F)

© Body Scientific International

Figure 2.13 Cryosurgery

Laser Surgery

A laser is a light beam that can be precisely focused on its target. It is used to treat diseased or damaged tissue by heating the targeted cells until they "burst."

Laser surgery is a medical procedure in which rapid pulses of light are used to remove diseased tissue or treat bleeding blood vessels. Laser surgery may also be used for cosmetic purposes, such as removing wrinkles, sunspots, birthmarks, tattoos, or enlarged blood vessels that are superficial (close to the skin's surface).

Onychectomy

An **onychectomy** is the surgical excision (removal) of a nail from a finger or toe. *Onychocryptosis* (ŎN-ĭ-kō-krĭp-TŌ-sĭs), more commonly known as an *ingrown toenail*, is a condition in which the nail grows into the soft flesh of the toe, causing pain, erythema, edema, and sometimes a fungal infection called *onychomycosis* (ŎN-ĭ-kō-mī-KŌ-sĭs). If onychomycosis is unresponsive to treatment, the physician may recommend removing all or part of the nail plate.

Diseases, Disorders, Procedures, and Treatments

Directions: Define each disease, disorder, procedure, or treatment. You can also complete this activity online using *EduHub*.

1. biopsy _____

_____

2. contact dermatitis _____

_____

3. malignant melanoma _____

_____

4. cryosurgery _____

_____

5. edema _____

_____

6. acne _____

_____

7. debridement _____

_____

8. onychectomy _____

_____

9. psoriasis _____

_____

10. alopecia _____

_____

11. laser surgery _____

_____

12. herpes _____

_____

13. incision and drainage (I&D) _____

_____

14. first-degree burn _____

_____

15. second-degree burn _____

_____

_____

16. third-degree burn _____

_____

_____

Assessment 2.8

Identifying Abbreviations

Directions: Supply the correct abbreviation for each medical term. You can also complete this activity online using *EduHub*.

Medical Term	Abbreviation
1. ultraviolet light	_____
2. biopsy	_____
3. herpes simplex virus 1	_____
4. incision and drainage	_____

Analyzing the Intern Experience

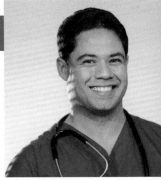

As you know, all professionals in the healthcare field speak the same language—medical terminology. Patients come to the doctor's office with a variety of signs and symptoms that must be translated and communicated to other medical professionals using correct terminology. As a healthcare professional, you will be expected to pronounce, spell, write, and understand medical terms.

In the Intern Experience at the beginning of this chapter, Kate arrived at the doctor's office with specific signs and symptoms. Kate's doctor obtained a history of her health problems, performed a medical examination, and ordered a diagnostic test to help determine the cause of her condition. He analyzed all of this information, made a medical diagnosis, and formulated a treatment plan. The physician then made a dictated recording of Kate's health information, which was later transcribed into a medical record. In an outpatient setting, a medical record is commonly known as a *chart note*.

We will now analyze the Intern Experience scenario from a clinical perspective, interpreting the medical terms in Kate's chart note to gain an understanding of her health condition.

Audio Activity: Kate Stephano's Chart Note

Directions: Access your *EduHub* subscription and listen to the recording of the physician reading Kate Stephano's chart note. Read along with the physician and pay attention to the pronunciation of each medical term.

CHART NOTE

Patient Name: Stephano, Kate
ID Number: 96453
Examination Date: January 23, 20xx

SUBJECTIVE
Kate was seen today for complaints of red and swollen, right great toe. Patient denies injury. She is extremely anxious about the appearance of her toe.

OBJECTIVE
Examination reveals **erythematous** right great toe with purulent (pertaining to pus) drainage around the nail bed. The nail is thickened and appears to be **mycotic** in nature. It involves the entire nail plate.

ASSESSMENT
Onychomycosis

PLAN
Onychectomy. This is deferred due to patient anxiety and her desire to discuss this plan with her parents. Will follow up with phone call on how she wants to proceed.

Interpret Kate Stephano's Chart Note

Directions: Access your *EduHub* subscription and listen to the recording of the physician reading Kate Stephano's chart note. After listening to the recording, supply the medical term that matches each definition.

Example: condition of dry skin   *Answer:* xeroderma

1. pertaining to fungus   _____

2. surgical removal/excision of the nail   _____

3. pertaining to redness of the skin   _____

4. condition of nail fungus   _____

SCORECARD: How Did You Do?

Number correct (_____), divided by 4 (_____), multiplied by 100 equals _____ (your score)

Working with Medical Records

In this activity, you will interpret the medical records (chart notes) of patients with health problems related to the integumentary system. These examples illustrate typical medical records prepared in a real-world healthcare environment. To interpret these chart notes, you will apply your knowledge of word elements (prefixes, combining forms, and suffixes), diseases and disorders, and procedures and treatments related to the integumentary system.

Audio Activity: Matthew Dixon's Chart Note

Directions: Access your *EduHub* subscription and listen to the recording of the physician reading Matthew Dixon's chart note. Read along with the physician and pay attention to the pronunciation of each medical term.

CHART NOTE

Patient Name: Dixon, Matthew
ID Number: 98651
Examination Date: February 16, 20xx

SUBJECTIVE
Patient presents with painful lump on right side of neck. Slight fever of 101°F, but denies any chills or sweating.

OBJECTIVE
There is an **erythematous** cystic lesion of the **epidermis** measuring 3×4 cm. The mass is fluctuant (movable and compressible) and slightly tender to the touch. No lymphadenomegaly (enlarged lymph glands) noted.

ASSESSMENT
Infected sebaceous cyst; right neck.

PLAN
Area was sterilely prepped and injected with 1% lidocaine (drug that numbs). A #11 scalpel blade was used to incise the **pyogenic** cyst. Copious amounts of purulent (pus-containing) material and sebum were extracted. Wound was irrigated with sterile saline solution and packed with ¼-inch gauze, and sterile dressing was applied. The **sebaceous** material was sent for culture. Prescribed cephalexin 250 mg q.i.d. × 10 days (take a 250 mg tablet of cephalexin, an antibiotic, 4 times per day for 10 days). Will return in 2 days for recheck.

Assessment 2.10

Interpret Matthew Dixon's Chart Note

Directions: Access your *EduHub* subscription and listen to the recording of the physician reading Matthew Dixon's chart note. After listening to the recording, supply the medical term that matches each definition.

Example: pertaining to within the skin   *Answer:* intradermal

1. pertaining to oil   _____

2. upon the skin   _____

3. pertaining to redness   _____

4. pertaining to producing pus   _____

SCORECARD: How Did You Do?

Number correct (_____), divided by 4 (_____), multiplied by 100 equals _____ (your score)

Audio Activity: Bennett Meira's Chart Note

Directions: Access your *EduHub* subscription and listen to the recording of the physician reading Bennett Meira's chart note. Read along with the physician and pay attention to the pronunciation of each medical term.

CHART NOTE

Patient Name: Meira, Bennett
ID Number: 94421
Examination Date: February 20, 20xx

SUBJECTIVE
Patient is a 19-year-old male who was brought to FedDes Urgent Care by friends. He states that he was "knifed" due to a dispute over the outcome of a pool game. He has **contusions** to the abdomen and forehead and a stab wound of the right thigh. His tetanus is up to date. No other injuries. Denies any allergies and is not on any medications.

OBJECTIVE
Patient has a 2.5-cm vertical laceration of the lateral aspect of the right thigh that goes through the **epidermis**, **dermis**, and **subcutaneous** tissue down to the vascular layer of the thigh muscles. There does not appear to be any muscle injury, and there is no active bleeding, so no muscular tissue repair is necessary. **Ecchymosis** of the lower right anterior abdomen. Small **hematoma** of the forehead.

ASSESSMENT
Laceration, right lateral thigh.

PLAN
Suture repair and dressing applied. Wound care sheet given. Patient to return in 8 days for suture removal or earlier if signs of infection occur. He can use ibuprofen for pain. He was released in stable condition.

Assessment 2.11

Interpret Bennett Meira's Chart Note

Directions: Access your *EduHub* subscription and listen to the recording of the physician reading Bennett Meira's chart note. After listening to the recording, supply the medical term that matches each definition.

Example: pertaining to redness of the skin   *Answer:* erythematous

1. upon the skin   _____

2. beneath the skin   _____

3. "true skin"   _____

4. tumor of blood   _____

5. condition of blood in tissue   _____

6. condition of bruising   _____

SCORECARD: How Did You Do?

Number correct (_____), divided by 6 (_____), multiplied by 100 equals _____ (your score)

Chapter Review

Word Elements Summary

Prefixes

Prefix	Meaning
epi-	upon
hypo-	below; below normal
intra-	within
per-	through
sub-	beneath; below
trans-	across

Combining Forms

Root Word/Combining Vowel	Meaning
carcin/o	cancer
contus/o	bruising
cry/o	cold
cutane/o	skin
cyan/o	blue
cyst/o	sac containing fluid
derm/a, derm/o, dermat/o	skin
ecchym/o	blood in the tissues
erythemat/o	redness
erythr/o	red
hemat/o	blood
lip/o	fat
malign/o	causing harm; cancer
melan/o	black
myc/o	fungus
necr/o	death
onych/o	nail
path/o	disease

(Continued)

Root Word/Combining Vowel	Meaning
prurit/o	itching
py/o	pus
schiz/o	split
seb/o	oil or sebum
squam/o	scale-like
topic/o	place
trich/o	hair
xer/o	dry

Suffixes

Suffix	Meaning
-al	pertaining to
-ancy	state of
-cyte	cell
-ectomy	surgical removal; excision
-gen	producing; originating; causing
-ia	condition
-ic	pertaining to
-ion	condition
-itis	inflammation
-logist	specialist in the study and treatment of
-logy	study of
-oid	like; resembling
-oma	tumor; mass
-osis	abnormal condition
-ous	pertaining to
-rrhea	flow; discharge
-tic	pertaining to
-tomy	incision; cut into

More Practice: Activities and Games

The following activities will help you reinforce your skills and check your mastery of the medical terminology you learned in this chapter. Access your *EduHub* subscription to complete more activities and vocabulary games for mastering the word parts and terms you have learned.

Multiple Choice: Diseases and Disorders

Directions: Choose the disease or disorder that matches each definition.

_____ 1. a disorder in which body tissues retain an excessive amount of fluid, causing them to swell
  a. edema   c. acne
  b. psoriasis   d. alopecia

_____ 2. a disorder that is typically prominent during puberty, when the sebaceous glands secrete large amounts of sebum on the face, shoulders, and back
  a. edema   c. acne
  b. psoriasis   d. contact dermatitis

_____ 3. a disorder associated with silvery-white, scaly patches and erythematous skin
  a. contact dermatitis   c. psoriasis
  b. edema   d. acne

_____ 4. an acute loss of scalp hair
  a. contact dermatitis   c. herpes
  b. alopecia   d. psoriasis

_____ 5. a condition produced by contact with an allergen or irritant, causing edema, pruritic skin, and in many cases, small vesicles on the skin
  a. psoriasis   c. alopecia
  b. shingles   d. contact dermatitis

_____ 6. an aggressive type of skin cancer that begins in the melanocytes of the epidermis and quickly metastasizes to other parts of the body; caused by chronic exposure to the sun's ultraviolet rays
  a. third-degree burn   c. malignant melanoma
  b. shingles   d. alopecia

Multiple Choice: Procedures and Treatments

Directions: Choose the procedure or treatment that matches each definition.

_____ 1. a surgical procedure in which liquid nitrogen is used to freeze and destroy abnormal cells
  a. biopsy   c. onychectomy
  b. cryosurgery   d. debridement

_____ 2. excision, or surgical removal, of the nail from a finger or toe
  a. cryosurgery
  b. debridement
  c. onychectomy
  d. incision and drainage

_____ 3. surgical removal of all or part of a skin lesion for pathological examination
  a. onychectomy   c. debridement
  b. cryosurgery   d. biopsy

_____ 4. removal of foreign material or necrotic tissue from a skin wound
  a. laser surgery
  b. incision and drainage
  c. debridement
  d. biopsy

_____ 5. a medical procedure performed to drain a cyst or abscess
  a. incision and drainage
  b. laser surgery
  c. debridement
  d. onychectomy

_____ 6. the use of rapid pulses of light to remove wrinkles, sunspots, tattoos, birthmarks, or enlarged blood vessels that are close to the skin's surface
  a. incision and drainage
  b. laser surgery
  c. debridement
  d. onychectomy

True or False

Directions: Indicate whether each statement is true or false.

True or False?

_____ 1. Sudoriferous glands produce an oily substance called *sebum*.

_____ 2. The skin is our first line of defense against microbes, harmful chemicals, and the sun's ultraviolet rays.

_____ 3. The skin is made up of five layers.

_____ 4. Skin color is determined by the amount of melanin produced by melanocytes.

_____ 5. A lipoma is a tumor of blood.

_____ 6. An onychoma is a fungus of the nail.

_____ 7. Vesicles are fluid-filled sacs.

_____ 8. First-degree burns involve only the dermis.

_____ 9. A benign melanoma is an aggressive form of skin cancer.

_____ 10. Fair-skinned individuals are less susceptible to UV damage from the sun.

_____ 11. *Psoriasis* is a Greek word meaning "creeping skin disease caused by a virus."

_____ 12. Laser surgery uses rapid pulses of light to remove diseased tissue.

_____ 13. Sebaceous glands cool the body by secreting perspiration, or sweat.

_____ 14. The outer layer of the skin is called the *dermis*.

_____ 15. Melanocytes are responsible for the production of melanin, a pigment in the skin.

_____ 16. The epidermis is sometimes referred to as the "true skin."

_____ 17. A dermatologist is a physician who specializes in the study and treatment of the skin.

_____ 18. A whitehead is a pustule that appears when a pore becomes clogged with sebum that cannot reach the skin's surface.

_____ 19. The medical terms *cutaneous* and *dermal* both mean "pertaining to the skin."

_____ 20. The term *intradermal* means "beneath the skin."

Break It Down

Directions: Dissect each medical term into its word parts (prefix, root word, combining vowel, and suffix) using one or more slashes. Then define each term.

Medical Term	Dissection
1. cystectomy	c y s t e c t o m y

Definition: _____

_____

Medical Term	Dissection
2. dermatologic	d e r m a t o l o g i c

Definition: _____

_____

3. transcutaneous	t r a n s c u t a n e o u s

Definition: _____

_____

4. carcinogen	c a r c i n o g e n

Definition: _____

_____

5. ecchymotic	e c c h y m o t i c

Definition: _____

_____

6. subdermal	s u b d e r m a l

Definition: _____

_____

7. seborrheic	s e b o r r h e i c

Definition: _____

_____

8. intracystic	i n t r a c y s t i c

Definition: _____

_____

9. carcinogenic	c a r c i n o g e n i c

Definition: _____

_____

Medical Term	Dissection
10. cyanotic	c y a n o t i c

Definition: _____

_____

11. dermatopathology   d e r m a t o p a t h o l o g y

Definition: _____

_____

12. hypotrichosis   h y p o t r i c h o s i s

Definition: _____

_____

13. necrogenic   n e c r o g e n i c

Definition: _____

_____

14. trichoid   t r i c h o i d

Definition: _____

_____

15. hypoliposis   h y p o l i p o s i s

Definition: _____

_____

Audio Activity: Gwenn Larson's Chart Note

Directions: Access your *EduHub* subscription and listen to the recording of the physician reading Gwenn Larson's chart note. Read along with the physician and pay attention to the pronunciation of each medical term.

CHART NOTE

Patient Name: Larson, Gwenn
ID Number: 94671
Examination Date: February 24, 20xx

SUBJECTIVE
Patient returns with continued complaints of redness, swelling, and flaking of the skin around the elbow, **etiology** unknown. Patient wishes to discuss the results of her **biopsy.**

OBJECTIVE
Erythematous rash over left posterior elbow. Multiple trials of topical steroid applications have been unsuccessful.

ASSESSMENT
Biopsy report indicates chronic **psoriasis**.

PLAN
Prescribed new topical corticosteroid to be applied 3–4 times daily. **Prognosis** is favorable if the patient is compliant.

Assessment

Interpret Gwenn Larson's Chart Note

Directions: Access your *EduHub* subscription and listen to the recording of the physician reading Gwenn Larson's chart note. After listening to the recording, supply the medical term that matches each definition.

    Example: condition of bruising   *Answer:* contusion

1. removal of tissue for microscopic examination   _____

2. pertaining to redness of the skin   _____

3. chronic skin disorder characterized by silvery-white, scaly patches   _____

4. expected outcome   _____

5. cause of a disease or disorder   _____

Chapter 3
The Digestive System

gastr / o / enter / o / logy: the study of the digestive system

Chapter Organization

- Intern Experience
- Overview of Digestive System Anatomy and Physiology
- Word Elements
- Breaking Down and Building Digestive System Terms
- Diseases and Disorders
- Procedures and Treatments
- Analyzing the Intern Experience
- Working with Medical Records
- Chapter Review

Chapter Objectives

After completing this chapter, you will be able to

1. label an anatomical diagram of the digestive system;
2. dissect and define common medical terminology related to the digestive system;
3. build terms used to describe digestive system diseases and disorders, diagnostic procedures, and therapeutic treatments;
4. pronounce and spell common medical terminology related to the digestive system;
5. understand that the process of building and dissecting a medical term based on its prefix, root word, and suffix enables you to analyze an extremely large number of medical terms beyond those presented in this chapter;
6. interpret the meaning of abbreviations associated with the digestive system; and
7. interpret medical records containing terminology and abbreviations related to the digestive system.

Your *EduHub* subscription that accompanies this text provides access to online assessments, assignments, activities, and resources. Throughout this chapter, access *EduHub* to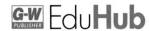

- use e-flash cards to review the medical terminology and word parts you learn;
- listen to the correct pronunciations of medical terms; and
- complete medical terminology activities and assignments.

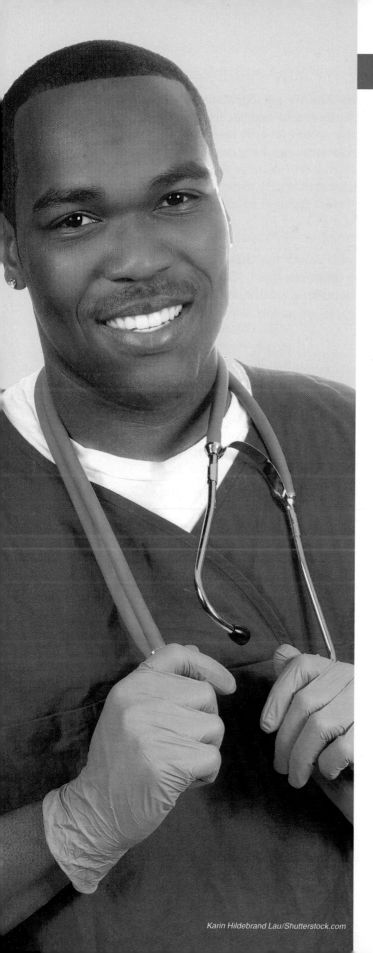

Intern Experience

Evan Walker, an intern with Gratz Urgent Care Clinic, is working with Dr. Emily Stomack this week. Evan accompanies Dr. Stomack to exam room 3, where a nervous, young female patient is waiting with her mother.

Evan and Dr. Stomack learn that the patient, Sue, had the lead role in her high school play. Too nervous to eat before the performance, she skipped dinner. After the play, Sue was very hungry, so her mother took Sue and her friend to the Brickhouse, a new restaurant in town. All three gobbled down the deluxe burger special and turkey noodle soup.

When Sue arrived home, she took her dog for a walk. While walking the dog, Sue suddenly felt like something was caught in her throat. She had difficulty swallowing, and the sensation would not go away. A few hours later, the symptoms persisted, so Sue's mother suggested that she make an appointment with their family doctor first thing the next morning.

Sue is experiencing a problem with her digestive system, the body system that breaks down food and converts it into the "fuel" that the body needs for physical and cellular processes. To help you understand what is happening to Sue, this chapter will present word elements (combining forms, prefixes, and suffixes) that make up medical terminology related to the digestive system. As you progress through this book, you will see many word parts that are also used in medical terms related to other body systems.

Before you begin this chapter, take some time to review the strategies presented in chapter 1 for analyzing medical terms. Reviewing these strategies will help you understand and recall the word elements and definitions of medical terms that you are about to learn, as well as those you learned previously.

After you have learned the medical terms presented in this chapter, you will practice analyzing patient chart notes. Accurate interpretation of these chart notes will demonstrate that you have a solid understanding of medical terminology related to the digestive system.

Let's begin our study with a brief overview of the anatomy and physiology of the digestive system.

Overview of Digestive System Anatomy and Physiology

Super Bowl parties are great fun. We get together with friends, watch the game, and of course eat our favorite snacks and beverages. While we're caught up in the excitement of cheering on our favorite team, our digestive systems are quietly working in the background, breaking down those snacks into life-sustaining chemical substances that will nourish the cells in our bodies and give us energy. In this section, we will briefly explore the major organs of the digestive system and how they work together to accomplish these tasks.

Major Organs of the Digestive System

The **digestive system** is also called the **digestive tract**, the **alimentary** (ăl-ĭ-MĔN-tăr-ē) **canal**, and the **gastrointestinal (GI) tract**. The digestive tract consists of a long, hollow tube that extends from the **pharynx** (FĂR-inks), more commonly known as the *throat*, to the anus. Major organs of the GI tract include the mouth, esophagus, stomach, small intestine, large intestine (colon), rectum, and anus (Figure 3.1). The liver, gallbladder, pancreas, salivary glands, and teeth are accessory organs that aid in digestion.

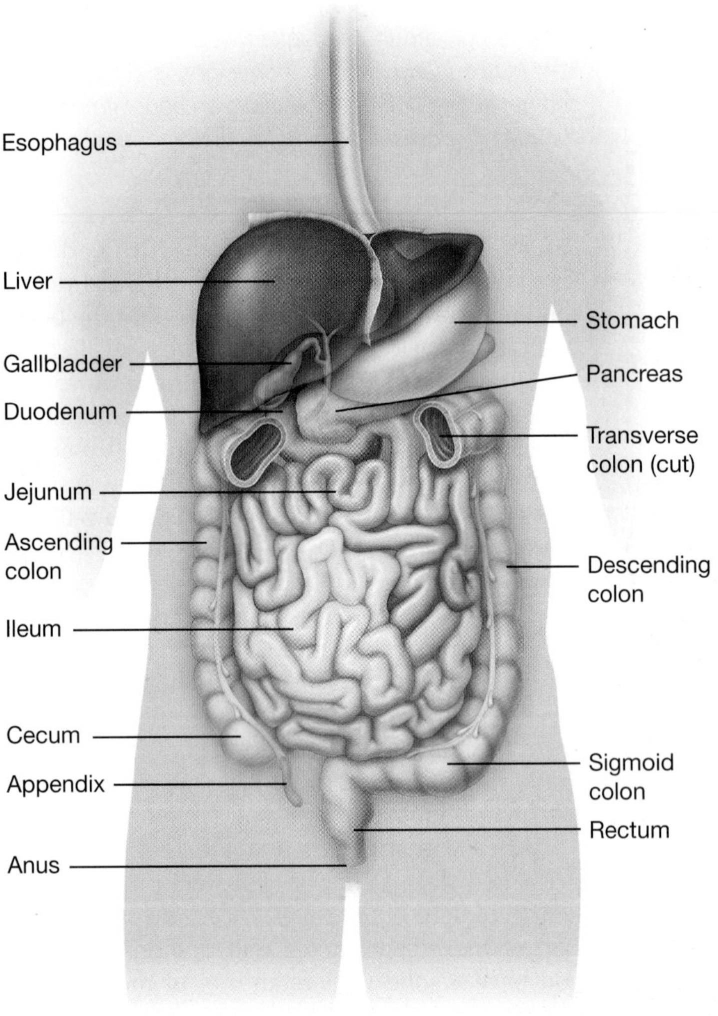

Main Functions of the Digestive System

The job of the digestive system is to ingest (take in), break down, and absorb nutrients from food and liquids and to eliminate waste products of the digestive process.

Digestion begins in the mouth, where the teeth and salivary glands work together to break down into smaller pieces the chicken wings, salsa, and chips consumed during the Super Bowl party. When the food is swallowed, it moves from the pharynx into the **esophagus** (ĕ-SŎF-ă-gŭs), a tubular structure that carries food into the stomach.

The **stomach** is an expandable organ, so it can accommodate a late-night pizza craving or a Super Bowl feeding frenzy. It acts like a blender by converting food into a paste-like mixture. Digestive juices and enzymes from the pancreas, liver, and gallbladder reduce the semi-digested food into

Esophagus

Liver

Gallbladder

Duodenum

Jejunum

Ascending colon

Ileum

Cecum

Appendix

Anus

Stomach

Pancreas

Transverse colon (cut)

Descending colon

Sigmoid colon

Rectum

© Body Scientific International

Figure 3.1 Organs of the digestive system

smaller molecules, allowing nutrients to be absorbed in the small intestine and transported throughout the body by the blood.

The activities of chemical digestion and nutrient absorption both occur in the **small intestine**. The **duodenum** is the first segment of the small intestine, the **jejunum** is the middle part, and the **ileum** is the last—and the longest— segment of the small intestine.

The **large intestine**, or **colon**, is the last section of the digestive system. It absorbs water and electrolytes and eliminates waste. The large intestine is so named because its diameter is wider than that of the small intestine. In comparison, the small intestine is much longer than the large intestine, but is smaller in diameter. The **rectum** receives waste products (feces) from the **sigmoid colon**, an S-shaped section of the large intestine, and stores feces prior to elimination from the anus.

The study of the digestive system is called **gastroenterology** (GĂS-trō-ĕn-tĕr-ŎL-ō-jē). Even though the medical term *gastroenterology* literally means "the study of the stomach and intestines," the term is used to refer to the study of the entire digestive system. A **gastroenterologist** (GĂS-trō-ĕn-tĕr-ŎL-ō-jĭst) is a physician who specializes in the study and treatment of the digestive system.

Anatomy and Physiology Vocabulary

Now that you have been introduced to the basic structure and functions of the digestive system, let's explore in more detail the key terms presented in the introduction.

Key Term	Definition
digestive tract (also called **alimentary canal** or **gastrointestinal tract**)	long, hollow tube that starts at the pharynx and ends at the anus
duodenum	first part of the small intestine
esophagus	tubular structure that carries food from the pharynx (throat) to the stomach
gastroenterologist	physician who specializes in the study and treatment of the digestive system
gastroenterology	the study of the digestive system
ileum	final and longest part of the small intestine
jejunum	middle part of the small intestine
large intestine	last section of the digestive system, which absorbs water and electrolytes and eliminates waste; the colon
pharynx	the throat
rectum	last part of the large intestine leading to the anus
sigmoid	S-shaped section of the large intestine
small intestine	long, narrow, folded tube that extends from the stomach to the large intestine; the site of chemical digestion and the absorption of food
stomach	an expandable organ that stores and breaks down food; located between the esophagus and small intestine

E-Flash Card Activity: Anatomy and Physiology Vocabulary

Directions: After you have reviewed the anatomy and physiology vocabulary related to the digestive system, access your *EduHub* subscription and practice with the e-flash cards until you are comfortable with the spelling and definition of each term.

Assessment 3.1

Identifying Major Organs of the Digestive System

Directions: Label the diagram of the digestive tract. You can also complete this activity online using *EduHub*.

16. _____ _____

15. _____ _____

14. _____ _____

13. _____ _____

12. _____

11. _____

10. _____

9. _____

8. _____

7. _____

1. _____

2. _____

3. _____

4. _____

5. _____

6. _____

© *Body Scientific International*

SCORECARD: How Did You Do?

Number correct (_____), divided by 16 (_____), multiplied by 100 equals _____ (your score)

Matching Anatomy and Physiology Vocabulary

Directions: Choose the correct vocabulary term for each meaning. You can also complete this activity online using *EduHub*.

_____ 1. physician who specializes in the study and treatment of the digestive system

_____ 2. tubular structure that carries food from the pharynx (throat) to the stomach

_____ 3. long, hollow tube that starts at the pharynx and extends to the anus

_____ 4. the study of the digestive system

_____ 5. the throat

_____ 6. last section of the digestive system, which absorbs water and electrolytes and eliminates waste; also called the colon

_____ 7. expandable organ that stores and breaks down food; located between the esophagus and small intestine

_____ 8. last (and longest) part of the small intestine

_____ 9. first part of the small intestine

_____ 10. middle part of the small intestine

_____ 11. part of the digestive tract in which chemical digestion and absorption occur

_____ 12. last part of the intestine leading to the anus

_____ 13. S-shaped section of the large intestine

A. large intestine

B. esophagus

C. alimentary canal

D. small intestine

E. pharynx

F. gastroenterology

G. gastroenterologist

H. stomach

I. ileum

J. jejunum

K. duodenum

L. sigmoid

M. rectum

SCORECARD: How Did You Do?

Number correct (_____), divided by 13 (_____), multiplied by 100 equals _____ (your score)

Word Elements

In this section, you will learn word elements—prefixes, combining forms, and suffixes—that are common to the digestive system. By learning these word parts and understanding how they are combined to build medical terms, you will be able to analyze Sue's health problem (described in the Intern Experience at the beginning of this chapter) and identify a large number of terms associated with the digestive system.

E-Flash Card Activity: Word Elements

Directions: Review the word elements in the tables that follow. Then, access your *EduHub* subscription and practice with the e-flash cards until you are able to quickly recognize the different word parts (prefixes, combining forms, and suffixes) and their meanings. The e-flash cards are grouped together by prefixes, combining forms, and suffixes, followed by a cumulative review of all the word elements you are learning in this chapter.

Prefixes

Let's start our study of digestive system word elements by looking at the prefixes listed in the table below. These prefixes appear not only in medical terms related to the digestive system, but also in many terms pertaining to other body systems.

Prefix	Meaning
a-	not; without
ad-	toward
anti-	against
brady-	slow
dia-	through
dys-	painful; difficult
epi-	upon; above
hyper-	above; above normal
pan-	all; everything
peri-	around
poly-	many
retro-	backward; behind

Combining Forms

Listed below are common combining forms used in medical terms related to the digestive system. As you progress through this book, you will discover that some of these combining forms are used in medical terms related to other body systems as well.

Root Word/Combining Vowel	Meaning
carcin/o	cancer
celi/o	abdomen
chol/e	bile; gall
cholecyst/o	gallbladder
col/o, colon/o	colon; large intestine
dist/o	away from the point of origin
diverticul/o	diverticulum
duoden/o	duodenum
enter/o	intestines
esophag/o	esophagus
gastr/o	stomach
gingiv/o	gums
gloss/o	tongue
hemat/o	blood
hepat/o	liver
herni/o	hernia; rupture; protrusion
ile/o	ileum
jejun/o	jejunum
lapar/o	abdomen
lith/o	stone
or/o	mouth
organ/o	organ
pancreat/o	pancreas
peps/o	digestion
polyp/o	polyp; small growth
proct/o	anus and rectum
proxim/o	nearest the point of origin
rect/o	rectum
sial/o	saliva
sigmoid/o	sigmoid colon

Suffixes

Listed below are suffixes used in medical terms pertaining to the digestive system. You will also encounter these suffixes in your study of many terms related to other body systems.

Suffix	Meaning
-al	pertaining to
-algia	pain
-cele	hernia; swelling; protrusion
-dynia	pain
-eal	pertaining to
-ectomy	surgical removal; excision
-emesis	vomiting
-gram	record; image
-graphy	process of recording an image
-ia	condition
-iasis	abnormal condition
-ic	pertaining to
-itis	inflammation
-logist	specialist in the study and treatment of
-logy	study of
-megaly	enlargement
-oma	tumor; mass
-osis	abnormal condition
-phagia	condition of eating or swallowing
-pharynx	pharynx; throat
-plasty	surgical repair
-ptosis	drooping; downward displacement
-rrhea	flow; discharge
-scope	instrument used to observe
-scopy	process of observing
-stomy	new opening
-tomy	incision; cut into
-tripsy	crushing
-y	condition; process

Matching Prefixes, Combining Forms, and Suffixes

Directions: Choose the correct meaning for each word element. Some meanings may be used more than once. You can also complete this activity online using *EduHub*.

Prefixes

_____ 1. peri-

_____ 2. a-

_____ 3. pan-

_____ 4. brady-

_____ 5. dys-

_____ 6. ad-

_____ 7. hyper-

_____ 8. dia-

_____ 9. poly-

_____ 10. anti-

_____ 11. retro-

_____ 12. epi-

A. toward

B. slow

C. against

D. painful; difficult

E. through

F. many

G. not; without

H. all; everything

I. around

J. backward; behind

K. upon; above

L. above; above normal

Combining Forms

_____ 1. sigmoid/o

_____ 2. carcin/o

_____ 3. hepat/o

_____ 4. chol/e

_____ 5. gloss/o

_____ 6. dist/o

_____ 7. diverticul/o

_____ 8. proxim/o

_____ 9. pancreat/o

_____ 10. duoden/o

_____ 11. hemat/o

_____ 12. esophag/o

_____ 13. gingiv/o

A. tongue

B. sigmoid colon

C. abdomen

D. saliva

E. blood

F. esophagus

G. jejunum

H. mouth

I. cancer

J. hernia; rupture; protrusion

K. stomach

L. anus and rectum

M. pancreas

_____ 14. lith/o

_____ 15. rect/o

_____ 16. jejun/o

_____ 17. col/o

_____ 18. colon/o

_____ 19. or/o

_____ 20. celi/o

_____ 21. enter/o

_____ 22. gastr/o

_____ 23. polyp/o

_____ 24. hern/o

_____ 25. sial/o

_____ 26. ile/o

_____ 27. proct/o

_____ 28. lapar/o

_____ 29. cholecyst/o

_____ 30. organ/o

_____ 31. peps/o

N. rectum

P. away from the point of origin

Q. polyp; small growth

R. duodenum

S. stone

T. ileum

U. gums

V. nearest the point of origin

W. diverticulum

X. liver

Y. gallbladder

Z. colon; large intestine

AA. bile; gall

BB. organ

CC. intestines

DD. digestion

Suffixes

_____ 1. -dynia

_____ 2. -gram

_____ 3. -logist

_____ 4. -osis

_____ 5. -scope

_____ 6. -tripsy

_____ 7. -al

_____ 8. -eal

_____ 9. -graphy

_____ 10. -logy

_____ 11. -megaly

A. pertaining to

B. record; image

C. vomiting

D. pain

E. crushing

F. specialist in the study and treatment of

G. incision; cut into

H. surgical removal; excision

I. surgical repair

J. tumor; mass

K. condition

_____ 12. -scopy	L. abnormal condition
_____ 13. -algia	M. process of recording an image
_____ 14. -ectomy	N. inflammation
_____ 15. -ia	O. study of
_____ 16. -phagia	P. drooping; downward displacement
_____ 17. -tomy	Q. process of observing
_____ 18. -cele	R. condition of eating or swallowing
_____ 19. -emesis	S. instrument used to observe
_____ 20. -iasis	T. new opening
_____ 21. -oma	U. flow; discharge
_____ 22. -stomy	V. enlargement
_____ 23. -ic	W. throat
_____ 24. -plasty	X. condition; process
_____ 25. -itis	Y. hernia; swelling; protrusion
_____ 26. -pharynx	
_____ 27. -ptosis	
_____ 28. -rrhea	
_____ 29. -y	

SCORECARD: How Did You Do?

Number correct (_____), divided by 72 (_____), multiplied by 100 equals _____ (your score)

Breaking Down and Building Digestive System Terms

Now that you have mastered the prefixes, combining forms, and suffixes for digestive system terminology, you have the ability to dissect and build a large number of medical terms related to this system.

Below is a list of common medical terms related to the study, diagnosis, and treatment of the digestive system. For each term, a dissection has been provided, along with the meaning of each word element and the definition of the term as a whole.

Term	Dissection	Word Part/Meaning	Term Definition
Note: *For simplification, combining vowels have been omitted from the Word Part/Meaning column.*			
1. **aphagia** (ă-FĀ-jē-ă)	a/phagia	**a** = not; without **phagia** = condition of eating or swallowing	condition of without swallowing
2. **carcinoma** (kär-sĭ-NŌ-mă)	carcin/oma	**carcin** = cancer **oma** = tumor; mass	cancerous tumor or mass
3. **celiectomy** (sē-lē-ĔK-tō-mē)	celi/ectomy	**celi** = abdomen **ectomy** = surgical removal; excision	excision of the abdomen
4. **cholecystitis** (KŌ-lĕ-sĭs-TĪ-tĭs)	cholecyst/itis	**cholecyst** = gallbladder **itis** = inflammation	inflammation of the gallbladder
5. **cholelithiasis** (KŌ-lĕ-lĭ-THĪ-ă-sĭs)	chol/e/lith/iasis	**chol** = bile; gall **lith** = stone **iasis** = abnormal condition	abnormal condition of gallstones
6. **colitis** (kō-LĪ-tĭs)	col/itis	**col** = colon **itis** = inflammation	inflammation of the colon
7. **colonoscopy** (kō-lŏn-ŎS-kō-pē)	colon/o/scopy	**colon** = colon **scopy** = process of observing	process of observing the colon
8. **colostomy** (kō-LŎS-tō-mē)	col/o/stomy	**col** = colon **stomy** = new opening	new opening in the colon
9. **diarrhea** (dī-ă-RĒ-ă)	dia/rrhea	**dia** = through **rrhea** = flow; discharge	flow through
10. **diverticulitis** (DĪ-vĕr-tĭk-ū-LĪ-tĭs)	diverticul/itis	**diverticul** = diverticulum **itis** = inflammation	inflammation of the diverticulum
11. **diverticulosis** (dī-vĕr-tĭk-ū-LŌ-sĭs)	diverticul/osis	**diverticul** = diverticulum **osis** = abnormal condition	abnormal condition of the diverticulum

Prefixes = Green   Root Words = **Red**   Suffixes = Blue

Term	Dissection	Word Part/Meaning	Term Definition
12. **duodenal** (dū-ŏ-DĒ-năl) (dū-ŎD-ĕn-ăl)	duoden/al	**duoden** = duodenum **al** = pertaining to	pertaining to the duodenum
13. **dysentery** (DĬS-ĕn-tĕr-ē)	dys/enter/y	**dys** = painful; difficult **enter** = intestine **y** = condition; process	painful condition of the intestines
14. **dyspepsia** (dĭs-PĔP-sē-ă)	dys/peps/ia	**dys** = painful; difficult **peps** = digestion **ia** = condition	condition of painful or difficult digestion
15. **dysphagia** (dĭs-FĀ-jē-ă)	dys/phagia	**dys** = painful; difficult **phagia** = condition of eating or swallowing	condition of painful or difficult swallowing
16. **enteritis** (ĕn-tĕr-Ī-tĭs)	enter/itis	**enter** = intestine **itis** = inflammation	inflammation of the intestines
17. **epigastric** (ĕp-ĭ-GĂS-trĭk)	epi/gastr/ic	**epi** = upon; above **gastr** = stomach **ic** = pertaining to	pertaining to (the area) above the stomach
18. **esophageal** (ē-SŎF-ă-jē-ăl)	esophag/eal	**esophag** = esophagus **eal** = pertaining to	pertaining to the esophagus
19. **esophagogastro-duodenoscopy** (ē-SŎF-ă-gō-GĂS-trō-dū-ŏ-dĕ-NŎS-kō-pē)	esophag/o/gastr/o/duoden/o/scopy	**esophag** = esophagus **gastr** = stomach **duoden** = duodenum **scopy** = process of observing	process of observing the esophagus, stomach, and duodenum
20. **gastritis** (găs-TRĪ-tĭs)	gastr/itis	**gastr** = stomach **itis** = inflammation	inflammation of the stomach
21. **gastrodynia** (găs-trō-DĬN-ē-ă)	gastr/o/dynia	**gastr** = stomach **dynia** = pain	pain in the stomach
22. **gastroenterologist** (GĂS-trō-ĕn-tĕr-ŎL-ō-jĭst)	gastr/o/enter/o/logist	**gastr** = stomach **enter** = intestines **logist** = specialist in the study and treatment of	specialist in the study and treatment of the stomach and intestines
23. **gastroenterology** (GĂS-trō-ĕn-tĕr-ŎL-ō-jē)	gastr/o/enter/o/logy	**gastr** = stomach **enter** = intestines **logy** = study of	study of the stomach and intestines
24. **gastroesophageal** (găs-trō-ĕ-SŎF-ă-jē-ăl)	gastr/o/esophag/eal	**gastr** = stomach **esophag** = esophagus **eal** = pertaining to	pertaining to the stomach and esophagus
25. **gingivitis** (jĭn-jĭ-VĪ-tĭs)	gingiv/itis	**gingiv** = gums **itis** = inflammation	inflammation of the gums
26. **glossalgia** (glŏs-ĂL-jē-ă)	gloss/algia	**gloss** = tongue **algia** = pain	pain in the tongue

Prefixes = Green   Root Words = Red   Suffixes = Blue

Term	Dissection	Word Part/Meaning	Term Definition
27. **hematemesis** (HĒ-mă-TĔM-ĕ-sĭs)	hemat/emesis	**hemat** = blood **emesis** = vomiting	vomiting of blood
28. **hepatitis** (hĕp-ă-TĪ-tĭs)	hepat/itis	**hepat** = liver **itis** = inflammation	inflammation of the liver
29. **hepatomegaly** (HĔP-ă-tō-MĔG-ă-lē)	hepat/o/megaly	**hepat** = liver **megaly** = enlargement	enlargement of the liver
30. **laparoscope** (LĂP-ă-rō-skōp)	lapar/o/scope	**lapar** = abdomen **scope** = instrument used to observe	instrument used to observe the abdomen
31. **laparoscopy** (lăp-ă-RŎS-kō-pē)	lapar/o/scopy	**lapar** = abdomen **scopy** = process of observing	process of observing the abdomen
32. **organomegaly** (ŏr-gă-nō-MĔG-ă-lē)	organ/o/megaly	**organ** = organ **megaly** = enlargement	enlargement of an organ
33. **oropharynx** (or-ō-FĂR-inks)	or/o/pharynx	**or** = mouth **pharynx** = pharynx; throat	mouth and throat
34. **pancreatography** (păn-krē-ă-TŎG-ră-fē)	pancreat/o/graphy	**pancreat** = pancreas **graphy** = process of recording an image	process of recording an image of the pancreas
35. **polyposis** (pŏl-ĭ-PŌ-sĭs)	polyp/osis	**polyp** = polyp **osis** = abnormal condition	abnormal condition of polyps
36. **proctoplasty** (PRŎK-tō-plăs-tē)	proct/o/plasty	**proct** = anus and rectum **plasty** = surgical repair	surgical repair of the anus and rectum
37. **rectoscope** (RĔK-tō-skōp)	rect/o/scope	**rect** = rectum **scope** = instrument used to observe	instrument used to observe the rectum
38. **sialorrhea** (sī-ă-lō-RĒ-ă)	sial/o/rrhea	**sial** = saliva **rrhea** = flow; discharge	flow or discharge of saliva
39. **sigmoidoscopy** (sĭg-moy-DŎS-kō-pē)	sigmoid/o/scopy	**sigmoid** = sigmoid colon **scopy** = process of observing	process of observing the sigmoid colon

Prefixes = Green   Root Words = Red   Suffixes = Blue

Using the pronunciation guide in the Breaking Down and Building chart, practice saying each medical term aloud. To hear the pronunciation of each term, complete the Pronounce It activity on the next page.

Studying medical terminology is similar to learning a foreign language. At first, pronouncing new medical terms can be challenging. To develop fluency, it is necessary to practice pronouncing the terms until you are comfortable saying them aloud.

Audio Activity: Pronounce It

Directions: Access your *EduHub* subscription and listen to the correct pronunciations of the following medical terms. Practice pronouncing the terms until you are comfortable saying them aloud.

aphagia
(ă-FĀ-jē-ă)

carcinoma
(kär-sĭ-NŌ-mă)

celiectomy
(sē-lē-ĔK-tō-mē)

cholecystitis
(KŌ-lĕ-sĭs-TĪ-tĭs)

cholelithiasis
(KŌ-lĕ-lĭ-THĪ-ă-sĭs)

colitis
(kō-LĪ-tĭs)

colonoscopy
(kō-lŏn-ŎS-kō-pē)

colostomy
(kō-LŎS-tō-mē)

diarrhea
(dī-ă-RĒ-ă)

diverticulitis
(DĪ-vĕr-tĭk-ū-LĪ-tĭs)

diverticulosis
(dī-vĕr-tĭk-ū-LŌ-sĭs)

duodenal
(dū-ŏ-DĒ-năl)
(dū-ŎD-ĕn-ăl)

dysentery
(DĬS-ĕn-tĕr-ē)

dyspepsia
(dĭs-PĔP-sē-ă)

dysphagia
(dĭs-FĀ-jē-ă)

enteritis
(ĕn-tĕr-Ī-tĭs)

epigastric
(ĕp-ĭ-GĂS-trĭk)

esophageal
(ē-SŎF-ă-jē-ăl)

esophagogastro-
duodenoscopy
(ē-SŎF-ă-gō-GĂS-trō-
dū-ŏ-dĕ-NŎS-kō-pē)

gastritis
(găs-TRĪ-tĭs)

gastrodynia
(găs-trō-DĬN-ē-ă)

gastroenterologist
(GĂS-trō-ĕn-tĕr-ŎL-ō-
jĭst)

gastroenterology
(GĂS-trō-ĕn-tĕr-ŎL-ō-
jē)

gastroesophageal
(găs-trō-ĕ-SŎF-ă-jē-ăl)

gingivitis
(jĭn-jĭ-VĪ-tĭs)

glossalgia
(glŏs-ĂL-jē-ă)

hematemesis
(HĒ-mă-TĔM-ĕ-sĭs)

hepatitis
(hĕp-ă-TĪ-tĭs)

hepatomegaly
(HĔP-ă-tō-MĔG-ă-lē)

laparoscope
(LĂP-ă-rō-skōp)

laparoscopy
(lăp-ă-RŎS-kō-pē)

organomegaly
(ŏr-gă-nō-MĔG-ă-lē)

oropharynx
(or-ō-FĂR-inks)

pancreatography
(păn-krē-ă-TŎG-ră-fē)

polyposis
(pŏl-ĭ-PŌ-sĭs)

proctoplasty
(PRŎK-tō-plăs-tē)

rectoscope
(RĔK-tō-skōp)

sialorrhea
(sī-ă-lō-RĒ-ă)

sigmoidoscopy
(sĭg-moy-DŎS-kō-pē)

Audio Activity: Spell It

Directions: Access your *EduHub* subscription and listen to the pronunciation for each number. As you hear each term, write its correct spelling.

1. _____

2. _____

3. _____

4. _____

5. _____

6. _____

7. _____

8. _____

9. _____

10. _____

11. _____

12. _____

13. _____

14. _____

15. _____

16. _____

17. _____   29. _____
18. _____   30. _____
19. _____   31. _____
20. _____   32. _____
21. _____   33. _____
22. _____   34. _____
23. _____   35. _____
24. _____   36. _____
25. _____   37. _____
26. _____   38. _____
27. _____   39. _____
28. _____

SCORECARD: How Did You Do?

Number correct (_____), divided by 39 (_____), multiplied by 100 equals _____ (your score)

Assessment 3.5

Break It Down

Directions: Dissect each medical term into its word parts (prefix, root word, combining vowel, and suffix) using one or more slashes. Then define each term. You can also complete this activity online using *EduHub*.

Example:

Medical Term: hepatomegaly

Dissection: hepat/o/megaly

Definition: enlargement of the liver

Medical Term   **Dissection**

1. dysphagia   d y s p h a g i a

Definition: _____

_____

2. aphagia   a p h a g i a

Definition: _____

_____

Medical Term	Dissection
3. laparoscopy	l a p a r o s c o p y

Definition: _____

_____

4. diverticulosis   d i v e r t i c u l o s i s

Definition: _____

_____

5. sialorrhea   s i a l o r r h e a

Definition: _____

_____

6. sigmoidoscopy   s i g m o i d o s c o p y

Definition: _____

_____

7. cholelithiasis   c h o l e l i t h i a s i s

Definition: _____

_____

8. hepatomegaly   h e p a t o m e g a l y

Definition: _____

_____

9. gastroesophageal   g a s t r o e s o p h a g e a l

Definition: _____

_____

10. gastrodynia   g a s t r o d y n i a

Definition: _____

_____

Medical Term	Dissection

11. organomegaly   o r g a n o m e g a l y

Definition: _____

_____

12. dyspepsia   d y s p e p s i a

Definition: _____

_____

13. oropharynx   o r o p h a r y n x

Definition: _____

_____

14. gastroenterology   g a s t r o e n t e r o l o g y

Definition: _____

_____

15. colitis   c o l i t i s

Definition: _____

_____

16. esophagogastroduodenoscopy   e s o p h a g o g a s t r o d u o d e n o s c o p y

Definition: _____

_____

17. enteritis   e n t e r i t i s

Definition: _____

_____

Medical Term	Dissection
18. hematemesis	h e m a t e m e s i s

Definition: _____

_____

19. epigastric	e p i g a s t r i c

Definition: _____

_____

20. duodenal	d u o d e n a l

Definition: _____

_____

SCORECARD: How Did You Do?

Number correct (_____), divided by 20 (_____), multiplied by 100 equals _____ (your score)

Assessment 3.6

Build It

Directions: Build the medical term that matches each definition by supplying the correct word parts. You can also complete this activity online using *EduHub*.

P (Prefixes) = Green
RW (Root Words) = Red
S (Suffixes) = Blue
CV (Combining Vowel) = Purple

1. pertaining to the esophagus

   _____ _____
   RW   S

2. cancerous tumor

   _____ _____
   RW   S

3. new opening in the colon

   _____ _____ _____
   RW   CV   S

4. process of observing the colon

_____ _____ _____
RW   CV   S

5. specialist in the study and treatment of the stomach and intestines

_____ _____ _____ _____ _____
RW   CV   RW   CV   S

6. inflammation of the intestines

_____ _____
RW   S

7. pertaining to the duodenum

_____ _____
RW   S

8. inflammation of the gallbladder

_____ _____ _____ _____
RW   CV   RW   S

9. condition of painful or difficult swallowing

_____ _____
P   S

10. process of observing the sigmoid colon

_____ _____ _____
RW   CV   S

11. enlargement of the liver

_____ _____ _____
RW   CV   S

12. inflammation of the colon

_____ _____
RW   S

13. pertaining to the stomach and esophagus

_____ _____ _____ _____
RW   CV   RW   S

14. painful digestion

_____ _____ _____
P   RW   S

15. process of observing the esophagus, stomach, and duodenum

_____   _____   _____   _____   _____   _____ _____
         RW   CV   RW   CV   RW   CV   S

16. pain in the stomach

_____   _____ _____
         RW   CV   S

17. vomiting of blood

_____   _____
         RW   S

18. instrument used to observe the abdomen

_____   _____ _____
         RW   CV   S

19. enlargement of an organ

_____   _____ _____
         RW   CV   S

20. flow through

_____ _____
   P   S

21. mouth and throat

_____   _____ _____
         RW   CV   S

22. process of recording the pancreas

_____   _____ _____
         RW   CV   S

23. inflammation of the liver

_____   _____
         RW   S

24. abnormal condition of polyps

_____   _____
         RW   S

SCORECARD: How Did You Do?

Number correct (_____), divided by 24 (_____), multiplied by 100 equals _____ (your score)

Diseases and Disorders

Diseases and disorders of the digestive system range from the mild to severe and have a wide variety of causes. We will now take a look at some problems that commonly affect the digestive system.

Crohn's Disease

Crohn's disease is a chronic **inflammatory bowel disease (IBD)** with clinical symptoms of bloody diarrhea, abdominal pain, weight loss, and fatigue. It is characterized by the thickening and gradual erosion of the inner lining of the intestinal wall (Figure 3.2). Ulcerations of the intestinal wall result in scar tissue formation, which can cause intestinal obstruction. Because the etiology (cause) is unknown, there is no cure for Crohn's disease.

Gastroesophageal Reflux Disease

Gastroesophageal reflux disease (GERD) is a chronic digestive disease that occurs when stomach acid flows back into the esophagus (Figure 3.3). The acidity of regurgitated food irritates the esophageal lining and may cause ulcerations. GERD produces heartburn after eating, dysphagia (condition of painful or difficult swallowing), and occasional hematemesis (vomiting of blood).

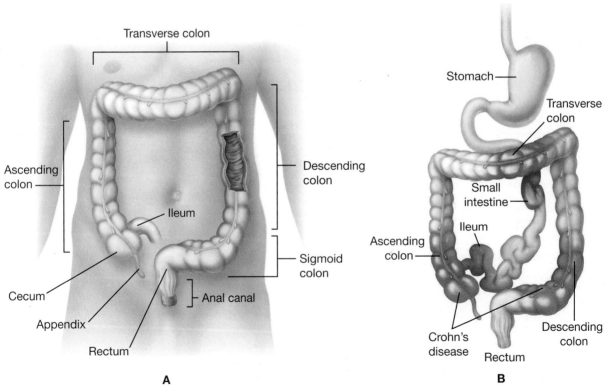

© Body Scientific International

Figure 3.2 A—Normal large intestine. B—Intestinal inflammation of Crohn's disease.

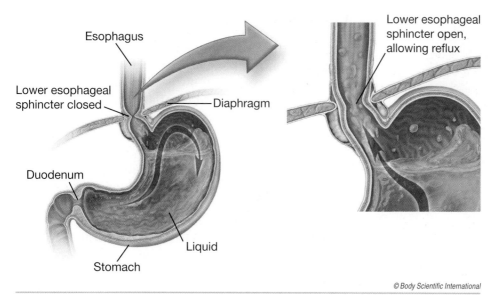

Figure 3.3 Gastroesophageal reflux disease (GERD) is characterized by backflow of stomach acids into the esophagus.

Hiatal Hernia

A **hiatal hernia** occurs when a portion of the stomach protrudes (bulges) through the diaphragm (Figure 3.4). The diaphragm, the major muscle involved in the breathing process, separates the thoracic (chest) cavity from the abdominal cavity.

The esophagus normally enters the abdominal cavity through an opening in the diaphragm. If the opening is weakened or enlarged, the stomach may herniate (bulge) upward through the diaphragm into the thoracic cavity. A large hiatal hernia causes heartburn, chest pain, belching, and nausea.

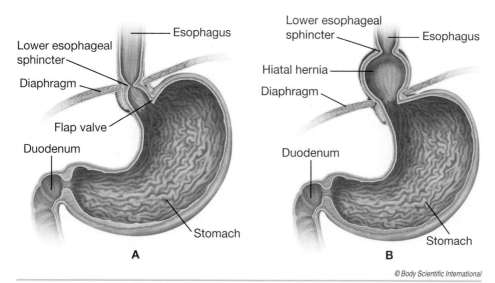

Figure 3.4 A—Normal muscle of the abdominal wall. B—In a hiatal hernia, a portion of the stomach bulges through the diaphragm.

Liver Disease

Hepatitis is an inflammation of the liver that causes abdominal pain, nausea, vomiting, and jaundice (yellowish discoloration of the skin and whites of the eyes). Most commonly, this inflammatory condition is caused by one of three viruses: hepatitis A, hepatitis B, or hepatitis C. Hepatitis can also result from chronic alcohol or drug abuse.

Cirrhosis is a chronic, irreversible liver disease in which normal liver cells are replaced with hard, fibrous scar tissue (Figure 3.5). Common symptoms include abdominal swelling, susceptibility to bruising, and renal failure. Cirrhosis is often associated with long-term alcoholism. There is no known cure.

Eating Disorders

Eating disorders are a group of serious conditions rooted in a negative or distorted self-image. Those affected are so preoccupied with food and weight that they can focus on little else in their lives. Anorexia nervosa and bulimia nervosa are two common types of behavioral eating disorders. Both involve weight loss achieved by different methods.

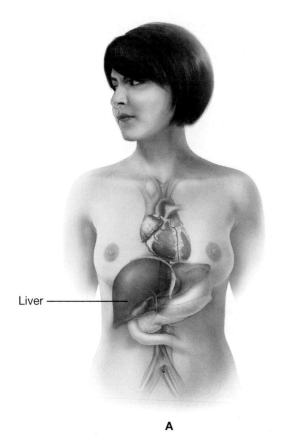

Liver

A

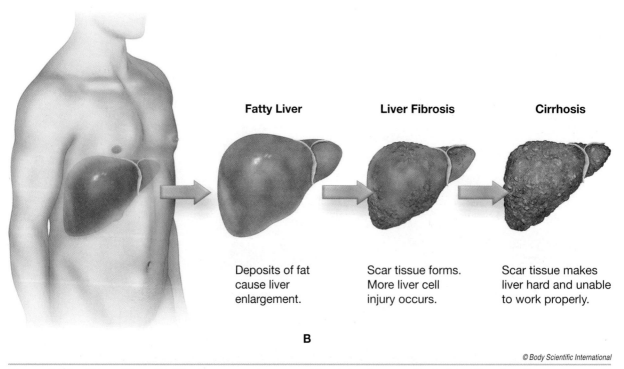

Fatty Liver

Liver Fibrosis

Cirrhosis

Deposits of fat cause liver enlargement.

Scar tissue forms. More liver cell injury occurs.

Scar tissue makes liver hard and unable to work properly.

B

© Body Scientific International

Figure 3.5 A—Normal liver. B—The tissue scarring caused by cirrhosis severely weakens liver function.

Anorexia nervosa is characterized by an extreme aversion to food that results in weight loss and may lead to malnutrition (Figure 3.6). **Bulimia nervosa** involves repeated gorging of food followed by intentional vomiting and/or laxative abuse. Severe eating disorders can be life-threatening.

Ulcers

An **ulcer**, or *peptic ulcer*, is a breakdown in the mucosal lining of the esophagus, stomach, or duodenum caused by chronic irritation (Figure 3.7). This breakdown is caused by hydrochloric acid and pepsin, the acidic chemicals involved in the digestion of food. Esophageal, gastric, and duodenal ulcers are types of peptic ulcers.

Most ulcers are caused by *Helicobacter pylori* (*H. pylori*), a bacterium that attacks the weakened mucosa. Dyspepsia (epigastric pain with bloating and nausea) is a common symptom. Factors that may contribute to ulcer formation include stress; excessive caffeine consumption;

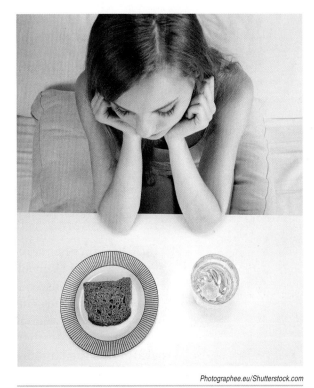

Photographee.eu/Shutterstock.com

Figure 3.6 Distorted body image is a major symptom of anorexia nervosa.

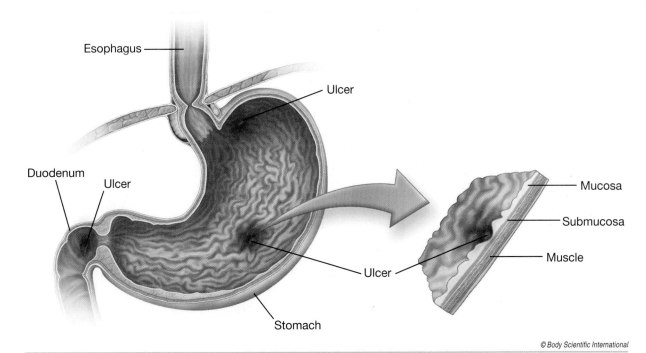

© Body Scientific International

Figure 3.7 A peptic ulcer is a breakdown in the mucosal lining of the stomach, esophagus, or duodenum. It is caused by chronic irritation from highly acidic gastric chemicals.

smoking; and drugs such as aspirin and ibuprofen, which irritate the mucosal lining of the esophagus, stomach, and duodenum.

H. pylori infections are treated with antibiotic drugs and antacids. The patient is also instructed to avoid taking any drugs that contain aspirin.

Procedures and Treatments

In this section, we will briefly describe some common diagnostic procedures used to help identify diseases and disorders of the digestive system, as well as therapeutic procedures used to treat certain conditions.

Barium Enema

A **barium enema** is a diagnostic procedure in which barium is used as a contrast agent to enable radiographic visualization of the large intestine. A barium enema is also called a **lower gastrointestinal (LGI) series** (Figure 3.8).

Before a barium enema test, the patient cleanses the bowels by following a special diet and taking a laxative. The procedure involves infusing the barium through a catheter (tube) inserted into the anus and rectum, until the barium fills the large intestine. X-rays are then taken of the entire length of the colon (Figure 3.9).

A barium enema is used to define normal and abnormal anatomy of the colon. The procedure is performed to help diagnose disorders such as diverticulosis

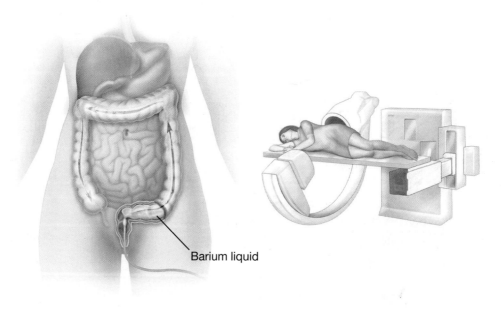

Barium liquid

Figure 3.8 During a barium enema, also called a *lower gastrointestinal (LGI) series*, a radioactive agent is introduced through a catheter inserted into the anus and rectum.

(the formation of pouches or sacs, called *diverticula*, in the colon wall), diverticulitis (inflammation of the diverticulum), polyps (small tissue masses that bulge or project outward or upward), intestinal blockages, abscesses, and cancer.

Colostomy

A **colostomy** is a surgical procedure in which one end of a healthy large intestine is brought out through the abdominal wall. The edges of the bowel are stitched to the skin of the abdominal wall (Figure 3.10). The surgically created opening is called a *stoma*.

A colostomy drains stool (feces) from the colon into a colostomy bag attached to the abdomen. Most colostomy stool is softer and contains more liquid than stool that is passed normally. The procedure is usually performed after partial or complete intestinal obstruction (blockage of the large intestine), a severe infection, cancer, or trauma to the colon such as from a penetrating wound. Whether a colostomy is temporary or permanent depends on the extent of the disease or injury.

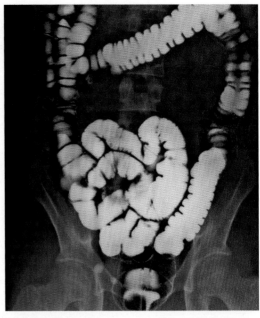

Praisaeng/Shutterstock.com

Figure 3.9 X-ray from a contrast barium enema. This diagnostic procedure allows doctors to look for a variety of abnormalities, such as intestinal blockages, polyps, diverticulosis, and cancer.

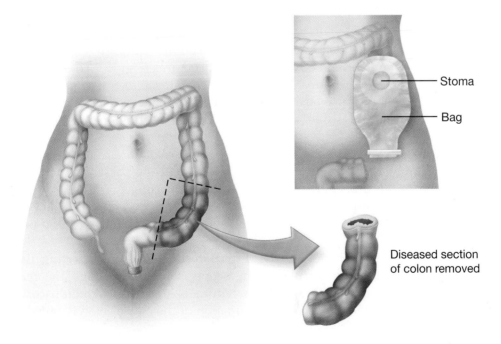

Stoma

Bag

Diseased section of colon removed

© Body Scientific International

Figure 3.10 A colostomy drains stool from the large intestine into a colostomy bag. The surgically created opening is called a *stoma*.

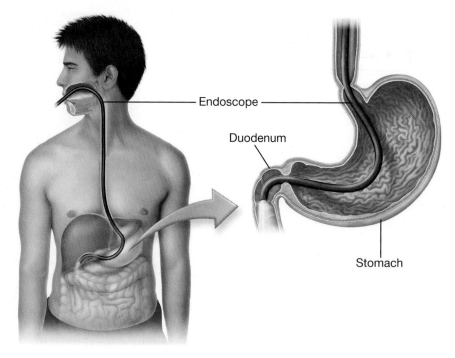

Endoscope

Duodenum

Stomach

© Body Scientific International

Figure 3.11 Endoscopy involves examination of internal body organs and structures with a flexible, fiber-optic instrument called an *endoscope*.

Endoscopy

An **endoscopy** (ĕn-DŎS-kō-pē) is a procedure in which an endoscope is used to examine internal body organs and structures (Figure 3.11). An *endoscope* is a flexible, fiber-optic instrument that contains a magnifying lens and a light source. It may also be equipped with a tool that can remove tissue for examination. The endoscope is inserted through an existing opening, such as the mouth or nose.

Esophagoscopy (ē-SŎF-a-GŎS-kō-pē) is examination of the esophagus with an *esophagoscope* (ē-SŎF-a-gō-skōp). If a scope passes farther into the stomach, the procedure is known as a **gastroscopy** (găs-TRŎS-kō-pē). If the scope is manipulated into the duodenum, the procedure is called an **esophagogastroduodenoscopy** (ē-SŎF-ă-gō-GĂS-trō-dū-ŏ-dĕ-NŎS-kō-pē), or **EGD**.

Endoscopic examination of the large intestine involves inserting the endoscope through the rectum. If the scope is passed through the rectum into the sigmoid colon, the procedure is called a **sigmoidoscopy** (sĭg-moy-DŎS-kō-pē). Endoscopic examination of the entire colon is called a **colonoscopy** (kō-lŏn-ŎS-kō-pē).

Upper Gastrointestinal Series

An **upper gastrointestinal (UGI) series** is a radiographic (X-ray) examination of the upper GI tract, which includes the esophagus, stomach, and duodenum (Figure 3.12). The patient drinks a milkshake-like mixture containing barium, a chemical element that serves as a contrast agent. The barium allows radiographic imaging of body organs and vessels that could not otherwise be seen on an X-ray. The barium mixture is flavored to make it more palatable to the patient.

During a UGI series, a radiologist views and records images as the barium flows through the esophagus and stomach. If the imaging procedure stops at the stomach, it is referred to as a **barium swallow**. If the entire small intestine also needs to be examined, the radiologist continues to record images of the duodenum, jejunum, and ileum until the barium reaches the beginning of the large intestine at the ileocecal valve. This valve prevents the backflow of waste from the large intestine into the small intestine. This diagnostic procedure is known as an **upper GI and small bowel series**.

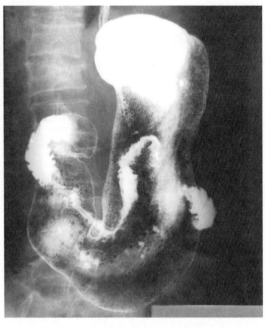

Santibhavank P/Shutterstock.com

Figure 3.12 This upper gastrointestinal (UGI) study of an adult female shows a close-up of the stomach and duodenum.

Gastric Bypass Surgery

Gastric bypass surgery is a type of weight-loss surgery that limits food consumption by reducing the size of the stomach (Figure 3.13). In addition to limiting the amount of food that can be consumed in one sitting, this surgery reduces the absorption of nutrients from food. Gastric bypass and other weight-loss surgeries are performed when diet and exercise methods alone have been ineffective or when obesity causes serious health problems.

Typically, gastric bypass surgery is performed with a *laparoscope* (LĂP-ă-rō-skōp) inserted through small incisions made in the abdomen. The laparoscope is linked to a video monitor, which enables the surgeon to see and operate inside the abdomen without making large incisions. Compared to open surgery, laparoscopy (lăp-ă-RŎS-kō-pē) involves a shorter hospitalization period and faster recovery.

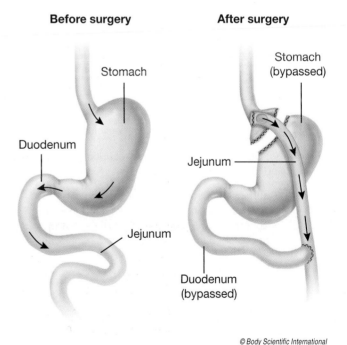

© Body Scientific International

Figure 3.13 Gastric bypass surgery limits food consumption by reducing the size of the stomach.

Multiple Choice: Diseases and Disorders

Directions: Choose the disease or disorder that matches each definition. You can also complete this activity online using *EduHub*.

_____ 1. disorder in which a portion of the stomach protrudes through the diaphragm
a. hiatal hernia
b. gastroesophageal reflux disease
c. Crohn's disease
d. ulcer

_____ 2. chronic disease in which stomach acid backs up into the esophagus
a. hiatal hernia
b. gastroesophageal reflux disease
c. Crohn's disease
d. ulcer

_____ 3. disorder resulting from breakdown of the mucosal lining in the stomach, esophagus, or duodenum due to chronic irritation
a. hiatal hernia
b. gastroesophageal reflux disease
c. Crohn's disease
d. ulcer

_____ 4. chronic inflammatory bowel disease characterized by thickening and a gradual erosion of the inner lining of the intestinal wall
a. hiatal hernia
b. gastroesophageal reflux disease
c. Crohn's disease
d. ulcer

_____ 5. chronic, irreversible liver disease in which normal cells are replaced with hard, fibrous scar tissue; associated with long-term alcoholism
a. hepatitis   c. Crohn's disease
b. cirrhosis   d. peptic ulcer

_____ 6. inflammation of the liver that causes abdominal pain, nausea, vomiting, and jaundice
a. bulimia nervosa   c. hepatitis
b. cirrhosis   d. Crohn's disease

_____ 7. eating disorder characterized by repeated gorging of food followed by intentional vomiting and/or laxative abuse
a. anorexia nervosa   c. reflux
b. bulimia nervosa   d. hepatitis

SCORECARD: How Did You Do?

Number correct (_____), divided by 7 (_____), multiplied by 100 equals _____ (your score)

Multiple Choice: Procedures and Treatments

Directions: Choose the procedure or treatment that matches each definition. You can also complete this activity online using *EduHub*.

_____ 1. surgical procedure in which one end of a healthy large intestine is drawn through the abdominal wall, and the edges of the bowel are stitched to the skin of the abdominal wall
a. gastric bypass surgery
b. colostomy
c. barium enema
d. endoscopy

_____ 2. endoscopic examination of the esophagus
a. upper gastrointestinal (UGI) series
b. esophagoscopy
c. barium swallow
d. sigmoidoscopy

_____ 3. radiographic examination of the esophagus, stomach, and duodenum using barium as a contrast agent
a. upper gastrointestinal (UGI) series
b. endoscopy
c. laparoscopy
d. colostomy

_____ 4. procedure in which an endoscope is used to examine internal body structures
a. barium enema
b. sigmoidoscopy
c. gastroscopy
d. endoscopy

_____ 5. surgical procedure that reduces the size of the stomach to limit food consumption
  a. colostomy
  b. endoscopy
  c. gastric bypass surgery
  d. esophagogastroduodenoscopy

_____ 6. diagnostic procedure in which barium is used as a contrast agent to enable radiographic visualization of the large intestine
  a. upper GI and small bowel series
  b. barium enema
  c. gastroscopy
  d. colostomy

_____ 7. upper GI imaging procedure that stops at the stomach
  a. esophagoscopy   c. barium swallow
  b. barium enema   d. sigmoidoscopy

_____ 8. another term for _barium enema_
  a. lower gastrointestinal (LGI) series
  b. upper gastrointestinal (UGI) series
  c. barium swallow
  d. barium flow

_____ 9. radiographic examination of all three parts of the small intestine (duodenum, jejunum, and ileum)
  a. lower gastrointestinal (LGI) series
  b. upper GI and small bowel series
  c. sigmoidoscopy
  d. colonoscopy

_____ 10. endoscopic examination of the sigmoid colon
  a. colonoscopy
  b. colostomy
  c. sigmoidoscopy
  d. esophagogastroduodenoscopy

_____ 11. endoscopic examination of the entire colon
  a. barium swallow
  b. lower gastrointestinal (LGI) series
  c. colostomy
  d. colonoscopy

_____ 12. examination procedure that involves the use of an endoscope
  a. gastroscopy
  b. esophagogastroduodenoscopy
  c. colonoscopy
  d. all of the above

SCORECARD: How Did You Do?

Number correct (_____), divided by 12 (_____), multiplied by 100 equals _____ (your score)

Assessment 3.9

Identifying Abbreviations

Directions: Supply the correct abbreviation for each medical term. You can also complete this activity online using _EduHub_.

Medical Term	Abbreviation
1. esophagogastroduodenoscopy	_____
2. gastroesophageal reflux disease	_____
3. lower gastrointestinal	_____
4. upper gastrointestinal	_____
5. inflammatory bowel disease	_____

SCORECARD: How Did You Do?

Number correct (_____), divided by 5 (_____), multiplied by 100 equals _____ (your score)

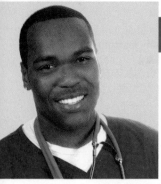

Analyzing the Intern Experience

In the Intern Experience described at the beginning of this chapter, Evan Walker encountered Sue, a young female patient who had difficulty swallowing. Sue was seen by Dr. Stomack, who obtained a history of her health problems and performed a physical examination. In addition, Dr. Stomack ordered a diagnostic test to help determine the cause of Sue's condition. When she received the test results, Dr. Stomack analyzed all the information that she had gathered, made a medical diagnosis, and developed a treatment plan. The physician then made a dictated recording of Sue's health information, which was later transcribed into a chart note.

We will now learn more about Sue's condition from a clinical perspective, interpreting the medical terms in her chart note as we analyze the scenario presented in the Intern Experience.

Audio Activity: Sue Resch's Chart Note

Directions: Access your *EduHub* subscription and listen to the recording of the physician reading Sue Resch's chart note. Read along with the physician and pay attention to the pronunciation of each medical term.

CHART NOTE

Patient Name: Resch, Sue
ID Number: 76554
Examination Date: March 1, 20xx

SUBJECTIVE
Sue came into our office complaining of a feeling that something is caught in her throat. She thinks it might be a turkey bone from the soup she ate last night.

OBJECTIVE
Sensation of a foreign body in the **proximal** esophagus, near the **oropharynx**. Vital signs are normal. No known allergies. She states that this has happened once before, but denies any regular symptoms of **dysphagia** or **gastroesophageal reflux**.

ASSESSMENT
Sensation of foreign body.

PLAN
Recommend immediate **esophagogastroduodenoscopy** to exclude an **esophageal** foreign body.

Interpret Sue Resch's Chart Note

Directions: Access your *EduHub* subscription and listen to the recording of the physician reading Sue Resch's chart note. After listening to the recording, supply the medical term that matches each definition.

> *Example:* inflammation of the intestine   *Answer:* enteritis

1. painful or difficult swallowing   _____

2. mouth and throat   _____

3. process of observing the esophagus, stomach, and duodenum   _____

4. nearest the point of origin   _____

5. backflow of stomach acid into the esophagus   _____

6. pertaining to the esophagus   _____

SCORECARD: How Did You Do?

Number correct (_____), divided by 6 (_____), multiplied by 100 equals _____ (your score)

Working with Medical Records

In this activity, you will interpret the medical records (chart notes) of patients with health problems related to the digestive system. These examples illustrate typical medical records prepared in a real-world healthcare environment. To interpret these chart notes, you will apply your knowledge of word elements (prefixes, combining forms, and suffixes), diseases and disorders, and procedures and treatments related to the digestive system.

Audio Activity: Ida Gundrum's Chart Note

Directions: Access your *EduHub* subscription and listen to the recording of the physician reading Ida Gundrum's chart note. Read along with the physician and pay attention to the pronunciation of each medical term.

CHART NOTE

Patient Name: Gundrum, Ida
ID Number: 98774
Examination Date: October 11, 20xx

SUBJECTIVE

29-year-old female complains of **epigastric** discomfort, which she describes as a constant burning for several weeks. Initial treatment was successful with Tagamet® (drug that reduces gastric acid secretions), but discomfort has recurred several times over a 2-week period. She complains of nausea. No vomiting or **hematemesis**. Tagamet® partially relieves her symptoms. She has been under considerable stress at work due to job downsizing and outsourcing of personnel. Headache relief in the form of Tylenol® or Motrin® has been unsuccessful and seems to exacerbate (worsen) her condition.

OBJECTIVE

Abdomen is soft, flat, and nontender with normal bowel sounds. No masses or **organomegaly**.

ASSESSMENT

Gastritis, probably exacerbated by NSAIDs (nonsteroidal anti-inflammatory drugs), and stress.

PLAN

We discussed several methods of stress reduction, including support group websites. She will stop using Motrin® and Tylenol® for headaches. She was given a sample of Prilosec® 20 mg q.i.d. (4 times a day) to be taken for one month. The patient will return in 3–4 weeks for a follow-up visit.

Assessment 3.11

Interpret Ida Gundrum's Chart Note

Directions: Access your *EduHub* subscription and listen to the recording of the physician reading Ida Gundrum's chart note. After listening to the recording, supply the medical term that matches each definition.

Example: abnormal condition of gallstones   *Answer:* cholelithiasis

1. enlargement of an organ   _____

2. vomiting blood   _____

3. inflammation of the stomach   _____

4. pertaining to the area above the stomach   _____

SCORECARD: How Did You Do?

Number correct (_____), divided by 4 (_____), multiplied by 100 equals _____ (your score)

Audio Activity: Sally Nguyen's Chart Note

Directions: Access your *EduHub* subscription and listen to the recording of the physician reading Sally Nguyen's chart note. Read along with the physician and pay attention to the pronunciation of each medical term.

CHART NOTE

Patient Name: Nguyen, Sally
ID Number: 22316
Examination Date: March 1, 20xx

PROCEDURE
Flexible **sigmoidoscopy**

INDICATIONS
Patient is an 81-year-old female for routine screening flexible sigmoidoscopy. Patient has a maternal history of Crohn's disease and a paternal history of diabetes.

PROCEDURE REPORT
The 60 cm **sigmoidoscope** was introduced to 40 cm and was well tolerated. **Erythematous**, nonbleeding polyp, less than 1 cm, was found between 35 and 40 cm. Retroflex (backward) viewing is negative. Patient tolerated the procedure well.

DIAGNOSIS
Polyp at 35–40 cm on flexible sigmoidoscopy screening examination.

PLAN
She is referred to a **gastroenterologist** for **colonoscopy**. We discussed the risks of colonoscopy, its benefits, and the procedure. The patient was provided with a brochure describing the procedure and instructed to contact the office with any questions.

Assessment 3.12

Interpret Sally Nguyen's Chart Note

Directions: Access your *EduHub* subscription and listen to the recording of the physician reading Sally Nguyen's chart note. After listening to the recording, supply the medical term that matches each definition.

Example: inflammation of the stomach   *Answer:* gastritis

1. process of observing the colon   _____

2. specialist in the study of the stomach and intestine   _____

3. instrument used to visualize the sigmoid colon   _____

4. process of observing the sigmoid colon   _____

SCORECARD: How Did You Do?

Number correct (_____), divided by 4 (_____), multiplied by 100 equals _____ (your score)

Chapter Review

Word Elements Summary

Prefixes

Prefix	Meaning
a-	not; without
ad-	toward
anti-	against
brady-	slow
dia-	through
dys-	painful; difficult
epi-	upon; above
hyper-	above; above normal
pan-	all; everything
peri-	around
poly-	many
retro-	backward; behind

Combining Forms

Root Word/Combining Vowel	Meaning
carcin/o	cancer
celi/o	abdomen
chol/e	bile; gall
cholecyst/o	gallbladder
col/o, colon/o	colon; large intestine
dist/o	away from the point of origin
diverticul/o	diverticulum
duoden/o	duodenum
enter/o	intestines
esophag/o	esophagus

(Continued)

Root Word/Combining Vowel	Meaning
gastr/o	stomach
gingiv/o	gums
gloss/o	tongue
hemat/o	blood
hepat/o	liver
herni/o	hernia; rupture; protrusion
ile/o	ileum
jejun/o	jejunum
lapar/o	abdomen
lith/o	stone
or/o	mouth
organ/o	organ
pancreat/o	pancreas
peps/o	digestion
polyp/o	polyp; small growth
proct/o	anus and rectum
proxim/o	nearest the point of origin
rect/o	rectum
sial/o	saliva
sigmoid/o	sigmoid colon

Suffixes

Suffix	Meaning
-al	pertaining to
-algia	pain
-cele	hernia; swelling; protrusion
-dynia	pain
-eal	pertaining to
-ectomy	surgical removal; excision
-emesis	vomiting

(Continued)

Suffix	Meaning
-gram	record; image
-graphy	process of recording an image
-ia	condition
-iasis	abnormal condition
-ic	pertaining to
-itis	inflammation
-logist	specialist in the study and treatment of
-logy	study of
-megaly	enlargement
-oma	tumor; mass
-osis	abnormal condition
-phagia	condition of eating or swallowing
-pharynx	pharynx; throat
-plasty	surgical repair
-ptosis	drooping; downward displacement
-rrhea	flow; discharge
-scope	instrument used to observe
-scopy	process of observing
-stomy	new opening
-tomy	incision; cut into
-tripsy	crushing
-y	condition; process

More Practice: Activities and Games

The following activities will help you reinforce your skills and check your mastery of the medical terminology you learned in this chapter. Access your *EduHub* subscription to complete more activities and vocabulary games for mastering the word parts and terms you have learned.

True or False

Directions: Indicate whether each statement is true or false.

True or False?

_____ 1. Major organs of the gastrointestinal (GI) tract include the mouth and stomach.

_____ 2. The liver, gallbladder, pancreas, salivary glands, and teeth are accessory organs that aid in digestion.

_____ 3. Chemical digestion and absorption of food occur in the stomach.

_____ 4. The small intestine is so named because its diameter is wider than that of the large intestine.

_____ 5. Crohn's disease is an acute inflammatory stomach disease.

_____ 6. A hiatal hernia occurs when a portion of the stomach protrudes through the diaphragm.

_____ 7. Hepatitis is an inflammation of the liver causing yellowish discoloration of the skin and eyes.

_____ 8. Ulcers can develop in the esophagus, stomach, or duodenum.

_____ 9. Gastric bypass is a type of weight-loss surgery.

_____ 10. Laparoscopic surgery involves a long, difficult recovery time.

_____ 11. The three parts of the small intestine are the duodenum, jejunum, and sigmoid.

_____ 12. The small intestine is known as the colon.

_____ 13. Anorexia nervosa and bulimia nervosa are two common types of behavioral eating disorders.

_____ 14. An endoscope is a flexible, fiber-optic instrument that has a magnifying lens and, in some cases, a tool for removing tissue for examination.

_____ 15. A colonoscopy drains stool from the colon into a colostomy bag attached to the abdomen.

_____ 16. A lower gastrointestinal (LGI) series can detect (for example) diverticulitis, polyps, abscesses, and cancer.

Dictionary Skills

Directions: Using a medical dictionary, such as *Taber's Cyclopedic Medical Dictionary*, look up the term *gastroparalysis*. For each medical term, indicate whether the term appears on the same page as *gastroparalysis* (*O*), before the page (*B*), or after the page (*A*). Then define each term.

Medical Term   **O, B, A**

  1. gastropulmonary   _____

Definition: _____

_____

  2. gastrology   _____

Definition: _____

_____

Medical Term	O, B, A
3. gastroptosis	_____

Definition: _____

_____

| 4. gastrulation | _____ |

Definition: _____

_____

| 5. gastroscope | _____ |

Definition: _____

_____

| 6. gastrolysis | _____ |

Definition: _____

_____

| 7. gastrogastrostomy | _____ |

Definition: _____

_____

| 8. gastrojejunostomy | _____ |

Definition: _____

_____

| 9. gastrostenosis | _____ |

Definition: _____

_____

| 10. gastromycosis | _____ |

Definition: _____

_____

Break It Down

Directions: Dissect each medical term into its word parts (prefix, root word, combining vowel, and suffix) using one or more slashes. Then define each term.

Medical Term	Dissection
1. sigmoiditis	s i g m o i d i t i s

Definition: _____

_____

2. rectocolitis	r e c t o c o l i t i s

Definition: _____

_____

3. celioscopy	c e l i o s c o p y

Definition: _____

_____

4. enterogram	e n t e r o g r a m

Definition: _____

_____

5. enterology	e n t e r o l o g y

Definition: _____

_____

6. gingival	g i n g i v a l

Definition: _____

_____

7. enteroplasty	e n t e r o p l a s t y

Definition: _____

_____

Medical Term	Dissection
8. pancreatitis	p a n c r e a t i t i s

Definition: _____

_____

9. gingivosis   g i n g i v o s i s

Definition: _____

_____

10. glossoplasty   g l o s s o p l a s t y

Definition: _____

_____

11. retrography   r e t r o g r a p h y

Definition: _____

_____

12. glossalgia   g l o s s a l g i a

Definition: _____

_____

Audio Activity: Shana Laquisha's Chart Note

Directions: Access your *EduHub* subscription and listen to the recording of the physician reading Shana Laquisha's chart note. Read along with the physician and pay attention to the pronunciation of each medical term.

RADIOLOGY REPORT

Patient Name: Laquisha, Shana
ID Number: 569801
Examination Date: March 1, 20xx

EXAMINATION
Upper GI

INDICATIONS
Patient has a history of **Crohn's disease** and uncontrolled diarrhea.

PROCEDURE
Swallowing mechanism appears normal. There is no evidence of aspiration (drawing of gastric contents into the throat). **Proximal esophagus** appears normal.
Fundus (base) of the **stomach** distends well. There is no suggestion of abnormal rugae (fold) pattern in the upper region of the stomach. The body and pyloris (passage at the lower end of the stomach that opens into the duodenum) of the stomach appear normal. There is a high-grade obstruction in the extreme distal end of the stomach. There is just a 2 to 3 mm passage of contrast agent beyond an "apple core" obstructing lesion. This certainly has to be considered a **carcinoma**; direct visualization is indicated. The **duodenal** bulb, loop, and proximal **jejunum** appear normal.

CONCLUSION
A 2 to 3 mm obstructing lesion in the distal end of the stomach, possibly carcinoma.

Assessment

Interpret Shana Laquisha's Chart Note

Directions: Access your *EduHub* subscription and listen to the recording of the physician reading Shana Laquisha's chart note. After listening to the recording, supply the medical term that matches each definition.

Example: inflammation of the diverticulum   *Answer:* diverticulitis

1. pertaining to the duodenum   _____

2. nearest the point of origin   _____

3. cancerous tumor   _____

4. an expandable organ that breaks food down for absorption by the body; located between the esophagus and small intestine   _____

5. tubular structure that carries food from the pharynx to the stomach   _____

6. the section of the small intestine between the duodenum and the ileum   _____

7. chronic, inflammatory bowel disease characterized by thickening and gradual erosion of the inner lining of the intestinal wall   _____

Chapter 4

The Musculoskeletal System

orth / o / ped / ics: the study of the musculoskeletal system

Chapter Organization

- Intern Experience
- Overview of Musculoskeletal System Anatomy and Physiology
- Word Elements
- Breaking Down and Building Musculoskeletal System Terms
- Diseases and Disorders
- Procedures and Treatments
- Analyzing the Intern Experience
- Working with Medical Records
- Chapter Review

Chapter Objectives

After completing this chapter, you will be able to

1. label anatomical diagrams of the musculoskeletal system;
2. dissect and define common medical terminology related to the musculoskeletal system;
3. build terms used to describe musculoskeletal system diseases and disorders, diagnostic procedures, and therapeutic treatments;
4. pronounce and spell common medical terminology related to the musculoskeletal system;
5. understand that the process of building and dissecting a medical term based on its prefix, root word, and suffix enables you to analyze an extremely large number of medical terms beyond those presented in this chapter;
6. interpret the meanings of abbreviations associated with the musculoskeletal system; and
7. interpret medical records containing terminology and abbreviations related to the musculoskeletal system.

Your *EduHub* subscription that accompanies this text provides access to online assessments, assignments, activities, and resources. Throughout this chapter, access *EduHub* to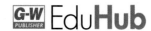

- use e-flash cards to review the medical terminology and word parts you learn;
- listen to the correct pronunciations of medical terms; and
- complete medical terminology activities and assignments.

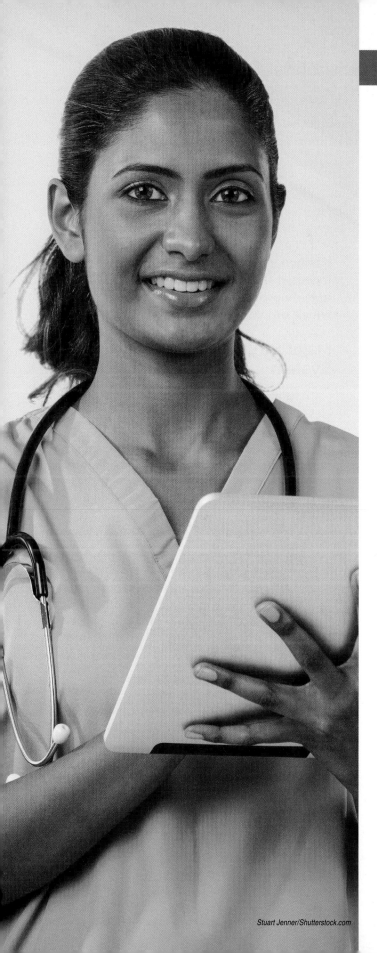

Intern Experience

Aishandi Koshy is serving an internship at the DesFed Urgent Care Center, a facility that offers treatment to patients of all ages for illnesses and injuries such as the flu, asthma attacks, broken bones, cuts requiring stitches, and other health issues requiring time-sensitive care.

Aishandi's assignment this week is to observe and assist Dr. Geiger. Aishandi accompanies the doctor to exam room 5, where the next patient is waiting. Bill, a high school sophomore, recounts for Dr. Geiger the details of his injury.

It was Bill's first football game of the season. He was running the play pattern that the coach had drilled into the team. The quarterback hurled the ball in his direction, and as Bill was about to catch it, the harsh glare of the setting sun blocked his view. Out of nowhere, his opponent tackled him, sliding sideways into his left knee. Dazed, Bill lay on the ground, clutching his knee in agony.

Bill is experiencing a problem with a part of his musculoskeletal system, the body system that provides a framework of support for muscles, ligaments, and tendons; protects delicate internal organs and tissues; and enables movement. To help you understand what is happening to Bill, this chapter will present word elements (combining forms, prefixes, and suffixes) that make up medical terminology related to the musculoskeletal system. As you progress through this book, you will see many word parts that are also used in medical terms related to other body systems.

We will begin our study of the musculoskeletal system with a brief overview of its anatomy and physiology. Major structures of both the muscular and skeletal systems will be covered, along with their main functions. Later in the chapter, you will learn about some common pathological conditions of the musculoskeletal system, tests and procedures used to diagnose these conditions, and common treatment methods.

Overview of Musculoskeletal System Anatomy and Physiology

The primary functions of the musculoskeletal system are to
1. provide the framework and support for the body;
2. protect the internal organs;
3. allow bodily movement;
4. store calcium, phosphorus, and other vital minerals;
5. manufacture red blood cells; and
6. provide body heat through energy produced by the muscles.

The musculoskeletal system is a combination of two body systems that work together: the muscular system, which provides movement, and the skeletal system, which supports and protects the body.

Major Structures of the Muscular System

The **muscular system** is made up of muscles, tendons, and ligaments (Figure 4.1A). These structures are attached to bones, enabling us to move, bend, and manipulate objects. Muscular tissue is unique in its ability to contract, or shorten. In fact, as much as 70 percent of our body heat is generated by muscle contractions.

Muscles are categorized as either *voluntary* or *involuntary*. **Voluntary muscle**, also called *skeletal muscle*, is under conscious control. During voluntary muscular action, your brain sends neural (nerve) impulses to certain muscles, directing them to move. Examples of voluntary muscular action include sending a text message, closing a door, or walking up a flight of stairs.

By contrast, **involuntary muscle** is not under conscious control. Examples of involuntary muscle are the smooth muscle of the digestive tract, and cardiac muscle, which contracts to move blood into and out of the heart. Involuntary muscular movement happens unconsciously. Can you imagine if you had to think about contracting your heart to beat or your diaphragm muscle to breathe?

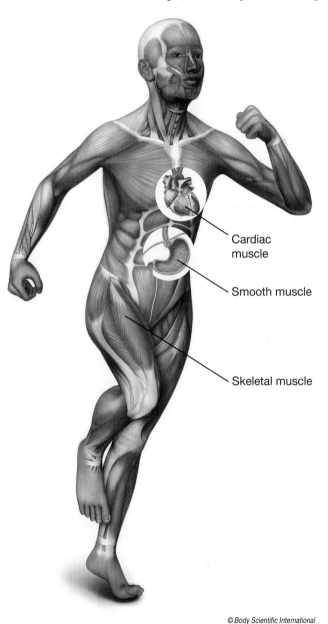

Cardiac muscle

Smooth muscle

Skeletal muscle

© Body Scientific International

Figure 4.1A The muscular system

Major Structures of the Skeletal System

The bones of the **skeletal system** provide a framework of support for the body and protect the internal organs (Figure 4.1B). Minerals such as calcium and phosphorus are stored in the bones, giving them their strength. The skeletal system also plays a crucial role in the production of red blood cells.

The adult skeletal system consists of 206 bones plus cartilage, ligaments, and tendons. **Cartilage** is connective tissue that acts as a shock absorber by cushioning bones that are linked together. This shock-absorbing function prevents friction between bones whenever we walk, run, or jump. The **meniscus** (mě-NĬS-kŭs) in the knee, for example, is a C-shaped disk of cartilage that cushions the knee joint. Actually, there are two *menisci* (mě-NĬS-ē) in each knee: one on the inner side of the knee and one on the outer side.

A **ligament** is a band of tissue that connects a bone to another bone. An example of a ligament is the **anterior cruciate** (KRŪ-shē-āt) **ligament** in the knee, which controls rotation and forward movement of the tibia (shin bone). A **tendon** is a cord of fibrous tissue that connects muscle to bone. Your Achilles tendon, for example, connects your heel bone to your calf (lower leg) muscles.

The point at which one bone meets another bone is called a **joint**. Joints make bodily motion possible. Without joints, your body movement would be limited and robotic.

Orthopedics is the study of the musculoskeletal system. The suffix **-ics** means "the organized knowledge, practice, or treatment" of a particular subject or field. An **orthopedist** is a physician who specializes in the study and treatment of the musculoskeletal system.

Anatomy and Physiology Vocabulary

Now that you have been introduced to the basic structure and functions of the musculoskeletal system, we will explore in more detail the key terms presented in the introduction.

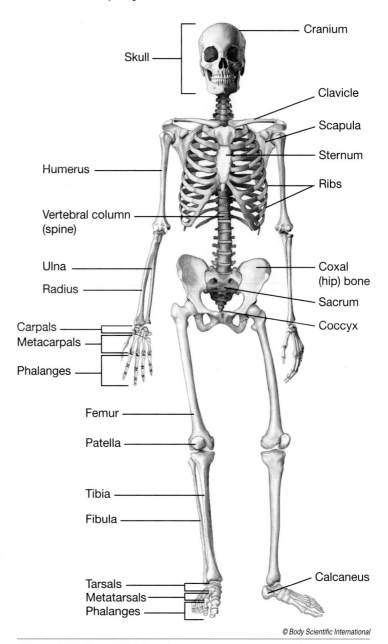

© Body Scientific International

Figure 4.1B The skeletal system

Key Term	Definition
cartilage	connective tissue that acts as a shock absorber by cushioning bones that are linked together
involuntary muscle	muscle that is not under conscious control; smooth muscle and cardiac muscle
joint	the point at which one bone meets another bone
ligament	band of tissue that connects a bone to another bone
meniscus (plural *menisci*)	C-shaped disk of cartilage that cushions the knee joint
muscular system	the body system made up of muscles, tendons, and ligaments, all of which control movement
orthopedics	the study of the musculoskeletal system
orthopedist	physician who specializes in the study and treatment of the musculoskeletal system
skeletal system	the body system that provides a framework of support for organs and tissues, protects the internal organs, stores minerals such as calcium and phosphorus, and plays a crucial role in the production of erythrocytes (red blood cells)
tendon	band of fibrous tissue that attaches muscle to bone
voluntary muscle	muscle that is under conscious control; skeletal muscle

E-Flash Card Activity: Anatomy and Physiology Vocabulary

Directions: After you have reviewed the anatomy and physiology vocabulary related to the musculoskeletal system, access your *EduHub* subscription and practice with the e-flash cards until you are comfortable with the spelling and definition of each term.

Identifying the Three Types of Muscle Tissue

Directions: Label the three types of muscular tissue in the diagram. You can also complete this activity online using *EduHub*.

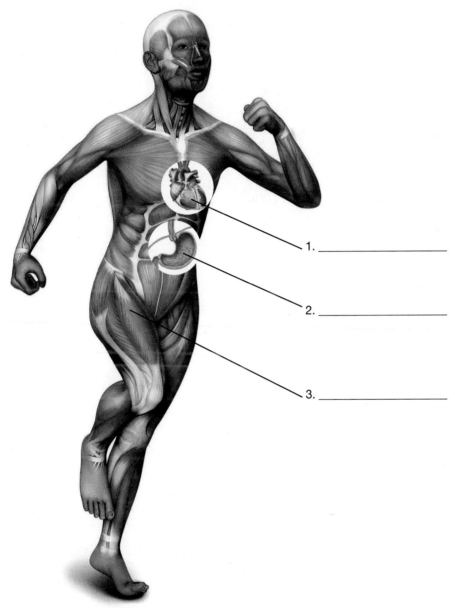

1. _____

2. _____

3. _____

© Body Scientific International

Identifying Major Bones of the Skeletal System

Directions: Label the diagram of the skeletal system. You can also complete this activity online using *EduHub*.

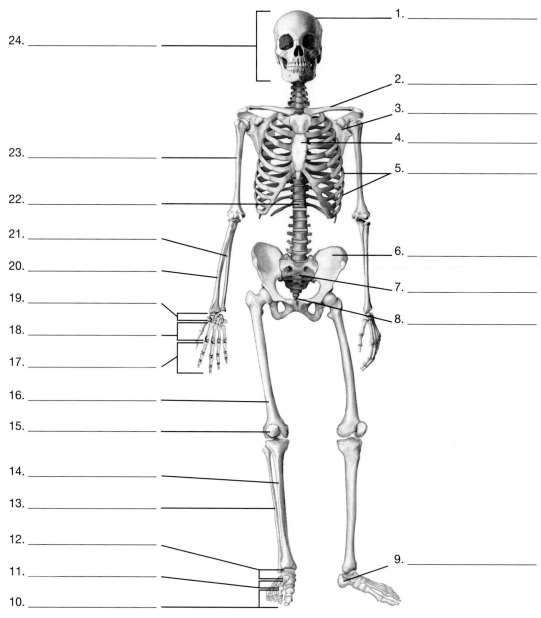

24. _____

23. _____

22. _____

21. _____

20. _____

19. _____

18. _____

17. _____

16. _____

15. _____

14. _____

13. _____

12. _____

11. _____

10. _____

1. _____

2. _____

3. _____

4. _____

5. _____

6. _____

7. _____

8. _____

9. _____

© Body Scientific International

SCORECARD: How Did You Do?

Number correct (_____), divided by 24 (_____), multiplied by 100 equals _____ (your score)

Matching Anatomy and Physiology Vocabulary

Directions: Choose the correct vocabulary term for each meaning. You can also complete this activity online using *EduHub*.

_____ 1. C-shaped disk of cartilage that cushions the knee joint

_____ 2. the body system that provides a framework of support for organs and tissues, protects the internal organs, stores minerals such as calcium and phosphorus, and plays a crucial role in the production of red blood cells

_____ 3. the study of the musculoskeletal system

_____ 4. physician who specializes in the study and treatment of the musculoskeletal system

_____ 5. band of fibrous tissue that attaches muscle to bone

_____ 6. muscle that is not under conscious control; smooth muscle and cardiac muscle

_____ 7. muscle that is under conscious control; skeletal muscle

_____ 8. the point at which one bone meets another bone

_____ 9. the body system made up of muscles, tendons, and ligaments, all of which control movement

_____ 10. connective tissue that acts as a shock absorber by cushioning bones that are linked together

_____ 11. band of tissue that connects a bone to another bone

A. cartilage

B. involuntary muscle

C. joint

D. ligament

E. meniscus

F. orthopedics

G. orthopedist

H. skeletal system

I. tendon

J. voluntary muscle

K. muscular system

SCORECARD: How Did You Do?

Number correct (_____), divided by 11 (_____), multiplied by 100 equals _____ (your score)

Word Elements

In this section, you will learn word elements—prefixes, combining forms, and suffixes—that are common to the musculoskeletal system. By learning these word elements and understanding how they are combined to build medical terms, you will be able to analyze Bill's musculoskeletal problem (described in the Intern Experience at the beginning of this chapter) and identify a large number of terms associated with the musculoskeletal system.

E-Flash Card Activity: Word Elements

Directions: Review the word elements in the tables that follow. Then, access your *EduHub* subscription and practice with the e-flash cards until you are able to quickly recognize the different word parts (prefixes, combining forms, and suffixes) and their meanings. The e-flash cards are grouped together by prefixes, combining forms, and suffixes, followed by a cumulative review of all the word elements you are learning in this chapter.

Prefixes

Let's begin our study of musculoskeletal system word elements by looking at the prefixes listed in the table below.

Prefix	Meaning
a-	not; without
an-	not; without
brady-	slow
dys-	painful; difficult
endo-	within
epi-	upon; above
hyper-	above; above normal
inter-	between
intra-	within
meta-	change; beyond
per-	through
peri-	around
poly-	many
quadri-	four
sub-	beneath; below
supra-	above
sym-, syn-	together; with

Combining Forms

Listed below are common combining forms used in medical terms related to the musculoskeletal system.

Root Word/Combining Vowel	Meaning
anter/o	front
arthr/o	joint
articul/o	joint
burs/a, burs/o	bursa; sac
cardi/o	heart
carp/o	carpals (wrist bones)
chondr/o	cartilage
clavicul/o	clavicle (collar bone)
coccyg/o	coccyx (tailbone)
cost/o	rib
crani/o	skull
dist/o	away from the point of origin
dors/o	back (of the body)
ecchym/o	blood in the tissues
electr/o	electrical activity
erythemat/o	redness
erythr/o	red
femor/o	femur (thigh bone)
fibul/o	fibula
herni/o	hernia; rupture; protrusion
humer/o	humerus (upper arm bone)
ili/o	ilium
infer/o	below; beneath
ischi/o	ischium (part of hip bone)
kines/o, kinesi/o	movement
kyph/o	hump
later/o	side
lord/o	curve
medi/o	middle
metacarp/o	metacarpals (bones of the hand)
metatars/o	metatarsals (bones of the foot)
muscul/o	muscle

(Continued)

Root Word/Combining Vowel	Meaning
my/o	muscle
myel/o	bone marrow; spinal cord
necr/o	death
neur/o	nerve
orth/o	straight
oste/o	bone
patell/a, patell/o	patella (kneecap)
path/o	disease
phalang/o	phalanges (bones of fingers/toes)
por/o	pore; duct; small opening
poster/o	back (of the body)
proxim/o	nearest the point of origin
pub/o	pubis (part of the hip bone)
radi/o	radius (bone of the forearm); X-ray
sacr/o	sacrum (bone at base of the spine)
scapul/o	scapula (shoulder blade)
scoli/o	crooked; bent
spondyl/o	vertebra; spine
stern/o	sternum (breastbone)
tars/o	ankle bones
ten/o	tendon
tendin/o, tendon/o	tendon
tibi/o	tibia (shin bone)
uln/o	ulna (bone of the forearm)
vascul/o	blood vessel
vertebr/o	vertebra; spine

Suffixes

Listed below are suffixes used in medical terms pertaining to the musculoskeletal system. Many of these prefixes are used in medical terms related to other body systems as well.

Suffix	Meaning
-ac	pertaining to
-al	pertaining to
-algia	pain

(Continued)

Suffix	Meaning
-ar	pertaining to
-ary	pertaining to
-asthenia	weakness
-centesis	surgical puncture to remove fluid
-clasia	surgical breaking
-cyte	cell
-desis	to bind or tie together surgically
-dynia	pain
-eal	pertaining to
-ectomy	surgical removal; excision
-edema	swelling
-ema	condition
-gen	producing; originating; causing
-gram	record; image
-graphy	process of recording an image
-ia	condition
-ic	pertaining to
-ior	pertaining to
-itis	inflammation
-kinesia	movement
-kinesis	movement
-logist	specialist in the study and treatment of
-logy	study of
-lysis	breakdown; loosening; dissolving
-malacia	softening
-metry	process of measuring
-oma	tumor; mass
-osis	abnormal condition
-ous	pertaining to
-pathy	disease
-penia	deficiency; abnormal reduction
-plasty	surgical repair
-plegia	paralysis
-rrhaphy	suture

(Continued)

Suffix	Meaning
-rrhexis	rupture
-scope	instrument used to observe
-scopy	process of observing
-tome	instrument used to cut
-tomy	incision; cut into
-trophy	development

Assessment 4.4

Matching Prefixes, Combining Forms, and Suffixes

Directions: Choose the correct meaning for each word element. Some meanings may be used more than once. You can also complete this activity online using *EduHub*.

Prefixes

_____ 1. quadri-

_____ 2. per-

_____ 3. a-

_____ 4. brady-

_____ 5. dys-

_____ 6. an-

_____ 7. poly-

_____ 8. hyper-

_____ 9. meta-

_____ 10. peri-

_____ 11. epi-

_____ 12. intra-

_____ 13. sub-

_____ 14. sym-

_____ 15. supra-

_____ 16. inter-

_____ 17. syn-

_____ 18. endo-

A. painful; difficult

B. not; without

C. upon; above

D. between

E. within

F. through

G. slow

H. many

I. above

J. four

K. together; with

L. above; above normal

M. around

N. beneath; below

O. change; beyond

Combining Forms

_____	1. orth/o	A. joint
_____	2. arthr/o	B. carpals
_____	3. oste/o	C. straight
_____	4. articul/o	D. skull
_____	5. patell/a, patell/o	E. clavicle
_____	6. phalang/o	F. rib
_____	7. carp/o	G. radius; X-ray
_____	8. femor/o	H. patella
_____	9. chondr/o	I. cartilage
_____	10. fibul/o	J. fibula
_____	11. clavicul/o	K. femur; thigh bone
_____	12. humer/o	L. phalanges
_____	13. cost/o	M. bone
_____	14. radi/o	N. vertebra; spine
_____	15. crani/o	O. tendon
_____	16. kines/o, kinesi/o	P. movement
_____	17. stern/o	Q. sternum
_____	18. tibi/o	R. ankle bones
_____	19. metatars/o	S. scapula
_____	20. my/o	T. metatarsals
_____	21. scapul/o	U. humerus
_____	22. spondyl/o	V. metacarpals
_____	23. tars/o	W. tibia
_____	24. tendin/o, tendon/o	X. muscle
_____	25. metacarp/o	

Suffixes

_____	1. -ar	A. surgical puncture to remove fluid
_____	2. -centesis	B. breakdown; loosening; dissolving
_____	3. -lysis	C. instrument used to cut
_____	4. -kinesis	D. pertaining to
_____	5. -metry	E. condition

_____	6. -ac	F.	pain
_____	7. -gen	G.	process of measuring
_____	8. -ior	H.	producing; originating; causing
_____	9. -kinesia	I.	surgical breaking
_____	10. -malacia	J.	weakness
_____	11. -trophy	K.	paralysis
_____	12. -ary	L.	softening
_____	13. -osis	M.	movement
_____	14. -ema	N.	development
_____	15. -algia	O.	deficiency; abnormal reduction
_____	16. -ic	P.	abnormal condition
_____	17. -plegia	Q.	to bind or tie together surgically
_____	18. -asthenia		
_____	19. -tome		
_____	20. -clasia		
_____	21. -desis		
_____	22. -ous		
_____	23. -penia		
_____	24. -ia		
_____	25. -dynia		

SCORECARD: How Did You Do?

Number correct (_____), divided by 68 (_____), multiplied by 100 equals _____ (your score)

Breaking Down and Building Musculoskeletal System Terms

Now that you have mastered the prefixes, combining forms, and suffixes for musculoskeletal system terminology, you have the ability to dissect and build a large number of medical terms related to this body system.

Below is a list of common medical terms related to the study and treatment of the musculoskeletal system. For each term, a dissection has been provided, along with the meaning of each word element and the definition of the term as a whole.

Term	Dissection	Word Part/Meaning	Term Definition
Note: *For simplification, combining vowels have been omitted from the Word Part/Meaning column.*			
1. **anterior** (ăn-TĒR-ē-or)	anter/ior	**anter** = front **ior** = pertaining to	pertaining to the front
2. **anteroinferior** (ĂN-tĕr-ō-ĭn-FĒR-ē-or)	anter/o/infer/ior	**anter** = front **infer** = below **ior** = pertaining to	pertaining to front and below
3. **arthralgia** (är-THRĂL-jē-ă)	arthr/algia	**arthr** = joint **algia** = pain	pain in the joint
4. **arthritis** (är-THRĪ-tĭs)	arthr/itis	**arthr** = joint **itis** = inflammation	inflammation of the joints
5. **arthrocentesis** (är-thrō-sĕn-TĒ-sĭs)	arthr/o/centesis	**arthr** = joint **centesis** = surgical puncture to remove fluid	surgical puncture to remove fluid from a joint
6. **arthrochondritis** (är-thrō-kŏn-DRĪ-tĭs)	arthr/o/chondr/itis	**arthr** = joint **chondr** = cartilage **itis** = inflammation	inflammation of the joint and cartilage
7. **arthrodesis** (är-thrō-DĒ-sĭs)	arthr/o/desis	**arthr** = joint **desis** = to bind or tie together surgically	to surgically bind/tie together joints
8. **arthrogram** (ÄR-thrō-grăm)	arthr/o/gram	**arthr** = joint **gram** = record; image	image of the joint
9. **arthroscope** (ÄR-thrō-skōp)	arthr/o/scope	**arthr** = joint **scope** = instrument used to observe	instrument used to observe the joints
10. **arthroscopy** (är-THRŎS-kō-pē)	arthr/o/scopy	**arthr** = joint **scopy** = process of observing	process of observing the joints
11. **arthrotome** (ÄR-thrō-tōm)	arthr/o/tome	**arthr** = joint **tome** = instrument used to cut	instrument used to cut joints
12. **atrophy** (ĂT-rō-fē)	a/trophy	**a** = not; without **trophy** = development	without development
13. **bradykinesia** (BRĂD-ē-kĭn-Ē-zē-ă)	brady/kinesia	**brady** = slow **kinesia** = movement	slow movement
14. **bursectomy** (bŭr-SĔK-tō-mē)	burs/ectomy	**burs** = bursa; sac **ectomy** = surgical removal; excision	excision of the bursa/sac
15. **bursitis** (bŭr-SĪ-tĭs)	burs/itis	**burs** = bursa; sac **itis** = inflammation	inflammation of the bursa/sac
16. **bursotomy** (bŭr-SŎT-ō-mē)	burs/o/tomy	**burs** = bursa; sac **tomy** = incision; cut into	incision to the bursa/sac

Prefixes = **Green**   Root Words = **Red**   Suffixes = **Blue**

Term	Dissection	Word Part/Meaning	Term Definition
17. **cardiorrhaphy** (kär-dē-OR-ă-fē)	cardi/o/rrhaphy	**cardi** = heart **rrhaphy** = suture	suture of the heart
18. **cardiorrhexis** (KĂR-dē-ō-RĔK-sĭs)	cardi/o/rrhexis	**cardi** = heart **rrhexis** = rupture	rupture of the heart
19. **carpal** (KĂR-păl)	carp/al	**carp** = carpals (wrist bones) **al** = pertaining to	pertaining to the carpals (wrist bones)
20. **chondrocostal** (kŏn-drō-KŎS-tăl)	chondr/o/cost/al	**chondr** = cartilage **cost** = rib **al** = pertaining to	pertaining to cartilage and ribs
21. **chondrogenic** (kŏn-drō-JĔN-ĭk)	chondr/o/gen/ic	**chondr** = cartilage **gen** = producing; originating; causing **ic** = pertaining to	pertaining to producing cartilage
22. **chondromalacia** (KŎN-drō-mă-LĀ-shē-ă)	chondr/o/malacia	**chondr** = cartilage **malacia** = softening	softening of the cartilage
23. **coccygeal** (kŏk-SĬJ-ē-ăl)	coccyg/eal	**coccyg** = coccyx (tailbone) **eal** = pertaining to	pertaining to the coccyx (tailbone)
24. **cranial** (KRĀ-nē-ăl)	crani/al	**crani** = skull **al** = pertaining to	pertaining to the skull
25. **craniotomy** (krā-nē-ŎT-ō-mē)	crani/o/tomy	**crani** = skull **tomy** = incision; cut into	incision to the skull
26. **dorsal** (DOR-săl)	dors/al	**dors** = back (of the body) **al** = pertaining to	pertaining to the back
27. **dyskinesia** (dĭs-kĭ-NĒ-zē-ă)	dys/kinesia	**dys** = painful; difficult **kinesia** = movement	painful or difficult movement
28. **dystrophy** (DĬS-trō-fē)	dys/trophy	**dys** = painful; difficult **trophy** = development	painful or difficult development
29. **ecchymosis** (ĕk-ĭ-MŌ-sĭs)	ecchym/osis	**ecchym** = blood in the tissues **osis** = abnormal condition	abnormal condition of blood in the tissues
30. **electromyogram** (ē-LĔK-trō-MĪ-ō-gram)	electr/o/my/o/gram	**electr** = electrical activity **my** = muscle **gram** = record; image	record/image of electrical activity in the muscle
31. **hypertrophy** (hī-PĔR-trō-fē)	hyper/trophy	**hyper** = above; above normal **trophy** = development	above-normal development
32. **intercostal** (ĭn-tĕr-KŎS-tăl)	inter/cost/al	**inter** = between **cost** = rib **al** = pertaining to	pertaining to between ribs
33. **intervertebral** (ĭn-tĕr-VĔR-tĕ-brăl)	inter/vertebr/al	**inter** = between **vertebr** = vertebra; spine **al** = pertaining to	pertaining to between vertebrae (plural form of *vertebra*)

Prefixes = Green   Root Words = Red   Suffixes = Blue

Term	Dissection	Word Part/Meaning	Term Definition
34. **kinesiology** (kĭ-nē-sē-ŎL-ō-jē)	kinesi/o/logy	**kinesi** = movement **logy** = study of	study of movement
35. **kyphosis** (kī-FŌ-sĭs)	kyph/osis	**kyph** = hump **osis** = abnormal condition	abnormal condition of a hump; humpback
36. **lateral** (LĂT-ĕr-ăl)	later/al	**later** = side **al** = pertaining to	pertaining to the side
37. **lordosis** (lor-DŌ-sĭs)	lord/osis	**lord** = curve **osis** = abnormal condition	abnormal condition of curve (of the spine)
38. **myalgia** (mī-ĂL-jē-ă)	my/algia	**my** = muscle **algia** = pain	pain in the muscle
39. **myasthenia** (mī-ăs-THĒ-nē-ă)	my/asthenia	**my** = muscle **asthenia** = weakness	weakness of the muscle
40. **myitis** (mī-Ī-tĭs)	my/itis	**my** = muscle **itis** = inflammation	inflammation of the muscle
41. **necrosis** (nĕ-KRŌ-sĭs)	necr/osis	**necr** = death **osis** = abnormal condition	abnormal condition of death
42. **osteoarthritis** (ŎS-tē-ō-är-THRĪ-tĭs)	oste/o/arthr/itis	**oste** = bone **arthr** = joint **itis** = inflammation	inflammation of the bone and joint
43. **osteochondritis** (ŎS-tē-ō-kŏn-DRĪ-tĭs)	oste/o/chondr/itis	**oste** = bone **chondr** = cartilage **itis** = inflammation	inflammation of the bone and cartilage
44. **osteomalacia** (ŎS-tē-ō-mă-LĀ-shē-ă)	oste/o/malacia	**oste** = bone **malacia** = softening	softening of the bone
45. **osteomyelitis** (ŎS-tē-ō-mī-ĕ-LĪ-tĭs)	oste/o/myel/itis	**oste** = bone **myel** = bone marrow; spinal cord **itis** = inflammation	inflammation of the bone and bone marrow
46. **osteonecrosis** (ŎS-tē-ō-nĕ-KRŌ-sĭs)	oste/o/necr/osis	**oste** = bone **necr** = death **osis** = abnormal condition	abnormal condition of death of the bone
47. **osteopathy** (ŏs-tē-ŎP-ă-thē)	oste/o/pathy	**oste** = bone **pathy** = disease	disease of the bone
48. **osteopenia** (ŏs-tē-ō-PĒ-nē-ă)	oste/o/penia	**oste** = bone **penia** = deficiency; abnormal reduction	deficiency/abnormal reduction of bone
49. **osteoporosis** (ŎS-tē-ō-por-Ō-sis)	oste/o/por/osis	**oste** = bone **por** = pore; duct; small opening **osis** = abnormal condition	abnormal condition of small openings in the bone

Prefixes = **Green**   Root Words = **Red**   Suffixes = **Blue**

Term	Dissection	Word Part/Meaning	Term Definition
50. **posterior** (pŏs-TĒR-ē-or)	poster/ior	**poster** = back (of the body) **ior** = pertaining to	pertaining to the back
51. **quadriplegia** (kwŏd-rĭ-PLĒ-jē-ă)	quadri/plegia	quadri = four **plegia** = paralysis	paralysis of four (extremities)
52. **scoliosis** (skō-lē-Ō-sĭs)	scoli/osis	**scoli** = crooked; bent **osis** = abnormal condition	abnormal condition of (being) crooked or bent
53. **spondylarthritis** (SPŎN-dĭl-är-THRĪ-tĭs)	spondyl/arthr/itis	**spondyl** = vertebra; spine **arthr** = joint **itis** = inflammation	inflammation of the vertebra and joint
54. **spondylodesis** (SPŎN-dĭ-lō-DĒ-sĭs)	spondyl/o/desis	**spondyl** = vertebra; spine **desis** = to bind or tie together surgically	to surgically bind/ tie together vertebrae (plural of *vertebra*)
55. **spondylolysis** (SPŎN-dĭ-lŏ-LĪ-sĭs)	spondyl/o/lysis	**spondyl** = vertebra; spine **lysis** = breakdown; loosening; dissolving	breakdown/ loosening/dissolving of the vertebra
56. **spondylosis** (spŏn-dĭ-LŌ-sĭs)	spondyl/osis	**spondyl** = vertebra; spine **osis** = abnormal condition	abnormal condition of the vertebra
57. **sternal** (STĔR-năl)	stern/al	**stern** = sternum (breastbone) **al** = pertaining to	pertaining to the sternum (breastbone)
58. **sternocostal** (stĕr-nō-KŎS-tăl)	stern/o/cost/al	**stern** = sternum (breastbone) **cost** = rib **al** = pertaining to	pertaining to the sternum (breastbone) and rib
59. **subcostal** (sŭb-KŎS-tăl)	sub/cost/al	sub = beneath; below **cost** = rib **al** = pertaining to	pertaining to below the rib
60. **synkinesis** (sĭn-kĭ-NĒ-sĭs)	syn/kinesis	syn = together; with **kinesis** = movement	movement together
61. **tendinitis** (tĕn-dĭ-NĪ-tĭs)	tendin/itis	**tendin** = tendon **itis** = inflammation	inflammation of the tendon
62. **vasculitis** (văs-kū-LĪ-tĭs)	vascul/itis	**vascul** = blood vessel **itis** = inflammation	inflammation of the blood vessel
63. **vertebral** (VĔR-tĕ-brăl)	vertebr/al	**vertebr** = vertebra; spine **al** = pertaining to	pertaining to the vertebra
64. **vertebrectomy** (vĕr-tĕ-BRĔK-tō-mē)	vertebr/ectomy	**vertebr** = vertebra **ectomy** = surgical removal; excision	excision of the vertebra

Prefixes = Green   Root Words = **Red**   Suffixes = Blue

Using the pronunciation guide in the Breaking Down and Building chart, practice saying each medical term aloud. To hear the pronunciation of each term, complete the Pronounce It activity on the next page.

Audio Activity: Pronounce It

Directions: Access your *EduHub* subscription and listen to the correct pronunciations of the following medical terms. Practice pronouncing the terms until you are comfortable saying them aloud.

anterior
(ăn-TĒR-ē-or)

anteroinferior
(ĂN-tĕr-ō-ĭn-FĒR-ē-or)

arthralgia
(är-THRĂL-jē-ă)

arthritis
(är-THRĪ-tĭs)

arthrocentesis
(är-thrō-sĕn-TĒ-sĭs)

arthrochondritis
(är-thrō-kŏn-DRĪ-tĭs)

arthrodesis
(är-thrō-DĒ-sĭs)

arthrogram
(ĂR-thrō-grăm)

arthroscope
(ĂR-thrō-skōp)

arthroscopy
(är-THRŎS-kō-pē)

arthrotome
(ĂR-thrō-tōm)

atrophy
(ĂT-rō-fē)

bradykinesia
(BRĂD-ē-kĭn-Ē-zē-ă)

bursectomy
(bŭr-SĔK-tō-mē)

bursitis
(bŭr-SĪ-tĭs)

bursotomy
(bŭr-SŎT-ō-mē)

cardiorrhaphy
(kär-dē-OR-ă-fē)

cardiorrhexis
(KÄR-dē-ō-RĔK-sĭs)

carpal
(KĂR-păl)

chondrocostal
(kŏn-drō-KŎS-tăl)

chondrogenic
(kŏn-drō-JĔN-ĭk)

chondromalacia
(KŎN-drō-mă-LĀ-shē-ă)

coccygeal
(kŏk-SĬJ-ē-ăl)

cranial
(KRĀ-nē-ăl)

craniotomy
(krā-nē-ŎT-ō-mē)

dorsal
(DOR-săl)

dyskinesia
(dĭs-kĭ-NĒ-zē-ă)

dystrophy
(DĬS-trō-fē)

ecchymosis
(ĕk-ĭ-MŌ-sĭs)

electromyogram
(ē-LĔK-trō-MĪ-ō-gram)

hypertrophy
(hī-PĔR-trō-fē)

intercostal
(ĭn-tĕr-KŎS-tăl)

intervertebral
(ĭn-tĕr-VĔR-tĕ-brăl)

kinesiology
(kĭ-nē-sē-ŎL-ō-jē)

kyphosis
(kī-FŌ-sĭs)

lateral
(LĂT-ĕr-ăl)

lordosis
(lor-DŌ-sĭs)

myalgia
(mī-ĂL-jē-ă)

myasthenia
(mī-ăs-THĒ-nē-ă)

myitis
(mī-Ī-tĭs)

necrosis
(nĕ-KRŌ-sĭs)

osteoarthritis
(ŎS-tē-ō-är-THRĪ-tĭs)

osteochondritis
(ŎS-tē-ō-kŏn-DRĪ-tĭs)

osteomalacia
(ŎS-tē-ō-mă-LĀ-shē-ă)

osteomyelitis
(ŎS-tē-ō-mī-ĕ-LĪ-tĭs)

osteonecrosis
(ŎS-tē-ō-nĕ-KRŌ-sĭs)

osteopathy
(ŏs-tē-ŎP-ă-thē)

osteopenia
(ŏs-tē-ō-PĒ-nē-ă)

osteoporosis
(ŎS-tē-ō-por-Ō-sis)

posterior
(pŏs-TĒR-ē-or)

quadriplegia
(kwŏd-rĭ-PLĒ-jē-ă)

scoliosis
(skō-lē-Ō-sĭs)

spondylarthritis
(SPŎN-dĭl-är-THRĪ-tĭs)

spondylodesis
(SPŎN-dĭ-lō-DĒ-sĭs)

spondylolysis
(SPŎN-dĭ-lŏ-LĪ-sĭs)

spondylosis
(spŏn-dĭ-LŌ-sĭs)

sternal
(STĔR-năl)

sternocostal
(stĕr-nō-KŎS-tăl)

subcostal
(sŭb-KŎS-tăl)

synkinesis
(sĭn-kĭ-NĒ-sĭs)

tendinitis
(tĕn-dĭ-NĪ-tĭs)

vasculitis
(văs-kū-LĪ-tĭs)

vertebral
(VĔR-tĕ-brăl)

vertebrectomy
(vĕr-tĕ-BRĔK-tō-mē)

Audio Activity: Spell It

Directions: Access your *EduHub* subscription and listen to the pronunciation for each number. As you hear each term, write its correct spelling.

1. _____
2. _____
3. _____
4. _____
5. _____
6. _____
7. _____
8. _____
9. _____
10. _____
11. _____
12. _____
13. _____
14. _____
15. _____
16. _____
17. _____
18. _____
19. _____
20. _____
21. _____
22. _____
23. _____
24. _____
25. _____
26. _____
27. _____
28. _____
29. _____
30. _____
31. _____
32. _____
33. _____
34. _____
35. _____
36. _____
37. _____
38. _____
39. _____
40. _____
41. _____
42. _____
43. _____
44. _____
45. _____
46. _____
47. _____
48. _____
49. _____
50. _____
51. _____
52. _____
53. _____
54. _____
55. _____
56. _____
57. _____
58. _____
59. _____
60. _____
61. _____
62. _____
63. _____
64. _____

SCORECARD: How Did You Do?

Number correct (_____), divided by 64 (_____), multiplied by 100 equals _____ (your score)

Break It Down

Directions: Dissect each medical term into its word parts (prefix, root word, combining vowel, and suffix) using one or more slashes. Then define each term. You can also complete this activity online using *EduHub*.

Example:

Medical Term: quadriplegia

Dissection: quadri/plegia

Definition: paralysis of four

Medical Term	Dissection
1. anterior	a n t e r i o r

Definition: _____

_____

2. arthritis   a r t h r i t i s

Definition: _____

_____

3. bradykinesia   b r a d y k i n e s i a

Definition: _____

_____

4. carpal   c a r p a l

Definition: _____

_____

5. anteroinferior   a n t e r o i n f e r i o r

Definition: _____

_____

Medical Term	Dissection

6. hypertrophy   h y p e r t r o p h y

Definition: _____

_____

7. arthralgia   a r t h r a l g i a

Definition: _____

_____

8. dorsal   d o r s a l

Definition: _____

_____

9. arthroscope   a r t h r o s c o p e

Definition: _____

_____

10. myasthenia   m y a s t h e n i a

Definition: _____

_____

11. osteoporosis   o s t e o p o r o s i s

Definition: _____

_____

12. chondrogenic   c h o n d r o g e n i c

Definition: _____

_____

13. arthrogram   a r t h r o g r a m

Definition: _____

_____

Medical Term	Dissection
14. atrophy	a t r o p h y

Definition: _____

_____

15. kyphosis	k y p h o s i s

Definition: _____

_____

16. osteochondritis	o s t e o c h o n d r i t i s

Definition: _____

_____

17. bursotomy	b u r s o t o m y

Definition: _____

_____

18. dyskinesia	d y s k i n e s i a

Definition: _____

_____

19. spondylodesis	s p o n d y l o d e s i s

Definition: _____

_____

20. bursitis	b u r s i t i s

Definition: _____

_____

21. chondromalacia	c h o n d r o m a l a c i a

Definition: _____

_____

Medical Term	Dissection
22. osteomyelitis	o s t e o m y e l i t i s

Definition: _____

_____

| 23. cranial | c r a n i a l |

Definition: _____

_____

| 24. sternocostal | s t e r n o c o s t a l |

Definition: _____

_____

| 25. arthrocentesis | a r t h r o c e n t e s i s |

Definition: _____

_____

| 26. coccygeal | c o c c y g e a l |

Definition: _____

_____

| 27. lateral | l a t e r a l |

Definition: _____

_____

SCORECARD: How Did You Do?

Number correct (_____), divided by 27 (_____), multiplied by 100 equals _____ (your score)

Build It

Directions: Build the medical term that matches each definition by supplying the correct word parts. You can also complete this activity online using *EduHub*.

P (Prefixes) = Green
RW (Root Words) = Red
S (Suffixes) = Blue
CV (Combining Vowel) = Purple

1. to surgically bind/tie together the joint

   _____ _____ _____
   RW   CV   S

2. pertaining to front and below

   _____ _____ _____ _____
   RW   CV   RW   S

3. abnormal condition of a hump; humpback

   _____ _____
   RW   S

4. abnormal condition of small openings in the bone

   _____ _____ _____ _____
   RW   CV   RW   S

5. inflammation of the joints

   _____ _____
   RW   S

6. incision to the skull

   _____ _____ _____
   RW   CV   S

7. surgical puncture to remove fluid from a joint

   _____ _____ _____
   RW   CV   S

8. abnormal condition of death

   _____ _____
   RW   S

9. incision to the bursa

_____ _____ _____
RW   CV   S

10. instrument used to observe the joints

_____ _____ _____
RW   CV   S

11. pertaining to the side

_____ _____
RW   S

12. pertaining to the back (of the body) **(two possible answers)**

_____ _____
RW   S

_____ _____
RW   S

13. inflammation of the joint and cartilage

_____ _____ _____ _____
RW   CV   RW   S

14. study of movement

_____ _____ _____
RW   CV   S

15. rupture of the heart

_____ _____ _____
RW   CV   S

16. image of the joint

_____ _____ _____
RW   CV   S

17. pertaining to the carpals (wrist bones)

_____ _____
RW   S

18. pertaining to the front

_____ _____
RW   S

19. abnormal condition of blood in the tissues

_____   _____
          RW   S

20. process of observing the joints

_____ _____ _____
          RW   CV   S

21. record/image of electrical activity in the muscle

_____ _____ _____ _____ _____
          RW   CV   RW   CV   S

22. pertaining to the cartilage and rib

_____ _____ _____ _____
          RW   CV   RW   S

23. painful or difficult development

_____ _____
   P   S

24. slow movement

_____ _____
   P   S

25. painful or difficult movement

_____ _____
   P   S

26. without development

_____ _____
   P   S

27. excision of the bursa/sac

_____ _____
          RW   S

28. abnormal condition of curve (of the spine)

_____ _____
          RW   S

29. pertaining to the coccyx (tailbone)

_____ _____
          RW   S

30. inflammation of the bursa/sac

_____ _____
        RW   S

31. above-normal development

_____ _____
  P   S

32. suture of the heart

_____ _____ _____
        RW   CV   S

33. pain in the joint

_____ _____
        RW   S

34. pertaining to producing cartilage

_____ _____ _____ _____
        RW   CV   S   S

35. inflammation of the bone and cartilage

_____ _____ _____ _____
        RW   CV   RW   S

36. weakness of the muscle

_____ _____
        RW   S

37. softening of the cartilage

_____ _____ _____
        RW   CV   S

38. disease of the bone

_____ _____ _____
        RW   CV   S

39. abnormal condition of (being) crooked or bent

_____ _____
        RW   S

40. pertaining to the skull

_____ _____
        RW   S

41. inflammation of the vertebra and joint

_____ _____ _____
        RW   RW   S

42. pertaining to between ribs

_____ _____ _____
  P   RW   S

43. inflammation of the bone and bone marrow

_____ _____ _____ _____
       RW   CV   RW   S

44. to surgically bind/tie together vertebrae

_____ _____ _____
       RW   CV   S

45. softening of the bone

_____ _____ _____
       RW   CV   S

46. breakdown/loosening/dissolving of the vertebra

_____ _____ _____
       RW   CV   S

47. pertaining to below the rib

_____ _____ _____
  P   RW   S

48. inflammation of the bone and joint

_____ _____ _____ _____
       RW   CV   RW   S

49. abnormal condition of death of the bone

_____ _____ _____ _____
       RW   CV   RW   S

SCORECARD: How Did You Do?

Number correct (_____), divided by 49 (_____), multiplied by 100 equals _____ (your score)

Diseases and Disorders

Diseases and disorders of the musculo-skeletal system range from the mild to the severe and have a wide variety of causes. We will briefly examine some problems that commonly affect this system.

Bursitis

Bursitis is an inflammation of the bursa, a pad-like sac filled with lubricating fluid (Figure 4.2). *Bursae* (plural form of *bursa*) are found in connective tissue near joints. These fluid-filled sacs reduce friction between tendons, muscles, and bones.

Bursitis most commonly develops in the shoulder, elbow, or hip, but it can also occur in the knee, heel, or base of the great (big) toe. This condition is the result of frequent repetitive motion, a sudden impact injury, or lack of elasticity in aging tendons.

Fracture

A **fracture** is a break in a bone. There are two categories of bone fractures: simple and compound (Figure 4.3). A bone fracture that does not penetrate the skin is called a *simple* or *closed fracture*. If the broken bone protrudes through the skin, it is called a *compound* or *open fracture*.

Car accidents, falls, and athletic injuries are common causes of fractures. Low bone density from osteoporosis (discussed later in this section) may also result in bone fractures.

Herniated Disk

Spinal disks (also called *vertebral disks*) are rubbery cushions between the **vertebrae**, the individual bones that make up the spinal column. They have a soft interior surrounded by a tough exterior. Spinal disks cushion the bones of the spinal column and allow forward and side-to-side movement between the vertebrae.

With age, spinal disks become less flexible and more vulnerable to injury. Injury

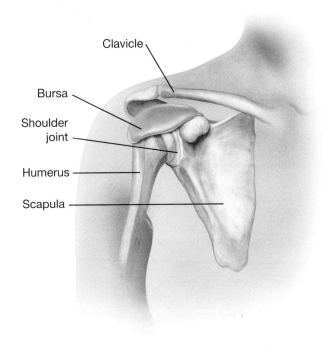

© Body Scientific International

Figure 4.2 Bursitis is an inflammation of the bursa, a pad-like sac filled with lubricating fluid, which reduces friction between tendons, muscles, and bones.

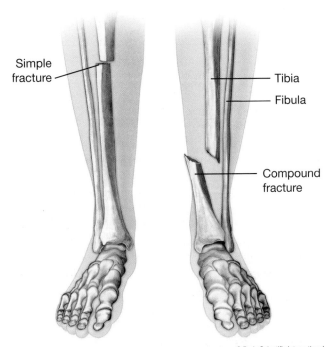

© Body Scientific International

Figure 4.3 A simple (closed) and compound (open) fracture

to a disk can cause it to slide out of place, resulting in what is commonly referred to as a *slipped disk*. As a spinal disk becomes less elastic, it may rupture. The result is a **herniated disk** (Figure 4.4). The rupture in the spinal disk causes a portion of the disk—the soft interior—to be forced through a weakened part of the tough, exterior part of the disk. When a herniated disk bulges out from between the vertebrae, it places pressure on nearby nerves. This can lead to pain, numbness, or weakness.

Joint Effusion

Joint effusion (ĕ-FYŪ-zhŭn) is an increase in the amount of fluid within the synovial (freely movable) compartment of a joint. Articular cartilage covers the ends of bones to prevent friction that would otherwise damage the bones during movement. A membrane encloses the joint in a capsule that contains synovial (lubricating) fluid. A small amount of synovial fluid exists in all freely movable joints.

When a joint has been affected by disease or trauma, synovial fluid buildup causes a freely movable joint to appear swollen. A doctor may drain the fluid to help relieve the pressure (Figure 4.5). If an infection is not suspected, a small amount of cortisone (anti-inflammatory medication) may be injected into the joint to provide pain relief and to help prevent the fluid from returning.

Knee Injuries

The knee joint contains four ligaments that provide stability and strength: the anterior and posterior cruciate ligaments (ACL and PCL, respectively) and the medial and lateral collateral ligaments (MCL and LCL, respectively). As you learned earlier in the chapter, the meniscus is a C-shaped cartilage pad that cushions the knee joint. Injury to the knee can affect any of the four stabilizing ligaments (Figure 4.6).

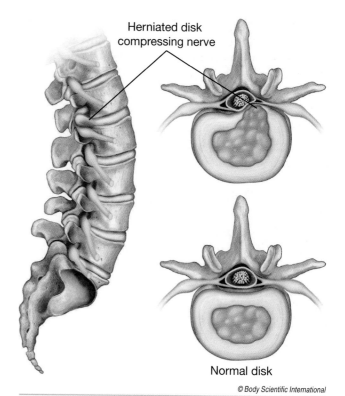

Herniated disk compressing nerve

Normal disk

© Body Scientific International

Figure 4.4 When a herniated disk bulges out between the vertebrae, it places pressure on nearby nerves, which can lead to pain, numbness, or weakness.

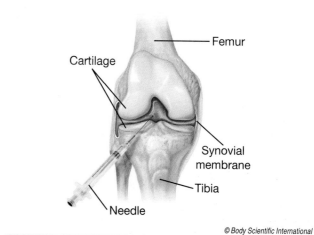

Femur

Cartilage

Synovial membrane

Tibia

Needle

© Body Scientific International

Figure 4.5 To treat joint effusion, a doctor may use a needle to remove excess synovial fluid. This procedure is called *arthrocentesis*.

One of the most common knee injuries is a sprained or torn ACL, which can result from overextension of the knee joint, a severe blow to the side of the knee (a common occurrence during football games), or coming to a sudden stop and then quickly changing direction while running. Likewise, when the knee is struck from the outside, it may buckle, causing the MCL to stretch or tear. As with ACL injuries, MCL injuries are often the result of "clipping" during a football game, when a player is struck behind the knee. Both ACL and MCL injuries are characterized by swelling, pain, tenderness, and the sensation that the knee will "give way" when standing or moving.

Meniscus tears are typically caused by twisting or overextending the knee joint. A torn meniscus causes pain, swelling, and stiffness.

Lateral Epicondylitis

Lateral epicondylitis (ĔP-ĭ-kŏn-dĭ-LĪ-tĭs), the formal term for *tennis elbow*, is inflammation and pain on the lateral (outside) part of the upper arm near the elbow (Figure 4.7). This condition is caused by activity in which repetitive twisting of the wrist is frequent. Lateral epicondylitis is common in people who play a lot of tennis or other racquet sports—thus the name "tennis elbow."

As you learned earlier, tendons attach muscle to bone. When the tendons of the elbow are overworked, small tears can develop. Over time, this leads to irritation and pain where the tendons of the forearm muscles attach to the *lateral epicondyle* (ĕp-ĭ-KŎN-dīl), the bony prominence on the outside of the elbow. Rest and over-the-counter pain relievers often help alleviate discomfort from lateral epicondylitis. Surgery is recommended only when the pain is incapacitating (interferes significantly with activities of daily living) and has lasted six months or more.

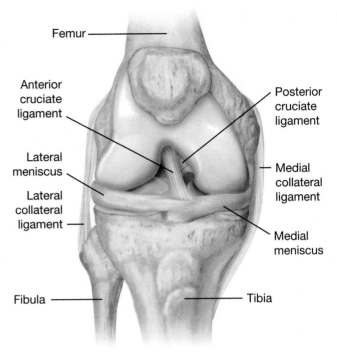

© Body Scientific International

Figure 4.6 Anterior view of the knee showing the major ligaments of the knee typically affected by injury

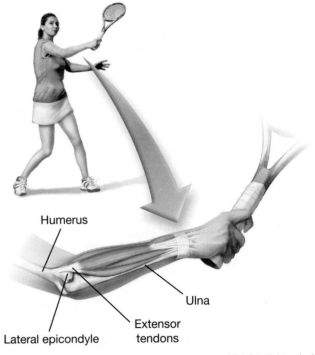

© Body Scientific International

Figure 4.7 Lateral epicondylitis, more commonly known as *tennis elbow*

Muscular Dystrophy

Muscular dystrophy (DĬS-trō-fē) is a group of inherited muscular disorders characterized by progressive muscle degeneration, weakness, and atrophy (wasting away) without nerve involvement (Figure 4.8).

Duchenne (dū-SHĔN) *muscular dystrophy* (DMD), the most common form of the disease, occurs primarily in boys. DMD is characterized by mild muscle weakness in the legs and difficulty walking. The first signs of DMD are apparent by three years of age and become more severe with age. Death from respiratory or cardiac muscle weakness may occur in early adulthood.

Osteomyelitis

Osteomyelitis (ŎS-tē-ō-mī-ĕ-LĪ-tĭs) is an acute or chronic bone infection usually caused by bacteria (Figures 4.9, 4.10, and 4.11). It produces fever, chills, and pain in the area of the infection. The area may appear swollen, warm, and red. Sometimes, however, osteomyelitis does not cause any signs or symptoms, or symptoms that are present may be difficult to distinguish from signs and symptoms of other health conditions.

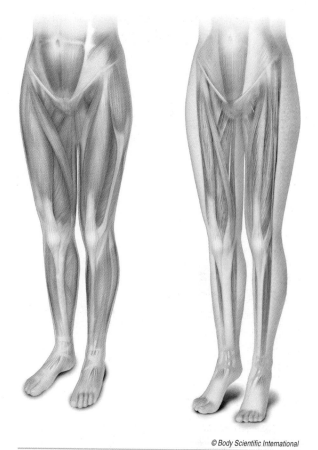

© Body Scientific International

Figure 4.8 Muscular dystrophy is marked by degeneration and atrophy (wasting away) of the muscles.

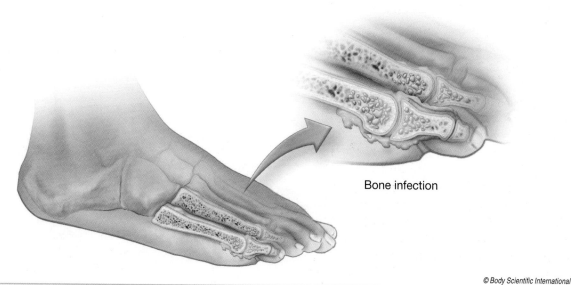

Bone infection

© Body Scientific International

Figure 4.9 Osteomyelitis, an acute or chronic bone infection, is usually caused by bacteria.

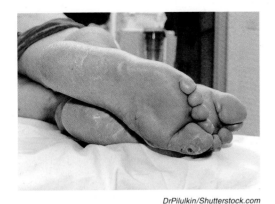

DrPilulkin/Shutterstock.com

Figure 4.10 Osteomyelitis

In osteomyelitis, bacteria may enter a bone via the bloodstream, from a nearby infection, or through direct contamination from an open fracture or surgery. Circulation problems can hinder leukocytes and lymphocytes (infection-fighting cells) from reaching the site of infection. (You will learn more about these infection-fighting microorganisms in Chapter 5: The Lymphatic and Immune Systems.) Thus, what begins as a small infection may intensify, exposing bone and deep tissue to infection. Patients typically undergo extended intravenous antibiotic therapy (four to eight weeks).

Osteoporosis

Osteoporosis (ŎS-tē-ō-por-Ō-sis) is the thinning of bone tissue and the gradual loss of bone density (Figure 4.12). It is the most common type of bone disease. Usually, the loss of bone occurs gradually over a period of years.

Osteoporosis develops when the body fails to form enough new bone, when too much calcium moves from the bone into the blood, or both. Calcium and phosphate are two minerals essential for healthy bone formation. A diet deficient in calcium causes a decrease in bone production, which can result in brittle, fragile bones that are more prone to fracture, even without injury (Figure 4.13).

The leading cause of osteoporosis in women is reduced production of the hormone estrogen during menopause. In men, decreased production of the hormone testosterone heightens the risk of developing osteoporosis.

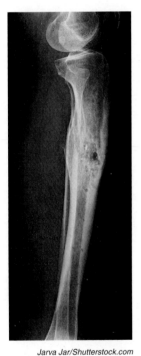

Jarva Jar/Shutterstock.com

Figure 4.11 Radiograph showing osteomyelitis in the leg

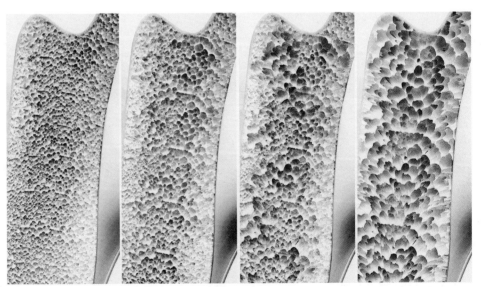

Crevis/Shutterstock.com

Figure 4.12 In osteoporosis, the thinning of bone tissue and gradual loss of bone density makes bones more fragile and prone to fracture.

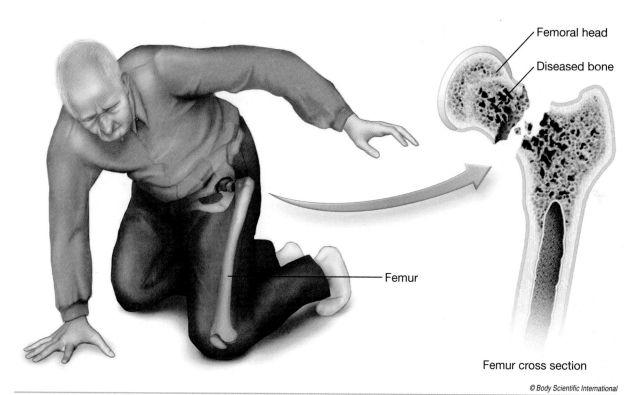

Femoral head

Diseased bone

Femur

Femur cross section

© Body Scientific International

Figure 4.13 Osteoporosis causes the bones to thin and decreases their density, making them more fragile and susceptible to fracture.

Rotator Cuff Tear

The rotator cuff is a group of muscles and tendons that attach the humerus (upper arm) to the scapula (shoulder blade). The rotator cuff stabilizes the shoulder joint and allows broad range of motion. It holds the proximal humerus (the upper part of the arm, where the shoulder and elbow meet) within the joint socket of the scapula. This joint is called the *ball-and-socket joint* because it allows the shoulder to rotate.

Falling, lifting, and repetitive arm motions can irritate or damage the muscles or tendons of the rotator cuff, or cause a **rotator cuff tear** (Figure 4.14). Pain may occur when the shoulder is raised overhead. When a rotator cuff tear is suspected, a doctor may order a computerized tomography (CT) or magnetic resonance imaging (MRI) scan. (You will learn about these diagnostic procedures in the next section.) Arthroscopic (är-thrō-SKŎP-ik) surgery is often performed to repair the tendons in a torn rotator cuff.

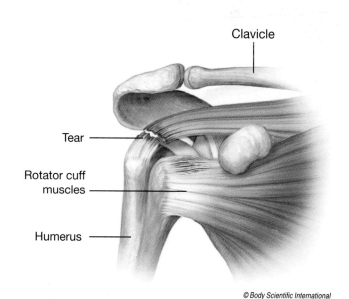

Clavicle

Tear

Rotator cuff muscles

Humerus

© Body Scientific International

Figure 4.14 Rotator cuff tear

Procedures and Treatments

We will now take a brief look at some common diagnostic tests and procedures used to help identify disorders and diseases of the musculoskeletal system, as well as some common therapeutic treatments.

Bone Scan

A **bone scan** is a type of nuclear medicine imaging (NMI) test. NMI involves the use of small amounts of radioactive materials called *radiopharmaceuticals* to generate images of bones, organs, soft tissues, and blood vessels. Bone scans are used to study body functions, analyze biological specimens, and help diagnose and treat a variety of musculoskeletal conditions. NMI technology aids doctors in determining the cause of a medical problem based on the *function* of a particular organ, tissue, or bone.

An NMI scan differs from a radiograph (X-ray), the latter of which helps doctors determine the presence of disease based on *structural appearance* rather than on the function of a particular organ, tissue, or bone. By contrast, nuclear medicine is an extremely sensitive technology; it can detect abnormalities in the very early stages of disease, long before other diagnostic tests might reveal their presence. Early detection means that treatment can be initiated immediately and a better prognosis can be achieved.

In a nuclear medicine bone scan, a special camera is used to capture images of the bone (Figure 4.15). A radioactive substance is injected into a vein and traced as it travels through the bloodstream and into the bones. The radioactive substance is referred to as a *tracer*. It often takes several hours for the entire procedure to be completed.

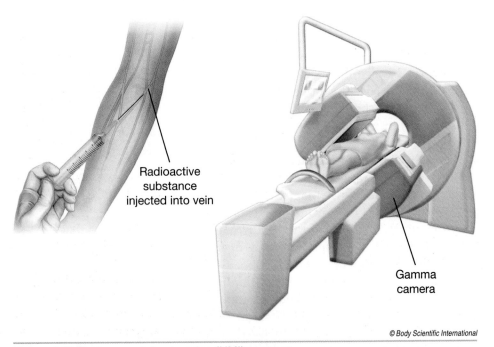

Radioactive substance injected into vein

Gamma camera

Figure 4.15 Nuclear medicine imaging (NMI) scanner

Bone scans are performed to help determine the cause of back pain, metastatic cancer (cancer that has spread, or moved to another site), or infection or trauma to the bones. An area of the body that absorbs little to no amount of the radioactive tracer appears as a dark area or "cold spot," indicating the presence of cancer or a decrease in blood supply to the bone. Conversely, an area of high bone activity, such as fast bone growth or repair, shows up as a bright area or "hot spot" on the scan. A hot spot on a bone scan can signify arthritis, a tumor, a fracture, or an infection. A bone scan can help identify certain health conditions days or even months earlier than a regular X-ray test.

Computerized Tomography

Computerized tomography (tō-MŎG-ră-fē), or CT, is a diagnostic procedure in which radiographs (X-rays) and a computer are used to display cross-sectional images of internal body structures (Figure 4.16). Computerized tomography is also called *computed tomography*. This cross-sectional imaging technique records details of human anatomy in the transverse (horizontal) or sagittal (right and left) planes. The CT scanner can be set to "image" (record images of) the body in different widths or sections. By contrast, plain-film radiographs or more current digital radiography techniques can image anatomical structures in anteroposterior (AP), lateral, and oblique planes. Computerized tomography is especially suited to imaging the bones, lungs, and chest and detecting cancerous growths.

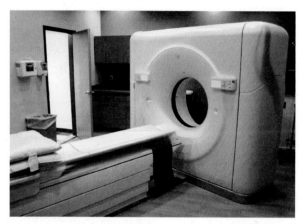

SNEHIT/Shutterstock.com

Figure 4.16 Computerized tomography (CT) scanner

CT scanning is similar to taking photographs of a friend or family member with a cell phone or digital camera. If a friend is facing you when you take a picture, she is in the anteroposterior position. If she is standing sideways, she is in the lateral position. In photography, we take photos in one dimension: from the front (AP) or the side (lateral). However, the human body is not one-dimensional. CT imaging is unique in its ability to view and record anatomy in the transverse and sagittal planes as well as in the anteroposterior and lateral planes.

If internal body structures were recorded only in one plane, then cancerous tumors, benign masses, and serious diseases could otherwise go undetected. Think of a sliced loaf of bread being photographed from the front and the side. We get the typical front and side views of the bread. Now remove a slice of bread, lay it down, and look at its internal structure. This view is what CT imaging allows us to see: internal "slices" of human anatomy.

A contrast agent, sometimes referred to as a *dye*, is often used during CT scanning to assist in visualizing body organs, blood vessels, and soft tissues (muscles, tendons, and ligaments). As you may recall from chapter 3, use of a contrast agent allows digital imaging of anatomical structures that are not dense enough to be viewed in an X-ray.

Electromyogram

An **electromyogram** (ē-lĕk-trō-MĪ-ō-gram), or **EMG**, is a test that records the electrical activity of muscles (Figure 4.17). It is used with patients who demonstrate impaired muscle strength. EMGs help detect various muscular diseases and conditions, including pinched nerves, herniated disks, inflamed muscles, muscular dystrophy, and peripheral muscle damage (damage to specific muscles rather than to the muscles as a whole).

In an EMG, a needle is inserted into the muscle. The needle acts as an electrode, detecting electrical activity that is visually displayed on an *oscilloscope*, a laboratory instrument that graphically represents and analyzes the waveform of electrical signals. Functioning muscles produce an electrical current proportional to the level of muscular activity they generate. An EMG can help distinguish between muscle weakness caused by injury to a nerve that is attached to a muscle and muscle weakness resulting from a neurological disorder. EMG technology is also used to identify the degree of nerve irritation or injury.

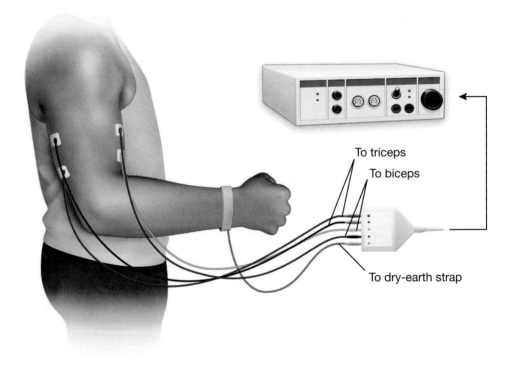

To triceps

To biceps

To dry-earth strap

© Body Scientific International

Figure 4.17 Electromyogram

Magnetic Resonance Imaging of the Bone

Magnetic resonance imaging, or **MRI**, is a diagnostic procedure in which a sophisticated magnet and a computer are used to generate cross-sectional images of blood vessels, bones, nerves, organs, and other internal body structures (Figure 4.18). MRI is typically performed to evaluate soft tissues, major body joints, the spine for disk disease, and bones of the extremities. This procedure often shows more anatomical detail than plain radiographs or even CT scans. Imaging performed with a contrast agent enhances the diagnostic process.

Cross-sectional imaging modalities such as MRI and CT scanning are now considered standard in diagnosing osteomyelitis, and a combination of these techniques may be used to confirm the presence of the disease. These modalities reveal superior anatomical detail of the infected area and the surrounding soft tissues. MRI allows early detection of osteomyelitis and, in cases of chronic bone infection, assessment of the extent of osteomyelitic involvement and activity. MRI also assists the surgeon in planning optimal surgical management for the treatment of osteomyelitis.

McMurray Test

The **McMurray test** is used to detect a meniscus tear in the knee (Figure 4.19). With the patient in the supine position (lying on the back with the face upward), the healthcare provider holds the heel of the injured leg with the knee flexed. The knee is gradually extended, and pressure is applied as the patient's lower leg is rotated both medially and laterally. The McMurray test is considered positive for meniscal injury if a clicking or cracking noise is heard.

Physical Therapy

Physical therapy (PT) is a form of rehabilitative treatment in which customized exercises and specially designed equipment are used to help patients regain or improve their mobility. Physical therapy benefits many different types of patients, from the infant born with a musculoskeletal condition to the adult recovering from a stroke, injury, or surgery. PT is a conservative treatment method often used prior to, in conjunction with, or following more aggressive treatment options such as surgery or certain kinds of medication.

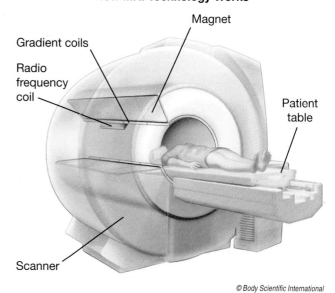

How MRI Technology Works

Magnet

Gradient coils

Radio frequency coil

Patient table

Scanner

© Body Scientific International

Figure 4.18 Magnetic resonance imaging (MRI) scanner

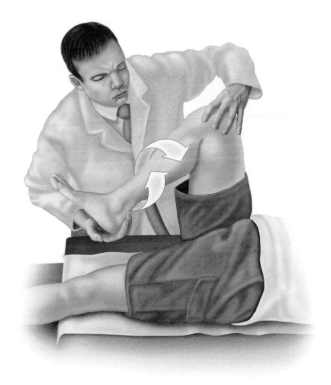

© Body Scientific International

Figure 4.19 McMurray test

Rest, Ice, Compression, and Elevation

Often expressed as the acronym **RICE**, this first-aid regimen stands for **Rest, Ice, Compression, and Elevation**. RICE is a commonly recommended treatment for strains and sprains.

A *strain* is a stretched or torn muscle or tendon. The most common types of strains occur in the back and hamstring muscles (the muscles in the back of the upper leg). A *sprain*, by contrast, is a stretched or torn ligament. Sprains often occur in the ankle, knee, or wrist.

Spinal Fusion

Spinal fusion, also known as *spondylodesis* (SPŎN-dĭ-lō-DĒ-sĭs), is a surgical procedure in which two or more vertebrae are fused, or joined together (Figure 4.20). Trauma, degenerative disease, or a spinal deformity causes pain due to abnormal motion of the vertebrae. Bone tissue derived from either the patient or a donor is used to fuse the vertebrae, thus alleviating the pain.

Spinal fusion is often facilitated by a process called *fixation*, during which metallic screws or rods are used to stabilize the vertebrae. Following injury to the cervical or lumbar region (lower back), spinal fusion can help stabilize the area and prevent fractures of the spinal column, which could damage the spinal cord. Spinal fusion is also performed to remove or reduce pressure on nerves.

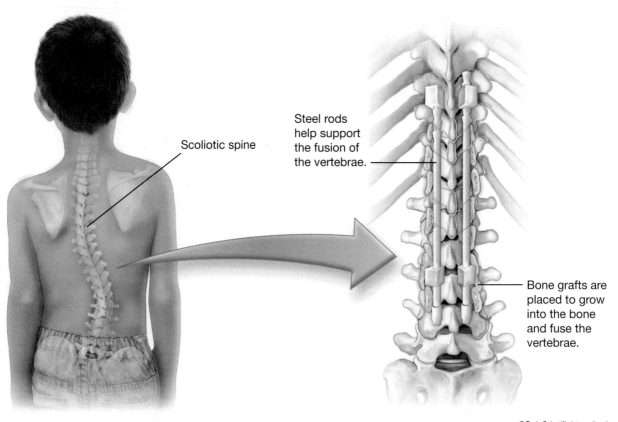

Scoliotic spine

Steel rods help support the fusion of the vertebrae.

Bone grafts are placed to grow into the bone and fuse the vertebrae.

© Body Scientific International

Figure 4.20 Spinal fusion

Multiple Choice: Diseases and Disorders

Directions: Choose the disease or disorder that matches each definition. You can also complete this activity online using *EduHub*.

_____ 1. the thinning of bone tissue and the gradual loss of bone density
a. osteoporosis   c. joint effusion
b. muscular dystrophy   d. bursitis

_____ 2. rupture of a vertebral disk that causes the soft interior of the disk to bulge between the vertebrae, creating pressure on nearby nerves
a. herniated disk   c. muscular dystrophy
b. bursitis   d. joint effusion

_____ 3. acute or chronic bone infection often caused by bacteria
a. muscular dystrophy   c. osteoporosis
b. bursitis   d. osteomyelitis

_____ 4. the leading cause of osteoporosis is
a. an increase in estrogen in women
b. a reduction in estrogen in women
c. a decrease in testosterone in men
d. both b and c

_____ 5. inflammation of a pad-like sac filled with lubricating fluid, found in connective tissue near joints
a. muscular dystrophy   c. bursitis
b. osteoporosis   d. osteomyelitis

_____ 6. a tear in one of the muscles or tendons that attaches the humerus (upper arm) to the scapula (shoulder blade)
a. meniscus tear   c. MCL tear
b. ACL tear   d. rotator cuff tear

_____ 7. an increase in the amount of fluid within the synovial compartment of a joint
a. osteoporosis   c. joint effusion
b. osteomyelitis   d. bursitis

_____ 8. a group of inherited muscular disorders characterized by progressive muscle degeneration, weakness, and atrophy without nerve involvement
a. joint effusion   c. muscular dystrophy
b. osteomyelitis   d. bursitis

_____ 9. a break in a bone
a. osteoporosis   c. joint effusion
b. fracture   d. bursitis

_____ 10. an injury caused by twisting or overextending the knee joint
a. ACL tear   c. lateral epicondylitis
b. bursitis   d. rotator cuff tear

_____ 11. inflammation of the lateral part of the upper arm due to repetitive twisting of the wrist
a. rotator cuff tear   c. lateral epicondylitis
b. bursitis   d. osteomyelitis

SCORECARD: How Did You Do?

Number correct (_____), divided by 11 (_____), multiplied by 100 equals _____ (your score)

Multiple Choice: Procedures and Treatments

Directions: Choose the procedure or treatment that matches each definition. You can also complete this activity online using *EduHub*.

_____ 1. procedure involving the use of radiographs and a computer to display cross-sectional images of internal body structures
a. magnetic resonance imaging (MRI)
b. bone scan
c. electromyogram (EMG)
d. computerized tomography (CT)

_____ 2. procedure in which a sophisticated magnet and a computer are used to generate cross-sectional images of bones, organs, nerves, blood vessels, and other structures; often shows more anatomical detail than other imaging tests
a. McMurray test
b. electromyogram (EMG)
c. computerized tomography (CT)
d. magnetic resonance imaging (MRI)

_____ 3. test that involves the use of a radioactive substance and a special camera to image the bone
a. bone scan
b. McMurray test
c. electromyogram (EMG)
d. spondylodesis

_____ 4. surgical procedure in which two or more vertebrae are fused
a. electromyogram (EMG)
b. spinal fusion
c. spondylodesis
d. both b and c

_____ 5. test that records the electrical activity of muscles
a. electromusculogram
b. electromusculography
c. McMurray test
d. electromyogram (EMG)

_____ 6. manual test used to detect a meniscus tear in the knee
a. meniscal laceration test
b. McMurray test
c. electromyogram
d. magnetic resonance imaging (MRI)

SCORECARD: How Did You Do?

Number correct (_____), divided by 6 (_____), multiplied by 100 equals _____ (your score)

Assessment 4.10

Identifying Abbreviations

Directions: Supply the correct abbreviation for each medical term. You can also complete this activity online using *EduHub*.

Medical Term	Abbreviation
1. computerized tomography	_____
2. magnetic resonance imaging	_____
3. Duchenne muscular dystrophy	_____
4. medial collateral ligament	_____
5. anterior cruciate ligament	_____
6. lateral collateral ligament	_____
7. rest, ice, compression, and elevation	_____
8. anteroposterior	_____
9. nuclear medicine imaging	_____
10. physical therapy	_____
11. electromyogram	_____

SCORECARD: How Did You Do?

Number correct (_____), divided by 11 (_____), multiplied by 100 equals _____ (your score)

In the Intern Experience described at the beginning of this chapter, we met Aishandi, an intern with the DesFed Urgent Care Center. Aishandi "shadowed" (that is, followed and observed) Dr. Geiger as he interacted with Bill, a teenage patient who had suffered a knee injury during a football game. Dr. Geiger examined Bill and obtained his personal and family health history. He then made a medical diagnosis and provided Bill with a treatment plan. He also referred the teenager to an orthopedic specialist for further examination. Later, Dr. Geiger made a dictated recording of Bill's health information, which was subsequently transcribed into a chart note.

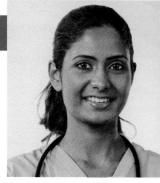

We will now learn more about Bill's injury from a clinical perspective, interpreting the medical terms in his chart note as we analyze the scenario presented in the Intern Experience.

Audio Activity: Bill Jesmann's Chart Note

Directions: Access your *EduHub* subscription and listen to the recording of the physician reading Bill Jesmann's chart note. Read along with the physician and pay attention to the pronunciation of each medical term.

CHART NOTE

Patient Name: Jesmann, William
ID Number: 42645
Date of Service: October 26, 20xx

SUBJECTIVE
This 16-year-old male was tackled during a football game, twisting his left knee. The pain is worse on the lateral and inferior aspect of the left knee. It's worse if he pivots. He states that he has sometimes noticed a "catch" in his knee after practice. It has responded well to ice and ibuprofen.

OBJECTIVE
There is slight tenderness with active and passive ROM (range of motion) of the knee. The knee is not **erythematous** or warm. There is no crepitus (crackling or grating sound) or **edema**. There is tenderness with palpation of the left medial collateral **ligament**. There is lateral collateral ligament laxity (looseness, slackness, or displacement), but no medial collateral laxity. **McMurray test** is negative.

ASSESSMENT
Left lateral collateral ligament **sprain**.

PLAN
He will be sent to an **orthopedist** for consultation and possible **MRI** and/or **arthroscopy**. Follow-up **PT** is recommended.

Interpret Bill Jesmann's Chart Note

Directions: Access your *EduHub* subscription and listen to the recording of the physician reading Bill Jesmann's chart note. After listening to the recording, supply the medical term that matches each definition.

Example: inflammation of the muscle   *Answer:* myitis

1. band of tissue that connects bone to bone   _____

2. specialist in the study and treatment of the musculoskeletal system   _____

3. test manually performed to detect a meniscus tear in the knee   _____

4. red   _____

5. diagnostic procedure in which a sophisticated magnet and a computer are used to generate cross-sectional images of body structures   _____

6. process of observing the joint   _____

7. swelling   _____

8. rehabilitative treatment in which customized exercises and specially designed equipment are used to help patients regain or improve their mobility   _____

9. stretched or torn ligament   _____

SCORECARD: How Did You Do?

Number correct (_____), divided by 9 (_____), multiplied by 100 equals _____ (your score)

Working with Medical Records

In this activity, you will interpret the medical records (chart notes) of patients with musculoskeletal conditions. These examples illustrate typical medical records prepared in a real-world healthcare environment. To interpret these chart notes, you will apply your knowledge of word elements (prefixes, combining forms, and suffixes), diseases and disorders, and procedures and treatments related to the musculoskeletal system.

Audio Activity: Ezilary Morales' Chart Note

Directions: Access your *EduHub* subscription and listen to the recording of the physician reading Ezilary Morales' chart note. Read along with the physician and pay attention to the pronunciation of each medical term.

CHART NOTE

Patient Name: Morales, Ezilary
ID Number: 93668
Date of Service: March 14, 20xx

SUBJECTIVE
This 15-year-old female suffered an injury to her left hand during a gymnastics tournament. She was splinted and sent to the office for evaluation.

OBJECTIVE
She has diffuse (spread out; scattered) **edema** and **ecchymosis** over the **dorsal** aspect of her left hand in the 3rd and 4th **metacarpal** region. She has full range of motion of her fingers. Neurological and sensory exam is normal. Peripheral circulation (blood flow to the upper and lower extremities) is normal. X-ray imaging shows evidence of a nondisplaced oblique (slanted) shaft **fracture** of the **metacarpals** without involvement of the joints.

ASSESSMENT
Right 3rd and 4th metacarpal fractures, nondisplaced.

PLAN
Her fingers were taped for immobilization and placed in a short-arm splint. She will keep it elevated and use Advil® for pain relief. She is scheduled for a follow-up visit with Orthopedic Specialists, Inc. in the next 3 to 7 weeks.

Assessment 4.12

Interpret Ezilary Morales' Chart Note

Directions: Access your *EduHub* subscription and listen to the recording of the physician reading Ezilary Morales' chart note. After listening to the recording, supply the medical term that matches each definition.

Example: inflammation of the bone and cartilage   *Answer:* osteochondritis

1. break in a bone   _____

2. pertaining to the back (of the body)   _____

3. bones of the hand   _____

4. swelling   _____

5. abnormal condition of blood in the tissues   _____

6. pertaining to the bones of the hand   _____

SCORECARD: How Did You Do?

Number correct (_____), divided by 6 (_____), multiplied by 100 equals _____ (your score)

Audio Activity: Amos Stoudt's Chart Note

Directions: Access your *EduHub* subscription and listen to the recording of the physician reading Amos Stoudt's chart note. Read along with the physician and pay attention to the pronunciation of each medical term.

CHART NOTE

Patient Name: Stoudt, Amos
ID Number: 12114
Date of Service: May 19, 20xx

SUBJECTIVE
This 23-year-old male presents with lower right arm pain. Two days ago he was helping his father cut up tree branches from last week's violent storm when he was struck by a falling limb. When he uses his right hand, he has swelling and pain with **pronation** (turning of the hand and forearm so the palm faces downward), **supination** (turning of the hand and forearm so the palm faces upward), and gripping.

OBJECTIVE
He has mild **edema** over the **distal radius** (outer lateral bone of the forearm), approximately 8 cm **proximal** to the radial styloid process (small protrusion of bone). Neurovascularly intact. He has full range of motion of his hand and **phalanges**. X-rays confirm a nondisplaced **fracture** of the distal forearm.

ASSESSMENT
Right radial shaft fracture in good alignment.

PLAN
Fiberglass cast applied. Patient provided with arm sling and told to keep the arm elevated. Advised use of Advil®, aspirin, or Tylenol® for pain. Follow follow-up appointment in 10 days.

Assessment 4.13

Interpret Amos Stoudt's Chart Note

Directions: Access your *EduHub* subscription and listen to the recording of the physician reading Amos Stoudt's chart note. After listening to the recording, supply the medical term that matches each definition.

Example: painful or difficult movement   *Answer:* dyskinesia

1. nearest the point of origin   _____

2. turning of the palm downward   _____

3. swelling   _____

4. fingers   _____

5. break in a bone   _____

6. outer lateral bone of the forearm   _____

7. turning of the palm upward   _____

SCORECARD: How Did You Do?

Number correct (_____), divided by 7 (_____), multiplied by 100 equals _____ (your score)

Chapter Review

Word Elements Summary

Prefixes

Prefix	Meaning
a-	not; without
an-	not; without
brady-	slow
dys-	painful; difficult
endo-	within
epi-	upon; above
hyper-	above; above normal
inter-	between
intra-	within
meta-	change; beyond
per-	through
peri-	around
poly-	many
quadri-	four
sub-	beneath; below
supra-	above
sym-, syn-	together; with

Combining Forms

Root Word/Combining Vowel	Meaning
anter/o	front
arthr/o	joint
articul/o	joint
burs/a, burs/o	bursa; sac
cardi/o	heart
carp/o	carpals (wrist bones)
chondr/o	cartilage
clavicul/o	clavicle (collar bone)

(Continued)

Root Word/Combining Vowel	Meaning
coccyg/o	coccyx (tailbone)
cost/o	rib
crani/o	skull
dist/o	away from the point of origin
dors/o	back (of the body)
ecchym/o	blood in the tissues
electr/o	electrical activity
erythemat/o	redness
erythr/o	red
femor/o	femur (thigh bone)
fibul/o	fibula
herni/o	hernia; rupture; protrusion
humer/o	humerus (upper arm bone)
ili/o	ilium
infer/o	below; beneath
ischi/o	ischium (part of hip bone)
kines/o, kinesi/o	movement
kyph/o	hump
later/o	side
lord/o	curve
medi/o	middle
metacarp/o	metacarpals (bones of the hand)
metatars/o	metatarsals (bones of the foot)
muscul/o	muscle
my/o	muscle
myel/o	bone marrow; spinal cord
necr/o	death
neur/o	nerve
orth/o	straight
oste/o	bone
patell/a, patell/o	patella (kneecap)
path/o	disease
phalang/o	phalanges (bones of the fingers and toes)

(Continued)

Root Word/Combining Vowel	Meaning
por/o	pore; duct; small opening
poster/o	back (of the body)
proxim/o	nearest the point of origin
pub/o	pubis (part of the hip bone)
radi/o	radius (bone of the forearm); X-ray
sacr/o	sacrum (bone at base of the spine)
scapul/o	scapula (shoulder blade)
scoli/o	crooked; bent
spondyl/o	vertebra; spine
stern/o	sternum (breastbone)
tars/o	ankle bones
ten/o	tendon
tendin/o, tendon/o	tendon
tibi/o	tibia (shin bone)
uln/o	ulna (bone of the forearm)
vascul/o	blood vessel
vertebr/o	vertebra; spine

Suffixes

Suffix	Meaning
-ac	pertaining to
-al	pertaining to
-algia	pain
-ar	pertaining to
-ary	pertaining to
-asthenia	weakness
-centesis	surgical puncture to remove fluid
-clasia	surgical breaking
-cyte	cell
-desis	to bind or tie together surgically
-dynia	pain
-eal	pertaining to
-ectomy	surgical removal; excision

(Continued)

Suffix	Meaning
-edema	swelling
-ema	condition
-gen	producing; originating; causing
-gram	record; image
-graphy	process of recording an image
-ia	condition
-ic	pertaining to
-ior	pertaining to
-itis	inflammation
-kinesia	movement
-kinesis	movement
-logist	specialist in the study and treatment of
-logy	study of
-lysis	breakdown; loosening; dissolving
-malacia	softening
-metry	process of measuring
-oma	tumor; mass
-osis	abnormal condition
-ous	pertaining to
-pathy	disease
-penia	deficiency; abnormal reduction
-plasty	surgical repair
-plegia	paralysis
-rrhaphy	suture
-rrhexis	rupture
-scope	instrument used to observe
-scopy	process of observing
-tome	instrument used to cut
-tomy	incision; cut into
-trophy	development

More Practice: Activities and Games

The following activities will help you reinforce your skills and check your mastery of the medical terminology you learned in this chapter. Access your *EduHub* subscription to complete more activities and vocabulary games for mastering the word parts and terms you have learned.

Break It Down

Directions: Dissect each medical term into its word parts (prefix, root word, combining vowel, and suffix) using one or more slashes. Then define each term.

Example:

Medical Term: arthritis

Dissection: arthr/itis

Definition: inflammation of the joint

Medical Term	Dissection
1. arthroscopy	a r t h r o s c o p y

Definition: _____

_____

2. arthrotomy	a r t h r o t o m y

Definition: _____

_____

3. costochondral	c o s t o c h o n d r a l

Definition: _____

_____

4. craniectomy	c r a n i e c t o m y

Definition: _____

_____

5. metacarpal	m e t a c a r p a l

Definition: _____

_____

6. myelography	m y e l o g r a p h y

Definition: _____

_____

Medical Term	Dissection

7. myocarditis   m y o c a r d i t i s

Definition: _____

_____

8. neuralgia   n e u r a l g i a

Definition: _____

_____

9. craniology   c r a n i o l o g y

Definition: _____

_____

10. polyneural   p o l y n e u r a l

Definition: _____

_____

11. supracostal   s u p r a c o s t a l

Definition: _____

_____

12. posterolateral   p o s t e r o l a t e r a l

Definition: _____

_____

13. iliocostal   i l i o c o s t a l

Definition: _____

_____

14. musculovascular   m u s c u l o v a s c u l a r

Definition: _____

_____

Medical Term	Dissection
15. ischiofemoral	i s c h i o f e m o r a l

Definition: _____

_____

16. costectomy	c o s t e c t o m y

Definition: _____

_____

17. supraclavicular	s u p r a c l a v i c u l a r

Definition: _____

_____

18. costotome	c o s t o t o m e

Definition: _____

_____

19. subscapular	s u b s c a p u l a r

Definition: _____

_____

20. dorsalgia	d o r s a l g i a

Definition: _____

_____

21. neuromuscular	n e u r o m u s c u l a r

Definition: _____

_____

22. humeral	h u m e r a l

Definition: _____

_____

Medical Term	Dissection
23. ecchymoma	e c c h y m o m a

Definition: _____

_____

24. femoral	f e m o r a l

Definition: _____

_____

25. iliococcygeal	i l i o c o c c y g e a l

Definition: _____

_____

Spelling

Directions: For each medical term, indicate the correct spelling.

1.	bradikinesia	bradikynesia	bradykinesia	bradykynesia
2.	artheralgia	arthralgia	arthralgea	artherelgia
3.	echymosis	ecchimosis	eccymosis	ecchymosis
4.	miasthenia	myasthenia	myaesthenia	miaesthenia
5.	condromalacia	chondromalacia	chondromalaysia	khondromalacia
6.	kyphosis	kyfosis	kifosis	kyphoses
7.	diskinesia	dyskinesia	dyskenesia	dyskenasia
8.	osteomyelitis	ostomyelitis	osteomielitis	osteomyalitis
9.	laterel	lateral	latteral	laterral
10.	epichondylitis	epicondilytis	epicondilitis	epicondylitis
11.	intevertebral	intervertebrel	intervertebral	intervertabral
12.	scoliosis	skoliosis	scholiosis	schoeliosis

True or False

Directions: Indicate whether each statement is true or false.

True or False?

_____ 1. The muscular system is made up of muscles and bones.

_____ 2. Voluntary muscles are under conscious control.

_____ 3. The skeletal system consists of bones plus cartilage, ligaments, and tendons.

_____ 4. The suffix **-gram** means "process of recording an image."

_____ 5. The prefix **inter-** means "within."

_____ 6. The prefix **per-** means "around."

_____ 7. The root word **articul** means "joint."

_____ 8. The term *dystrophy* contains a prefix and a suffix.

_____ 9. Skeletal muscle is an example of involuntary muscle.

_____ 10. The root word **clavicul** means "collar bone."

_____ 11. The rotator cuff is a group of muscles and ligaments that attach the humerus to the scapula.

_____ 12. The term *bradykinesia* contains a prefix, root word, and suffix.

_____ 13. The McMurray test is used to detect a meniscus tear in the elbow.

_____ 14. The root words **spondyl** and **vertebr** mean "vertebra" or "spine."

_____ 15. The suffixes **-ac, -al, -ar,** and **-ary** mean "pertaining to."

_____ 16. A small amount of synovial fluid exists in all freely movable joints.

_____ 17. The suffix **-oma** means "abnormal condition."

_____ 18. The root word **oste** means "muscle."

_____ 19. The suffix **-rrhexis** means "suture."

_____ 20. The term *intervertebral* contains a prefix, root word, and suffix.

_____ 21. The term *anteroinferior* contains two root words and a suffix.

_____ 22. The acronym **RICE** stands for *rest, ice, contraction, and elevation.*

_____ 23. The term *spondylarthritis* contains a prefix, root word, and suffix.

_____ 24. Spinal disks cushion the bones of the spinal column.

_____ 25. The prefix **brady-** means "slow."

_____ 26. The root word **metacarp** means "bones of the feet."

_____ 27. Lateral epicondylitis is commonly known as "tennis elbow."

_____ 28. The suffixes **-ic** and **-ior** mean "posterior."

_____ 29. Duchenne muscular dystrophy is the most common form of muscular dystrophy.

_____ 30. The term *arthrocentesis* contains a root word and a suffix.

_____ 31. Cardiac muscle is an example of involuntary muscle.

_____ 32. There are three major ligaments that provide stability and strength to the knee joint.

Audio Activity: Emma Almondo's Chart Note

Directions: Access your *EduHub* subscription and listen to the recording of the physician reading Emma Almondo's chart note. Read along with the physician and pay attention to the pronunciation of each medical term.

CHART NOTE

Patient Name: Almondo, Emma
ID Number: 14288
Date of Service: January 8, 20xx

SUBJECTIVE
Emma was babysitting her neighbor's 7-year-old son when he threw his spaghetti onto the floor. As she was cleaning the spaghetti off the floor, Emma slipped and fell to the floor, injuring her left wrist and left knee.

OBJECTIVE
The left wrist is swollen with obvious deformity. There is normal sensation of the fingers with normal motion of the fingers. Patient has pain with movement of the wrist. Left **patella** is tender to palpation (examination with the hands). There is **joint effusion** of the knee. Sensation and movement **distal** to the knee are both normal. X-rays of the left wrist reveal a **fracture** of the **distal radius** with approximately a 20-degree **dorsal** angulation, which is displaced about 30 percent from its normal position. There is no **ulna** (inner medial bone of the forearm) fracture. X-ray of the left patella shows a fracture with no displacement of the fragments.

ASSESSMENT
1. Fracture, left wrist
2. Patellar fracture, left knee

PLAN
Knee immobilizer was placed. She should bear as little weight as possible on the left knee. **Posterior** splint with elastic bandage was placed on the forearm. Patient was given acetaminophen with codeine for pain. An appointment with Orthopedic Specialists was made for Wednesday. Possible open reduction internal fixation (surgical realignment of bones with implants to guide the healing process).

Interpret Emma Almondo's Chart Note

Directions: Access your *EduHub* subscription and listen to the recording of the physician reading Emma Almondo's chart note. After listening to the recording, supply the medical term that matches each definition.

     Example: weakness in the muscle   *Answer:* myasthenia

1. increase in the amount of fluid in the synovial compartment of a joint

   _____

2. pertaining to the back (of the body) **(two possible answers)**

   _____

   _____

3. break in a bone

   _____

4. outer lateral bone of the forearm

   _____

5. kneecap

   _____

6. inner medial bone of the forearm

   _____

7. pertaining to away from the point of origin

   _____

Cumulative Review

Chapters 2–4: Integumentary, Digestive, and Musculoskeletal Systems

Directions: Check your mastery of word elements used in medical terminology related to the integumentary, digestive, and musculoskeletal systems by defining the following prefixes, combining forms, and suffixes.

Prefixes

ad- _____

an- _____

anti- _____

brady- _____

dia- _____

dys- _____

endo- _____

epi- _____

hyper- _____

hypo- _____

inter- _____

intra- _____

meta- _____

pan- _____

per- _____

peri- _____

poly- _____

quadri- _____

retro- _____

sub- _____

supra- _____

sym-, syn- _____

trans- _____

Combining Forms

arthr/o _____

articul/o _____

cardi/o _____

celi/o _____

chol/e _____

cholecyst/o _____

col/o, colon/o _____

contus/o _____

crani/o _____

cyst/o _____

derm/a, derm/o, dermat/o _____

dist/o _____

duoden/o _____

ecchym/o _____

electr/o _____

enter/o _____

esophag/o _____

femor/o _____

fibul/o _____

gastr/o _____

gingiv/o _____

gloss/o _____

hepat/o _____

herni/o _____

humer/o _____

ile/o _____

ili/o _____

infer/o _____

ischi/o _____

lapar/o _____

melan/o _____

metacarp/o _____

myel/o _____

necr/o _____

onych/o _____

orth/o _____

pancreat/o _____

phalang/o _____

por/o _____

poster/o _____

proct/o _____

proxim/o _____

prurit/o _____

sacr/o _____

scapul/o _____

schiz/o _____

scoli/o _____

squam/o _____

stern/o _____

tars/o _____

topic/o _____

uln/o _____

vertebr/o _____

xer/o _____

Suffixes

-algia   _____

-ar   _____

-ary   _____

-cele   _____

-centesis   _____

-clasia   _____

-cyte   _____

-edema   _____

-ema   _____

-gen   _____

-graphy   _____

-ia   _____

-iasis   _____

-ic   _____

-ior   _____

-itis   _____

-kinesia   _____

-kinesis   _____

-lysis   _____

-malacia   _____

-metry   _____

-penia   _____

-phagia   _____

-pharynx   _____

-plasty   _____

-ptosis   _____

-rrhea   _____

-scopy   _____

-stomy   _____

Chapter 5

The Lymphatic and Immune Systems

immun / o / logy: the study of the immune system

Chapter Organization

- Intern Experience
- Overview of Lymphatic and Immune System Anatomy and Physiology
- Word Elements
- Breaking Down and Building Terms Related to the Lymphatic and Immune Systems
- Diseases and Disorders
- Procedures and Treatments
- Analyzing the Intern Experience
- Working with Medical Records
- Chapter Review

Chapter Objectives

After completing this chapter, you will be able to

1. label an anatomical diagram of the lymphatic system;

2. dissect and define common medical terminology related to the lymphatic and immune systems;

3. build terms used to describe lymphatic and immune system diseases and disorders, diagnostic procedures, and therapeutic treatments;

4. pronounce and spell common medical terminology related to the lymphatic and immune systems;

5. understand that the process of building and dissecting a medical term based on its prefix, root word, and suffix enables you to analyze an extremely large number of medical terms beyond those presented in this chapter;

6. interpret the meaning of abbreviations associated with the lymphatic and immune systems; and

7. interpret medical records containing terminology and abbreviations related to the lymphatic and immune systems.

Your *EduHub* subscription that accompanies this text provides access to online assessments, assignments, activities, and resources. Throughout this chapter, access *EduHub* to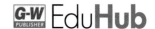

- use e-flash cards to review the medical terminology and word parts you learn;
- listen to the correct pronunciations of medical terms; and
- complete medical terminology activities and assignments.

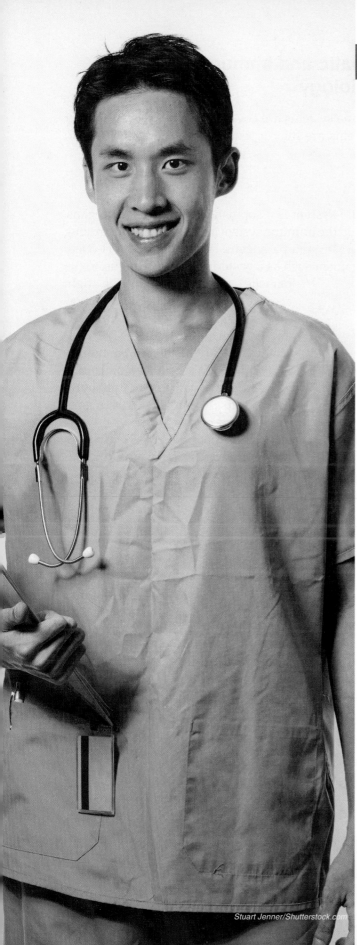

Intern Experience

Sean, an intern with the Cassel County Clinic, is asked by the nurse manager to assist Dr. Rymus in exam room 2. His patient is William Shumaker, a 57-year-old accountant. Mr. Shumaker tells Sean that lately he has been feeling excessively fatigued, which he attributes to working long hours during the tax season. About a week ago, he noticed a small lump on the right side of his neck. Mr. Shumaker is also concerned about two other symptoms: persistent night sweats and weight loss.

Mr. Shumaker is experiencing a problem with his lymphatic system, which plays a vital role in protecting the body from infection. To help you understand what is happening to him, this chapter will present medical terms consisting of word elements (combining forms, prefixes, and suffixes) related to the lymphatic and immune systems.

By now, you recognize that many of the same medical word elements appear in terms used to describe different body systems. This systematic use of combining forms, prefixes, and suffixes helps make the study of medical terminology logical, consistent, and predictable.

We will begin our study of the lymphatic and immune systems with a brief overview of their anatomy and physiology. Later in the chapter, you will learn about some common pathological conditions of the lymphatic and immune systems, tests and procedures used to diagnose these conditions, and common treatment methods.

Overview of Lymphatic and Immune System Anatomy and Physiology

The lymphatic and immune systems are covered together in this chapter because these two body systems are interdependent and complementary in structure and function.

The Lymphatic System

The **lymphatic** (lĭm-FĂT-ĭk) **system** is a sophisticated network of organs, glands, vessels, and cells that aid the immune system in filtering and destroying dead blood cells, particulate waste, and pathogens. A **pathogen** (PĂTH-ō-jĕn) is a disease-causing microorganism such as a bacterium, virus, fungus, toxin, parasite, or cancer cell. The fight against pathogens is a complex, coordinated effort between the immune and lymphatic systems. The lymphatic system manufactures **lymph**, or *lymphatic fluid*, a clear or milky-white fluid that contains **lymphocytes** (LĬM-fō-sīts). Lymphocytes are specialized **leukocytes** (LŪ-kō-sīts), white blood cells that protect the body from infection and disease by attacking foreign substances in the blood.

In addition to supporting the immune system, the lymphatic system supplements the functions of the cardiovascular system, also called the *circulatory system*. (You will learn more about the cardiovascular system in chapter 10.) Besides seeking out and destroying foreign "invaders" in the body, the lymphatic system also works to maintain proper fluid balance and blood volume.

The organs that make up the lymphatic system are the tonsils, adenoids, thymus gland, and spleen (Figure 5.1). The **tonsils** are two small, oval-shaped masses of lymphoid tissue in the back of the pharynx (throat). The tonsils protect the body from infection by trapping pathogens that enter through the mouth or nose. The **adenoids** (ĂD-ĕ-noyds) are small masses of lymphoid tissue located posterior to

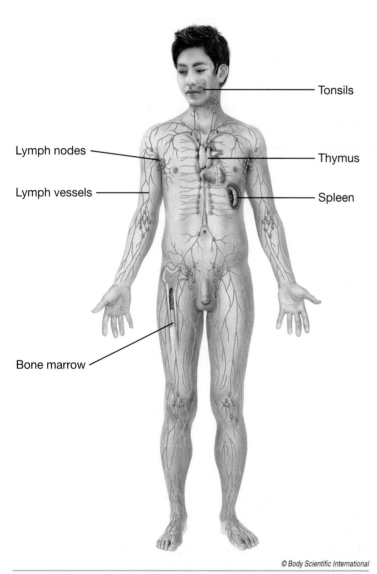

Tonsils

Lymph nodes

Lymph vessels

Thymus

Spleen

Bone marrow

© Body Scientific International

Figure 5.1 Major organs and structures of the lymphatic system

the nasal cavity. The difference between tonsils and adenoids is that you can see your tonsils when you stand before a mirror and open your mouth very wide. Because your adenoids are situated in your nasopharynx (where the throat meets the nasal cavity), you cannot easily see them. Adenoids perform the same function as tonsils: they trap bacteria and viruses that enter through the nose or mouth. When infected, adenoids can enlarge and interfere with breathing.

The **thymus** (THĪ-mŭs) **gland**, or **thymus**, is a butterfly-shaped gland in the upper chest beneath the sternum (breastbone). The thymus receives from the bone marrow a specialized type of leukocytes called *T lymphocytes*, which are critical to a properly functioning immune system. T lymphocytes, or *T cells*, originate in the bone marrow and mature in the thymus. After they have matured, T cells reproduce and then differentiate into *helper T cells*, which control immune responses.

The **spleen** is a fist-sized organ that lies above the stomach and beneath the ribs on the left side of the body. The spleen contains infection-fighting leukocytes. The spleen also performs two other important functions: It controls the amount of blood in the body, and it destroys old or damaged red blood cells.

Immunology is the study of the immune system. An **immunologist** is a physician who specializes in the study and treatment of diseases and disorders of the immune system.

The Immune System

The **immune system** is a network of organs, tissues, and cells that work in tandem with those of the lymphatic system to protect the body from pathogenic invasion. For the immune system to function properly, it must distinguish between those cells that are part of the body ("self" cells) and cells that are foreign to the body ("non-self" cells). Once this distinction has been made, the immune system takes steps to attack the foreign cells.

When the immune system fails to differentiate between "self" and "non-self" cells, the body attacks its own cells and tissues. This is known as an **autoimmune disorder**. Examples of autoimmune disorders include allergies, rheumatoid arthritis, type 1 diabetes, and thyroid disease. You were introduced to some common autoimmune disorders in chapter 2, and you will learn about others as you continue to read this text.

The defense mechanisms of the immune system are classified as *nonspecific* or *specific* based on the ways in which they respond to pathogenic invasion. **Nonspecific immunity** confers general protection against many different types of pathogens, such as viruses, bacteria, and fungi. A nonspecific immune response is one in which the body does not target a specific foreign substance. **Phagocytes** are an example of a nonspecific protective mechanism. These specialized cells (literally, "eating or swallowing cells") engulf and destroy pathogens in the body.

The first line of defense in nonspecific immunity is the skin. Intact skin serves as a barrier that keeps harmful microorganisms and other foreign substances from entering the body. Other nonspecific defense systems include the coughing and sneezing reflexes, which help dislodge irritants from the respiratory tract; mucous membranes, which trap bacteria and tiny particles; enzymes in our tears; and the lubricating oils in our skin.

By contrast, **specific immunity** affords protection against an **antigen**, a specific substance that, when introduced into the body, stimulates the production of an antibody. An **antibody** is a special kind of protein that the body produces to destroy or inactivate an antigen. The antibody confers protection against one specific substance and no others. Specific immunity involves "cell memory," the ability of cells in the body to recognize and respond to a specific harmful substance.

Anatomy and Physiology Vocabulary

Now that you have been introduced to the basic structure and functions of the lymphatic and immune systems, we will explore in more detail the key terms presented in the overview.

Key Term	Definition
adenoids	small masses of lymphoid tissue located posterior to the nasal cavity; when infected, can become enlarged and interfere with breathing
antibody	a special kind of protein that the body produces to destroy or inactivate an antigen
antigen	a specific substance that, when introduced into the body, stimulates the production of an antibody
autoimmune disorder	a disorder that arises when the immune system fails to differentiate between "self" and "non-self" cells, causing the body to attack its own cells and tissues
immune system	network of organs, tissues, and cells that work together to protect the body from disease-causing pathogens such as bacteria, viruses, toxins, and cancer cells
immunologist	physician who specializes in the study and treatment of diseases and disorders of the immune system
immunology	the study of the immune system
lymph	a clear or milky-white fluid that contains *lymphocytes*, or specialized leukocytes (white blood cells) that protect the body from infection and disease; lymphatic fluid

Key Term	Definition
lymphatic system	body system that works with the immune system to filter and destroy dead blood cells, particulate waste, and pathogens such as bacteria, viruses, toxins, and cancer cells
lymphocytes	specialized leukocytes (white blood cells) that protect the body from infection and disease by attacking foreign substances in the blood
nonspecific immunity	general protection provided by the immune system against many different types of pathogens
pathogen	a microorganism capable of causing disease; examples include bacteria, viruses, fungi, parasites, toxins, and cancer cells
phagocyte	a specialized type of disease-fighting cell that engulfs and destroys bacteria and other harmful microorganisms in the body
specific immunity	the ability of the body to recognize and respond to a specific pathogen, such as a bacterium or virus
spleen	the organ above the stomach that contains infection-fighting leukocytes, controls the amount of blood in the body, and destroys old or damaged red blood cells
thymus	small, butterfly-shaped gland in the upper chest beneath the sternum (breastbone); receives specialized leukocytes called *T lymphocytes (T cells)* from the bone marrow
tonsils	two small, oval-shaped tissue masses that lie at the back of the pharynx (throat); protect the body from infection by trapping pathogens that enter through the mouth or nose

E-Flash Card Activity: Anatomy and Physiology Vocabulary

Directions: After you have reviewed the anatomy and physiology vocabulary related to the lymphatic and immune systems, access your *EduHub* subscription and practice with the e-flash cards until you are comfortable with the spelling and definition of each term.

Identifying Major Organs of the Lymphatic System

Directions: Label the diagram of the lymphatic system. You can also complete this activity online using *EduHub*.

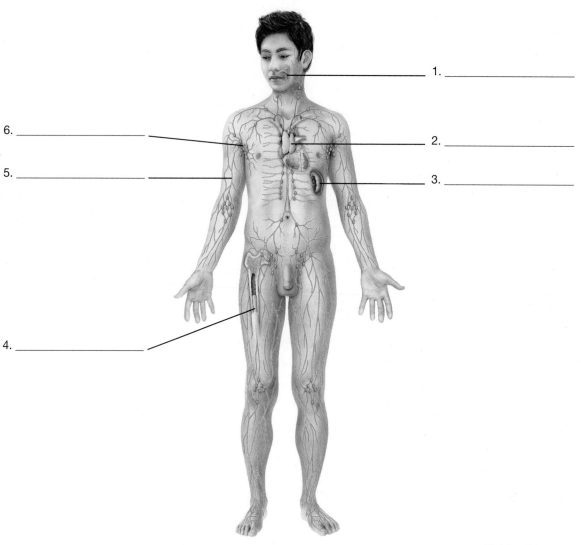

1. _____

6. _____

2. _____

5. _____

3. _____

4. _____

© Body Scientific International

SCORECARD: How Did You Do?

Number correct (_____), divided by 6 (_____), multiplied by 100 equals _____ (your score)

Matching Anatomy and Physiology Vocabulary

Directions: Choose the correct vocabulary term for each meaning. You can also complete this activity online using *EduHub*.

_____ 1. a specific substance that, when introduced into the body, stimulates the production of an antibody

_____ 2. network of organs, tissues, and cells that work together to protect the body from disease-causing pathogens such as bacteria, viruses, toxins, and cancer cells

_____ 3. specialized leukocytes (white blood cells) that protect the body from infection and disease by attacking foreign substances in the blood

_____ 4. a disorder that arises when the immune system fails to differentiate between "self" and "non-self" cells, causing the body to attack its own cells and tissues

_____ 5. physician who specializes in the study and treatment of diseases and disorders of the immune system

_____ 6. the study of the immune system

_____ 7. a clear or milky-white fluid that contains *lymphocytes*, or specialized white blood cells that protect the body from infection and disease; lymphatic fluid

_____ 8. body system that works with the immune system to filter and destroy dead blood cells, particulate waste, and pathogens

_____ 9. general protection provided by the immune system against many different types of foreign substances

_____ 10. small masses of lymphoid tissue located posterior to the nasal cavity; when infected, can become enlarged and interfere with breathing

_____ 11. a microorganism capable of causing disease; examples include bacteria, viruses, fungi, parasites, toxins, and cancer cells

_____ 12. a specialized type of disease-fighting cell that engulfs and destroys bacteria and other harmful microorganisms

_____ 13. the ability of the body to recognize and respond to a specific harmful substance, such as a bacterium or virus

_____ 14. the organ above the stomach that contains infection-fighting leukocytes, controls the amount of blood in the body, and destroys old or damaged cells

_____ 15. small, butterfly-shaped gland in the upper chest beneath the sternum (breastbone); produces *T lymphocytes* (*T cells*)

_____ 16. two small, oval-shaped tissue masses that lie at the back of the pharynx (throat); protect the body from infection by trapping pathogens that enter through the mouth or nose

_____ 17. a special kind of protein that the body produces to destroy or inactivate an antigen

A. specific immunity

B. spleen

C. nonspecific immunity

D. pathogen

E. adenoids

F. antibody

G. immune system

H. lymphocytes

I. immunologist

J. thymus

K. tonsils

L. phagocyte

M. lymphatic system

N. immunology

O. antigen

P. autoimmune disorder

Q. lymph

SCORECARD: How Did You Do?

Number correct (_____), divided by 17 (_____), multiplied by 100 equals _____ (your score)

Word Elements

In this section, you will learn word elements—prefixes, combining forms, and suffixes—that are common to study of the lymphatic and immune systems. By learning these word elements and understanding how they are combined to build medical terms, you will be able to analyze Mr. Shumaker's health condition (described in the Intern Experience at the beginning of this chapter) and identify a large number of terms associated with the lymphatic and immune systems.

E-Flash Card Activity: Word Elements

Directions: Review the word elements in the tables that follow. Then, access your *EduHub* subscription and practice with the e-flash cards until you are able to quickly recognize the different word parts (prefixes, combining forms, and suffixes) and their meanings. The e-flash cards are grouped together by prefixes, combining forms, and suffixes, followed by a cumulative review of all the word elements you are learning in this chapter.

Prefixes

Let's start our study of word elements by looking at the prefixes listed in the table below. As you know by now, these prefixes appear not only in medical terms related to the lymphatic and immune systems, but also in many terms used to describe other body systems.

Prefix	Meaning
auto-	self
hyper-	above; above normal
inter-	between
intra-	within

Combining Forms

Listed below are combining forms common in medical terminology used to describe the anatomy and physiology of the lymphatic and immune systems, as well as clinical conditions, diagnostic procedures, and therapeutic treatments related to these systems. You have already encountered some of these combining forms in previous chapters.

Root Word/Combining Vowel	Meaning
aden/o	gland
adenoid/o	adenoids
angi/o	vessel

(Continued)

Root Word/Combining Vowel	Meaning
cyt/o	cell
immun/o	protection
leuk/o	white
lymph/o	lymph
path/o	disease
phag/o	eat; swallow; engulf
splen/o	spleen
thym/o	thymus
tonsill/o	tonsils

Suffixes

Listed below are suffixes that appear in medical terms used to describe the lymphatic and immune systems. You are already familiar with these suffixes, which were introduced in previous chapters.

Suffix	Meaning
-ac	pertaining to
-ar	pertaining to
-atic	pertaining to
-cyte	cell
-ectomy	surgical removal; excision
-edema	swelling
-gen	producing; originating; causing
-ic	pertaining to
-itis	inflammation
-logist	specialist in the study and treatment of
-logy	study of
-malacia	softening
-megaly	enlargement
-oid	like; resembling
-oma	tumor; mass
-osis	abnormal condition
-pathy	disease
-pexy	surgical fixation
-rrhaphy	suture
-trophy	development

Matching Prefixes, Combining Forms, and Suffixes

Directions: Choose the correct meaning for each word element. Some meanings may be used more than once. You can also complete this activity online using *EduHub*.

Prefixes

_____	1. auto-	A.	above; above normal
_____	2. hyper-	B.	within
_____	3. inter-	C.	self
_____	4. intra-	D.	between

Combining Forms

_____	1. lymph/o	A.	gland
_____	2. tonsill/o	B.	adenoids
_____	3. cyt/o	C.	vessel
_____	4. thym/o	D.	cell
_____	5. aden/o	E.	protection
_____	6. splen/o	F.	white
_____	7. angi/o	G.	lymph
_____	8. phag/o	H.	disease
_____	9. adenoid/o	I.	eat; swallow; engulf
_____	10. immun/o	J.	spleen
_____	11. path/o	K.	thymus
_____	12. leuk/o	L.	tonsils

Suffixes

_____	1. -rrhaphy	A.	pertaining to
_____	2. -ac	B.	cell
_____	3. -trophy	C.	surgical removal; excision
_____	4. -atic	D.	swelling
_____	5. -osis	E.	producing; originating; causing
_____	6. -ectomy	F.	inflammation
_____	7. -logist	G.	specialist in the study and treatment of
_____	8. -oma	H.	study of

_____ 9. -ar   I.   softening

_____ 10. -pexy   J.   enlargement

_____ 11. -cyte   K.   like; resembling

_____ 12. -malacia   L.   tumor; mass

_____ 13. -edema   M.   abnormal condition

_____ 14. -pathy   N.   disease

_____ 15. -itis   O.   surgical fixation

_____ 16. -oid   P.   suture

_____ 17. -gen   Q.   development

_____ 18. -megaly

_____ 19. -ic

_____ 20. -logy

SCORECARD: How Did You Do?

Number correct (_____), divided by 36 (_____), multiplied by 100 equals _____ (your score)

Breaking Down and Building Terms Related to the Lymphatic and Immune Systems

Now that you have mastered the prefixes, combining forms, and suffixes used to describe the lymphatic and immune systems, you have the ability to dissect and build a large number of terms related to these body systems.

Below is a list of medical terms common to the study and treatment of the lymphatic and immune systems. For each term, a dissection has been provided, along with the meaning of each word element and the definition of the term as a whole.

Term	Dissection	Word Part/Meaning	Term Definition
Note: *For simplification, combining vowels have been omitted from the Word Part/Meaning column.*			
1. **adenoidectomy** (ĂD-ĕ-noy-DĔK-tō-mē)	adenoid/ectomy	**adenoid** = adenoids **ectomy** = surgical removal; excision	excision of the adenoids
2. **adenoiditis** (ĂD-ĕ-noy-DĪ-tĭs)	adenoid/itis	**adenoid** = adenoids **itis** = inflammation	inflammation of the adenoids
3. **autoimmune** (AW-tō-ĭ-MYŪN)	auto/immune	**auto** = self **immun** = protection	self-protection
Prefixes = **Green** Root Words = **Red** Suffixes = **Blue**			

Term	Dissection	Word Part/Meaning	Term Definition
4. **immunologist** (ĬM-yū-NŎL-ō-jĭst)	immun/o/logist	**immun** = protection **logist** = specialist in the study and treatment of	specialist in the study and treatment of protection
5. **immunology** (ĬM-yū-NŎL-ō-jē)	immun/o/logy	**immun** = protection **logy** = study of	study of protection
6. **lymphadenitis** (lĭm-FĂD-ĕ-NĪ-tĭs)	lymph/aden/itis	**lymph** = lymph **aden** = gland **itis** = inflammation	inflammation of the lymph glands
7. **lymphadenopathy** (lĭm-FĂD-ĕ-NŎP-ă-thē)	lymph/aden/o/pathy	**lymph** = lymph **aden** = gland **pathy** = disease	disease of the lymph glands
8. **lymphadenosis** (lĭm-FĂD-ĕ-NŌ-sĭs)	lymph/aden/osis	**lymph** = lymph **aden** = gland **osis** = abnormal condition	abnormal condition of the lymph glands
9. **lymphangiopathy** (lĭm-FĂN-jē-ŎP-ă-thē)	lymph/angi/o/pathy	**lymph** = lymph **angi** = vessel **pathy** = disease	disease of the lymph vessels
10. **lymphatic** (lĭm-FĂT-ĭk)	lymph/atic	**lymph** = lymph **atic** = pertaining to	pertaining to lymph
11. **lymphedema** (lĭm-fĕ-DĒ-mă)	lymph/edema	**lymph** = lymph **edema** = swelling	swelling of lymph
12. **lymphocyte** (LĬM-fō-sīt)	lymph/o/cyte	**lymph** = lymph **cyte** = cell	lymph cell
13. **lymphocytoma** (LĬM-fō-sī-TŌ-mă)	lymph/o/cyt/oma	**lymph** = lymph **cyt** = cell **oma** = tumor; mass	tumor of the lymph cells
14. **lymphoid** (LĬM-foyd)	lymph/oid	**lymph** = lymph **oid** = like; resembling	like or resembling lymph
15. **lymphoma** (lĭm-FŌ-mă)	lymph/oma	**lymph** = lymph **oma** = tumor; mass	tumor of the lymph
16. **pathogenic** (păth-ō-JĔN-ĭk)	path/o/gen/ic	**path** = disease **gen** = producing; originating; causing **ic** = pertaining to	pertaining to causing disease
17. **pathologist** (pă-THŎL-ō-jĭst)	path/o/logist	**path** = disease **logist** = specialist in the study and treatment of	specialist in the study and treatment of disease
18. **pathology** (pă-THŎL-ō-jē)	path/o/logy	**path** = disease **logy** = study of	study of disease
19. **phagocyte** (FĂG-ō-sīt)	phag/o/cyte	**phag** = eat; swallow; engulf **cyte** = cell	cell that eats, swallows, or engulfs

Prefixes = Green   Root Words = **Red**   Suffixes = Blue

Term	Dissection	Word Part/Meaning	Term Definition
20. **phagocytic** (făg-ō-SĬT-ĭk)	phag/o/cyt/ic	**phag** = eat; swallow; engulf **cyt** = cell **ic** = pertaining to	pertaining to a cell that eats, swallows, or engulfs
21. **splenectomy** (splē-NĔK-tō-mē)	splen/ectomy	**splen** = spleen **ectomy** = surgical removal; excision	excision of the spleen
22. **splenic** (SPLĔN-ĭk)	splen/ic	**splen** = spleen **ic** = pertaining to	pertaining to the spleen
23. **splenitis** (splē-NĪ-tĭs)	splen/itis	**splen** = spleen **itis** = inflammation	inflammation of the spleen
24. **splenoid** (SPLĒ-noyd)	splen/oid	**splen** = spleen **oid** = like; resembling	like or resembling the spleen
25. **splenoma** (splē-NŌ-mă)	splen/oma	**splen** = spleen **oma** = tumor; mass	tumor of the spleen
26. **splenomalacia** (SPLĒ-nō-mă-LĀ-shē-ă)	splen/o/malacia	**splen** = spleen **malacia** = softening	softening of the spleen
27. **splenomegaly** (SPLĒ-nō-MĔG-ă-lē)	splen/o/megaly	**splen** = spleen **megaly** = enlargement	enlargement of the spleen
28. **splenopexy** (SPLĒ-nō-PĔK-sē)	splen/o/pexy	**splen** = spleen **pexy** = surgical fixation	surgical fixation of the spleen
29. **splenorrhaphy** (splē-NOR-ă-fē)	splen/o/rrhaphy	**splen** = spleen **rrhaphy** = suture	suture of the spleen
30. **thymectomy** (thī-MĔK-tō-mē)	thym/ectomy	**thym** = thymus **ectomy** = surgical removal; excision	excision of the thymus
31. **thymic** (THĪ-mĭk)	thym/ic	**thym** = thymus **ic** = pertaining to	pertaining to the thymus
32. **thymoma** (thī-MŌ-mă)	thym/oma	**thym** = thymus **oma** = tumor; mass	tumor of the thymus
33. **tonsillar** (TŎN-sĭ-lăr)	tonsill/ar	**tonsill** = tonsils **ar** = pertaining to	pertaining to the tonsils
34. **tonsillectomy** (TŎN-sĭl-ĔK-tō-mē)	tonsill/ectomy	**tonsill** = tonsils **ectomy** = surgical removal; excision	excision of the tonsils
35. **tonsillitis** (TŎN-sĭl-Ī-tĭs)	tonsill/itis	**tonsill** = tonsils **itis** = inflammation	inflammation of the tonsils

Prefixes = Green   Root Words = **Red**   Suffixes = Blue

Using the pronunciation guide in the Breaking Down and Building chart, practice saying each medical term aloud. To hear the pronunciation of each term, complete the Pronounce It activity on the next page.

Audio Activity: Pronounce It

Directions: Access your *EduHub* subscription and listen to the correct pronunciations of the following medical terms. Practice pronouncing the terms until you are comfortable saying them aloud.

adenoidectomy
(ĂD-ĕ-noy-DĔK-tō-mē)

adenoiditis
(ĂD-ĕ-noy-DĪ-tĭs)

autoimmune
(AW-tō-ĭ-MYŪN)

immunologist
(ĬM-yū-NŎL-ō-jĭst)

immunology
(ĬM-yū-NŎL-ō-jē)

lymphadenitis
(lĭm-FĂD-ĕ-NĪ-tĭs)

lymphadenopathy
(lĭm-FĂD-ĕ-NŎP-ă-thē)

lymphadenosis
(lĭm-FĂD-ĕ-NŌ-sĭs)

lymphangiopathy
(lĭm-FĂN-jē-ŎP-ă-thē)

lymphatic
(lĭm-FĂT-ĭk)

lymphedema
(lĭm-fĕ-DĒ-mă)

lymphocyte
(LĬM-fō-sīt)

lymphocytoma
(LĬM-fō-sī-TŌ-mă)

lymphoid
(LĬM-foyd)

lymphoma
(lĭm-FŌ-mă)

pathogenic
(păth-ō-JĔN-ĭk)

pathologist
(pă-THŎL-ō-jĭst)

pathology
(pă-THŎL-ō-jē)

phagocyte
(FĂG-ō-sīt)

phagocytic
(făg-ō-SĬT-ĭk)

splenectomy
(splē-NĔK-tō-mē)

splenic
(SPLĔN-ĭk)

splenitis
(splē-NĪ-tĭs)

splenoid
(SPLĒ-noyd)

splenoma
(splē-NŌ-mă)

splenomalacia
(SPLĒ-nō-mă-LĀ-shē-ă)

splenomegaly
(SPLĒ-nō-MĔG-ă-lē)

splenopexy
(SPLĒ-nō-PĔK-sē)

splenorrhaphy
(splē-NOR-ă-fē)

thymectomy
(thī-MĔK-tō-mē)

thymic
(THĪ-mĭk)

thymoma
(thī-MŌ-mă)

tonsillar
(TŎN-sĭ-lăr)

tonsillectomy
(TŎN-sĭl-ĔK-tō-mē)

tonsillitis
(TŎN-sĭl-Ī-tĭs)

Audio Activity: Spell It

Directions: Access your *EduHub* subscription and listen to the pronunciation for each number. As you hear each term, write its correct spelling.

1. _____

2. _____

3. _____

4. _____

5. _____

6. _____

7. _____

8. _____

9. _____

10. _____

11. _____

12. _____

13. _____

14. _____

15. _____

16. _____

17. _____

18. _____

19. _____

20. _____

21. _____

22. _____

23. _____

24. _____

25. _____

26. _____

27. _____   32. _____

28. _____   33. _____

29. _____   34. _____

30. _____   35. _____

31. _____

Assessment 5.5

Break It Down

Directions: Dissect each medical term into its word parts (prefix, root word, combining vowel, and suffix) using one or more slashes. Then define each term. You can also complete this activity online using **EduHub**.

Example:

Medical Term: lymphadenopathy

Dissection: lymph/aden/o/pathy

Definition: disease of the lymph glands

Medical Term	Dissection
1. tonsillectomy	t o n s i l l e c t o m y

Definition: _____

_____

| 2. autoimmune | a u t o i m m u n e |

Definition: _____

_____

| 3. lymphadenitis | l y m p h a d e n i t i s |

Definition: _____

_____

| 4. pathogenic | p a t h o g e n i c |

Definition: _____

_____

Medical Term	Dissection
5. splenic	s p l e n i c

Definition: _____

_____

6. adenoidectomy	a d e n o i d e c t o m y

Definition: _____

_____

7. lymphangiopathy	l y m p h a n g i o p a t h y

Definition: _____

_____

8. pathology	p a t h o l o g y

Definition: _____

_____

9. immunologist	i m m u n o l o g i s t

Definition: _____

_____

10. splenorrhaphy	s p l e n o r r h a p h y

Definition: _____

_____

11. adenoiditis	a d e n o i d i t i s

Definition: _____

_____

12. splenomegaly	s p l e n o m e g a l y

Definition: _____

_____

Medical Term	Dissection
13. tonsillitis	t o n s i l l i t i s

Definition: _____

_____

| 14. lymphocytoma | l y m p h o c y t o m a |

Definition: _____

_____

| 15. lymphadenopathy | l y m p h a d e n o p a t h y |

Definition: _____

_____

| 16. splenitis | s p l e n i t i s |

Definition: _____

_____

| 17. lymphadenosis | l y m p h a d e n o s i s |

Definition: _____

_____

| 18. splenopexy | s p l e n o p e x y |

Definition: _____

_____

| 19. pathologist | p a t h o l o g i s t |

Definition: _____

_____

SCORECARD: How Did You Do?

Number correct (_____), divided by 19 (_____), multiplied by 100 equals _____ (your score)

Build It

Directions: Build the medical term that matches each definition by supplying the correct word parts. You can also complete this activity online using *EduHub*.

P (Prefixes) = Green
RW (Root Words) = Red
S (Suffixes) = Blue
CV (Combining Vowel) = Purple

1. abnormal condition of the lymph glands

   _____   _____   _____
            RW   RW   S

2. pertaining to causing disease

   _____   ____ ____ ____
           RW   CV   S   S

3. study of protection

   _____   ____ _____
           RW   CV   S

4. inflammation of the tonsils

   _____   _____
           RW   S

5. excision of the adenoids

   _____   _____
           RW   S

6. disease of the lymph glands

   _____   _____   ____ _____
           RW   RW   CV   S

7. self-protection

   _____   _____
     P   RW

8. enlargement of the spleen

   _____   ____ _____
           RW   CV   S

9. tumor of the lymph

_____ _____
　　　　RW　　　　　　　　　S

10. excision of the tonsils

_____ _____
　　　　RW　　　　　　　　　S

11. inflammation of the adenoids

_____ _____
　　　　RW　　　　　　　　　S

12. suture of the spleen

_____ _____ _____
　　　　RW　　　　　　CV　　　S

13. inflammation of the lymph glands

_____ _____ _____
　　　　RW　　　　　　　　　RW　　　　　　　　S

14. disease of the lymph vessels

_____ _____ _____ _____
　　　　RW　　　　　　　　　RW　　　　　CV　　　S

15. pertaining to the spleen

_____ _____
　　　　RW　　　　　　　　　S

16. pertaining to the tonsils

_____ _____
　　　　RW　　　　　　　　　S

17. like or resembling lymph

_____ _____
　　　　RW　　　　　　　　　S

18. excision of the spleen

_____ _____
　　　　RW　　　　　　　　　S

19. softening of the spleen

_____   _____   _____
           RW   CV   S

20. pertaining to lymph

_____   _____
           RW   S

21. specialist in the study and treatment of disease

_____   _____   _____
           RW   CV   S

22. specialist in the study and treatment of protection

_____   _____   _____
           RW   CV   S

23. surgical fixation of the spleen

_____   _____   _____
           RW   CV   S

24. swelling of lymph

_____   _____
           RW   S

25. tumor of the spleen

_____   _____
           RW   S

SCORECARD: How Did You Do?

Number correct (_____), divided by 25 (_____), multiplied by 100 equals _____ (your score)

Diseases and Disorders

Diseases and disorders of the lymphatic and immune systems run the spectrum from the mild to the severe and have a number of different causes. This section presents a brief overview of some common pathological conditions of the lymphatic and immune systems.

Acquired Immunodeficiency Syndrome

Acquired immunodeficiency syndrome (AIDS) is caused by the *human immunodeficiency virus (HIV)*, which attacks the body's infection-fighting helper T cells. The first signs of HIV infection often are swollen glands and flu-like symptoms. Onset of more severe symptoms occurs months or years later (Figure 5.2). AIDS typically spreads through unprotected sexual contact with an infected person. It can also be spread through contact with the blood of an infected person or by sharing drug needles.

As we learned earlier in the chapter, specific immunity depends on helper T cells to activate an immune response. Destruction of helper T cells by HIV impairs immune function and compromises the body's ability to fight infection. Unable to defend itself against foreign invaders, the body becomes vulnerable to many different kinds of infections that a healthy immune system could easily fend off.

Allergies

An **allergy** is a hypersensitive response (exaggerated reaction) by the immune system to an **allergen**, a substance that usually is recognized by the immune system as harmless. Contact with the allergen may occur through inhalation, injection (as by a bee sting), ingestion (eating or drinking), or skin contact (Figure 5.3). Common allergens include dust, mold, pollen, pet dander, insect stings, certain kinds of foods, and drugs (over-the-counter medicines or prescription pharmaceuticals).

An allergic response is characterized as "exaggerated" because the substance that provokes the hyperreactive immune response does not cause a reaction in nonallergic individuals. During an allergic response, certain cells in the body release histamine and other allergy-mediating chemicals.

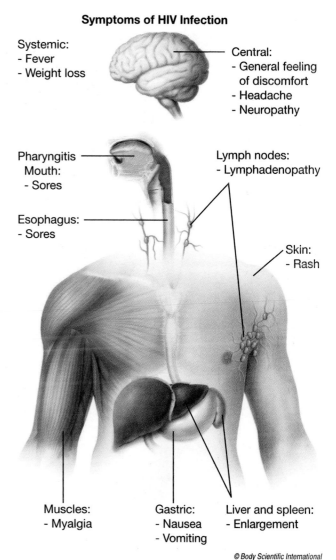

Symptoms of HIV Infection

Systemic:
- Fever
- Weight loss

Central:
- General feeling of discomfort
- Headache
- Neuropathy

Pharyngitis
Mouth:
- Sores

Lymph nodes:
- Lymphadenopathy

Esophagus:
- Sores

Skin:
- Rash

Muscles:
- Myalgia

Gastric:
- Nausea
- Vomiting

Liver and spleen:
- Enlargement

© Body Scientific International

Figure 5.2 Major symptoms of acute HIV infection

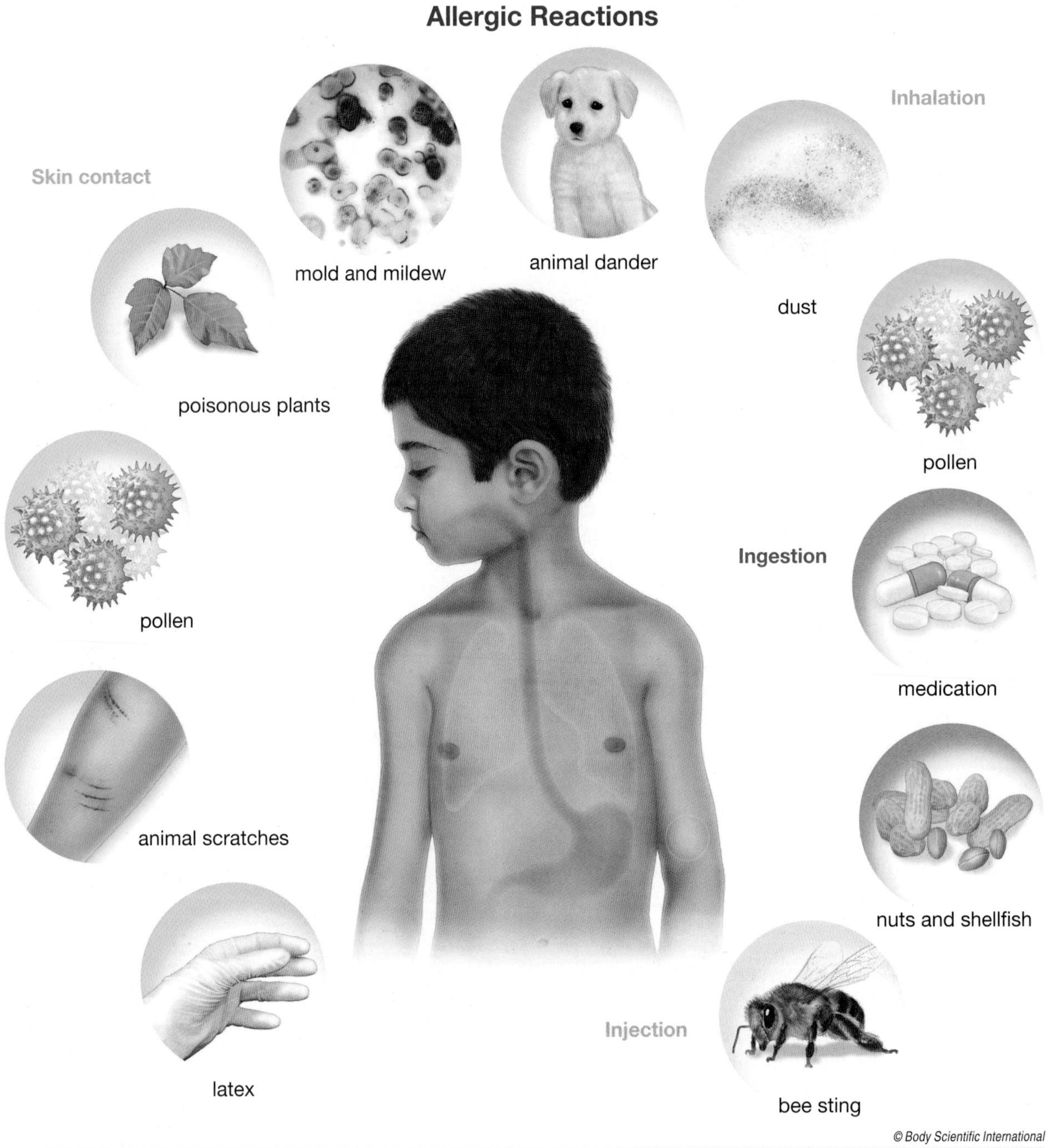

Allergic Reactions

Skin contact

mold and mildew

animal dander

Inhalation

dust

poisonous plants

pollen

pollen

Ingestion

medication

animal scratches

nuts and shellfish

latex

Injection

bee sting

© Body Scientific International

Figure 5.3 Common allergens

Depending on the allergen, these chemicals can cause symptoms such as nasal congestion, sneezing, coughing, wheezing, itching, burning, and swelling.

People who have allergies often are sensitive to more than one substance. Although a cure for allergies does not exist, allergies usually can be controlled with medication (over-the-counter or prescription) and by avoiding the allergen. However, a severe, systemic (whole-body) allergic reaction called **anaphylaxis** is life-threatening. The most serious signs of anaphylaxis are an abrupt decrease in blood pressure and difficulty breathing. Common causes of anaphylaxis include insect bites, certain foods such as shellfish, latex, and medications.

Individuals who are susceptible to systemic allergic reactions often carry an epinephrine auto-injector. Epinephrine is a chemical that constricts (narrows) the blood vessels and opens the airways in the lungs. The patient uses the device to quickly self-inject epinephrine during an anaphylactic reaction before receiving aid at an emergency facility.

Asthma

Asthma is a disorder that causes the bronchi (tubes that conduct air into the lungs) to narrow and swell and produce extra mucus. This leads to wheezing, shortness of breath, tightness in the chest, and coughing.

An asthmatic response is a hypersensitivity reaction, an exaggerated immune response to an environmental substance that the body perceives as foreign. During an asthma attack, the muscles surrounding the bronchi tighten, and the lining of the bronchial tubes becomes swollen. This tightening and swelling reduces the amount of air that can travel to the lungs. In sensitized people, asthma symptoms can be triggered by inhaling allergens. Typical asthma triggers include dust, mold, pollen, animal dander, chemicals in the air or in food, smoke, and stress. Asthma is not curable, but its symptoms can be controlled.

Autoimmune Disorders

As mentioned earlier in the chapter, an autoimmune disorder is a condition that causes the immune system to produce antibodies that attack the body's own tissues. In people with an autoimmune disorder, the immune system can't tell the difference between healthy body tissue ("self" tissue) and antigens ("nonself" substances). As a result, the immune system attacks and destroys normal body tissues. It is not yet known what mechanisms interfere with the body's ability to distinguish between healthy tissues and antigens.

There are many different types of autoimmune disorders. For example, **rheumatoid arthritis (RA)** is a chronic, systemic disease that affects the joints (Figure 5.4). This autoimmune disease causes inflammation and edema of the synovial membranes surrounding the joints. Over time, RA destroys cartilage, causes joint deformity, and erodes adjacent bone.

Autoimmune hemolytic anemia (AIHA) is a condition in which **erythrocytes** (red blood cells, or RBCs) are destroyed by antibodies. **Systemic lupus erythematosus (SLE)** is a chronic inflammatory disease that affects many different systems throughout the body. The term *erythematosus* refers to the red rash that often develops on the faces of those afflicted with the disease.

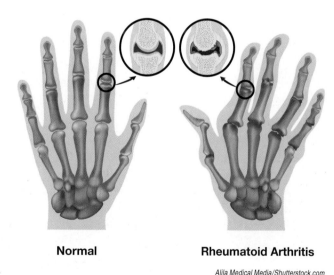

Normal　　　　　**Rheumatoid Arthritis**

Alila Medical Media/Shutterstock.com

Figure 5.4 Rheumatoid arthritis is an autoimmune disease that destroys cartilage, causes joint deformity, and erodes adjacent bone.

Multiple sclerosis (MS) is an inflammatory autoimmune disease of the central nervous system (brain and spinal cord). MS is caused by damage to the myelin sheath, a layer of white fatty matter that covers most of the nerves in the brain and spinal cord. Ultimately, MS causes sclerosis (hardening) that slows down or stops the transmission of nerve impulses.

Hodgkin's Disease

Hodgkin's disease (also called *Hodgkin lymphoma*) is a malignant lymphoma characterized by painless and progressive enlargement of lymphoid tissue followed by anemia, fever, persistent fatigue, and unexplained weight loss. In Hodgkin lymphoma, cells in the lymphatic system grow abnormally and may spread beyond the lymphatic system. As Hodgkin lymphoma progresses, it compromises the body's ability to fight infection. Treatment involves radiation and chemotherapy.

Mononucleosis

Mononucleosis, or **mono**, is a viral infection characterized by enlarged lymph nodes, atypical (abnormal) lymphocytes, pharyngitis (sore throat), fever, splenomegaly (enlarged spleen), and severe fatigue (Figure 5.5). Most cases of infectious mononucleosis are caused by the Epstein-Barr virus.

Mononucleosis is often called the "kissing disease" because the virus is carried in the saliva of infected individuals. Treatment includes bed rest, increased fluid intake, and acetaminophen or ibuprofen for pain and fever. The infection is generally self-limiting; that is, it resolves itself in about four to six weeks.

Sarcoidosis

Sarcoidosis is an inflammatory disease that can affect almost any body part or system, but most commonly affects the lungs. The cause of the disease is unknown. Symptoms of pulmonary (lung) sarcoidosis include chest pain, dry cough, and dyspnea (difficulty breathing), along with general symptoms of fatigue, fever, and arthralgia (joint pain).

Tests used to diagnose sarcoidosis include chest X-rays, a computerized tomography (CT) scan of the chest, pulmonary function tests, and a biopsy of the lung tissue. Biopsies of other body tissues are also helpful in diagnosing the condition. In many cases, sarcoidosis abates spontaneously with no treatment. Severe symptoms may be relieved with corticosteroids (drugs that reduce inflammation) and

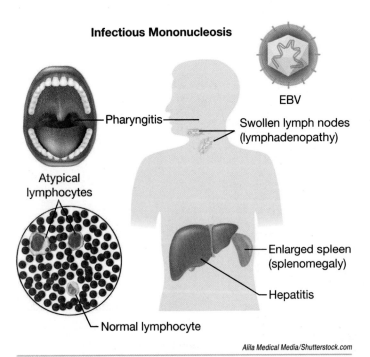

Infectious Mononucleosis

EBV

Pharyngitis

Swollen lymph nodes (lymphadenopathy)

Atypical lymphocytes

Enlarged spleen (splenomegaly)

Hepatitis

Normal lymphocyte

Alila Medical Media/Shutterstock.com

Figure 5.5 Infectious mononucleosis is characterized by atypical lymphocytes, lymphadenopathy, splenomegaly, and pharyngitis.

immunosuppressants, which inhibit the body's immune response, preventing the immune system from attacking the body's own cells.

Tonsillitis

Tonsillitis is an inflammation of the tonsils (Figure 5.6). The condition most often occurs in childhood. While a bacterial or viral infection can cause tonsillitis, the *Streptococcus* ("strep") bacterium is the most common cause.

Symptoms of tonsillitis include sore throat, chills, fever, and pain. Lymph nodes in the jaw and throat are tender and enlarged. The tonsils usually are red and may have white spots on them. Treatment for tonsillitis includes bed rest, a liquid diet, saline irrigation for the throat, and antibiotic therapy. Surgery may be recommended for persistent, chronic tonsillitis.

Procedures and Treatments

We will now take a brief look at some common diagnostic tests and procedures used to help identify disorders and diseases of the lymphatic and immune systems, as well as some common therapeutic treatments.

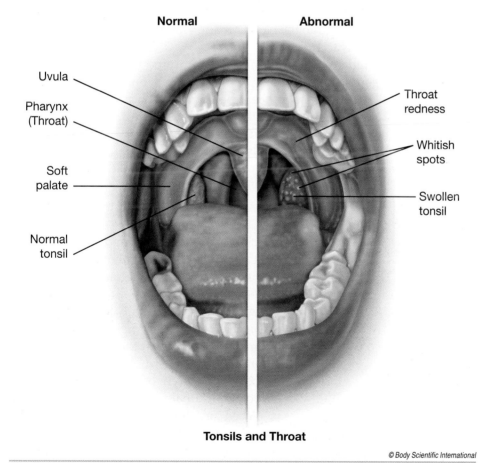

Normal   **Abnormal**

Uvula

Pharynx (Throat)

Soft palate

Normal tonsil

Throat redness

Whitish spots

Swollen tonsil

Tonsils and Throat

© Body Scientific International

Figure 5.6 Symptoms of tonsillitis include redness in the throat, swollen tonsils, and white spots in the back of the throat.

Enzyme-Linked Immunosorbent Assay

Enzyme-linked immunosorbent assay (ELISA) is a common laboratory test in which a blood sample is drawn and examined for the presence of antibodies. This test is often performed to determine whether or not a person has been exposed to viruses or other substances that cause infection. It can be used to screen for current or past infections.

The ELISA test is typically the first one used to detect infection by the human immunodeficiency virus (HIV). If antibodies to HIV are present, the test is positive. The test is usually repeated to confirm the diagnosis.

The ELISA test is a good screening tool; however, it can produce "false positive" results, indicating the presence of HIV when it is nonexistent. Therefore, the ELISA test alone cannot be used to make a definitive diagnosis of HIV infection. The presence of HIV must be confirmed by a Western blot test (discussed later in this section) or other more specific tests.

Immunization

Immunization is a procedure that provides immunity against a disease-causing pathogen without inducing infection. This is accomplished through **vaccination**, the injection of a substance containing dead or attenuated (weakened) pathogens directly into the bloodstream. The substance that contains the pathogens is called a **vaccine**.

A vaccine stimulates the immune system to produce antibodies against a specific pathogen. Immunizations against measles, mumps, rubella, polio, diphtheria, and pertussis help to keep the population healthy. Vaccines are a successful, cost-effective public health tool for preventing the spread of diseases that can be dangerous and even deadly.

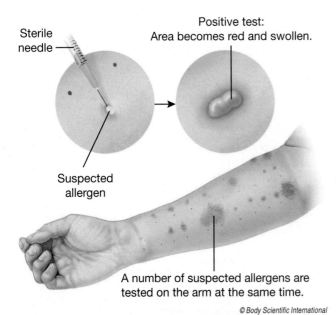

Sterile needle

Positive test: Area becomes red and swollen.

Suspected allergen

A number of suspected allergens are tested on the arm at the same time.

© Body Scientific International

Figure 5.7 A scratch test is used to identify substances that provoke an allergic reaction.

Scratch Test

A **scratch test** is a skin test used to identify the substance causing an allergy. An extract of an allergen is applied to the skin by scratching or pricking the skin's surface so that the extract can penetrate the epidermis (outer layer of skin).

A scratch test is usually performed on the forearm or back (Figure 5.7). Areas on the skin are marked with a pen to identify each allergen that will be tested. A very small amount of extract for each potential allergen (such as pollen, animal dander, or insect venom) is placed on the corresponding mark. The reaction of the skin is then evaluated. If the scratch test is positive for a particular allergen, the skin in that area will become raised, red, and pruritic (itchy).

Splenectomy

A **splenectomy** is the surgical removal of a diseased or damaged spleen. The spleen is located in the left upper quadrant of the abdomen, just underneath the ribs. The most common reason for splenectomy is to treat a ruptured spleen, often caused by traumatic abdominal injury, such as from an automobile accident. This procedure may also be performed to treat some blood disorders, certain cancers, infection, cysts, or tumors.

Splenectomy is most commonly performed by **laparoscopy**, also called *laparoscopic splenectomy* (Figure 5.8). The patient is placed under general anesthesia. The surgeon directs a *cannula* (hollow tube) into the abdomen, where it is inflated with carbon dioxide gas to create a space within which to operate. A **laparoscope**, a tiny telescope connected to a video camera, is inserted through the cannula and into the abdomen. The camera projects a video image of the spleen and surrounding internal organs onto a TV monitor.

During laparoscopic splenectomy, the surgeon views the operative site with the camera. Several other cannulas are placed in different locations inside the abdomen, allowing the surgeon to insert instruments, detach the spleen from other body structures, and remove it. When the spleen has been freed from surrounding tissues, it is placed in a sterile bag and then pulled out of the body through an incision.

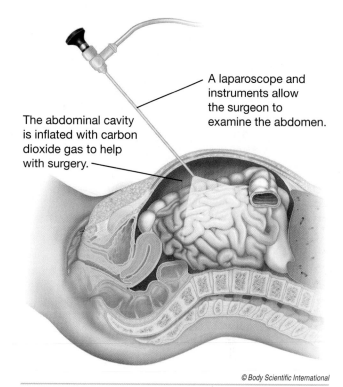

A laparoscope and instruments allow the surgeon to examine the abdomen.

The abdominal cavity is inflated with carbon dioxide gas to help with surgery.

© Body Scientific International

Figure 5.8 Splenectomy is commonly performed using a laparoscopic surgical method.

Tonsillectomy

A **tonsillectomy** is the surgical removal of the tonsils. It is used to treat severe, chronic, or recurring tonsillitis or complications due to enlarged tonsils.

At one time, tonsillectomy was a common procedure for treating inflammation and infection of the tonsils. Now it is generally reserved for the removal of enlarged tonsils that interfere with breathing or cause recurrent ear infections. It is also performed to treat tonsillitis that occurs frequently and does not improve with antibiotic treatment.

Western Blot Test

A **Western blot test** is a laboratory blood test that detects the presence of antibodies to specific antigens. It is used to diagnose chronic infection with human immunodeficiency virus (HIV). It is regarded as more precise than the enzyme-linked immunosorbent assay (ELISA) and is sometimes used to check the validity of the ELISA test. A positive Western blot confirms an HIV infection.

Multiple Choice: Diseases and Disorders

Directions: Choose the disease or disorder that matches each definition. You can also complete this activity online using *EduHub*.

_____ 1. an inflammatory autoimmune disease of the central nervous system
   a. multiple sclerosis
   b. rheumatoid arthritis
   c. systemic lupus erythematosus
   d. autoimmune hemolytic anemia

_____ 2. a viral infection characterized by enlarged lymph nodes, atypical lymphocytes, sore throat, fever, splenomegaly, and severe fatigue
   a. tonsillitis
   b. sarcoidosis
   c. mononucleosis
   d. asthma

_____ 3. a malignant lymphoma characterized by enlargement of lymphoid tissue, anemia, fatigue, fever, and weight loss
   a. asthma
   b. Hodgkin's disease
   c. multiple sclerosis
   d. sarcoidosis

_____ 4. a condition in which erythrocytes are destroyed by antibodies
   a. rheumatoid arthritis
   b. autoimmune hemolytic anemia
   c. systemic lupus erythematosus
   d. multiple sclerosis

_____ 5. an inflammatory disease that can affect almost any body part or organ, but most commonly affects the lungs
   a. mononucleosis
   b. tonsillitis
   c. asthma
   d. sarcoidosis

_____ 6. inflammation of the tonsils
   a. mononucleosis
   b. sarcoidosis
   c. tonsillitis
   d. asthma

_____ 7. a chronic inflammatory disease that affects many different body systems and often causes a red rash on the face
   a. multiple sclerosis
   b. autoimmune hemolytic anemia
   c. systemic lupus erythematosus
   d. rheumatoid arthritis

_____ 8. an exaggerated reaction by the immune system to a substance ordinarily recognized by the immune system as harmless
   a. mononucleosis
   b. autoimmune hemolytic anemia
   c. allergy
   d. sarcoidosis

_____ 9. a chronic, systemic autoimmune disease that causes inflammation of the joints
   a. rheumatoid arthritis
   b. systemic lupus erythematosus
   c. Hodgkin's disease
   d. sarcoidosis

_____ 10. a life-threatening, systemic (whole-body) reaction to an allergy
   a. allergic response
   b. antigen intolerance
   c. systemic lupus erythematosus
   d. anaphylaxis

_____ 11. a disorder that causes the bronchi to narrow, swell, and produce extra mucus
   a. mononucleosis
   b. asthma
   c. allergy
   d. anaphylaxis

SCORECARD: How Did You Do?

Number correct (_____), divided by 11 (_____), multiplied by 100 equals _____ (your score)

Multiple Choice: Procedures and Treatments

Directions: Choose the procedure or treatment that matches each definition. You can also complete this activity online using *EduHub*.

_____ 1. a procedure that provides immunity against a specific disease-causing pathogen without inducing infection
   a. scratch test
   b. Western blot test
   c. immunization
   d. enzyme-linked immunosorbent assay

_____ 2. a skin test used to identify the substance that is causing an allergy
   a. immunization
   b. scratch test
   c. enzyme-linked immunosorbent assay
   d. Western blot test

_____ 3. surgical removal of a diseased or damaged spleen
   a. splenorrhaphy   c. splenotomy
   b. splenectomy   d. splenoplasty

_____ 4. a laboratory test in which a blood sample is taken to detect the presence of antibodies; typically the first test used to detect HIV infection
   a. scratch test
   b. immunization
   c. enzyme-linked immunosorbent assay
   d. Western blot test

_____ 5. surgical removal of the tonsils
   a. tonsillotomy   c. tonsillorrhaphy
   b. tonsillectomy   d. tonsilloplasty

_____ 6. a laboratory test used to detect the presence of antibodies to specific antigens; used to definitively diagnose HIV
   a. immunization
   b. scratch test
   c. Western blot test
   d. enzyme-linked immunosorbent assay

SCORECARD: How Did You Do?

Number correct (_____), divided by 6 (_____), multiplied by 100 equals _____ (your score)

Identifying Abbreviations

Directions: Supply the correct abbreviation for each medical term. You can also complete this activity online using *EduHub*.

Medical Term	Abbreviation
1. multiple sclerosis	_____
2. acquired immunodeficiency syndrome	_____
3. enzyme-linked immunosorbent assay	_____
4. human immunodeficiency virus	_____
5. computerized tomography	_____
6. systemic lupus erythematosus	_____
7. rheumatoid arthritis	_____
8. mononucleosis	_____
9. autoimmune hemolytic anemia	_____

SCORECARD: How Did You Do?

Number correct (_____), divided by 9 (_____), multiplied by 100 equals _____ (your score)

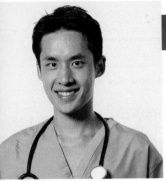

Analyzing the Intern Experience

In the Intern Experience described at the beginning of this chapter, we met Sean, an intern with the Cassel County Clinic. Sean "shadowed" (that is, followed and observed) Dr. Rymus as he interacted with William Shumaker, a 57-year-old accountant who described symptoms of extreme fatigue, persistent night sweats, weight loss, and a lump on the right side of his neck. Dr. Rymus examined William and obtained his personal and family health history. He then made a medical diagnosis and provided William with a treatment plan. Later, Dr. Rymus made a dictated recording of William's health information, which was subsequently transcribed into a chart note.

We will now learn more about William Shumaker's condition from a clinical perspective, interpreting the medical terms in his chart note as we analyze the scenario presented in the Intern Experience.

Audio Activity: William Shumaker's Chart Note

Directions: Access your *EduHub* subscription and listen to the recording of the physician reading William Shumaker's chart note. Read along with the physician and pay attention to the pronunciation of each medical term.

CHART NOTE

Patient Name: Shumaker, William
ID Number: WS3671
Examination Date: May 2, 20xx

SUBJECTIVE
Mr. William Shumaker is a 57-year-old accountant who is new to this practice. He has noticed a painless lump on the right side of his neck. He states that he is very tired, has been experiencing night sweats, and has lost about 8 pounds in the past 2 months.

OBJECTIVE
Low-grade fever. **BP** (blood pressure), pulse, and respiration within normal limits. There are 2 firm, enlarged lymph nodes on the right side of the neck, to the right and just below the **laryngeal prominence** (Adam's apple).

ASSESSMENT
Lymphadenopathy. Rule out **Hodgkin's disease**.

PLAN
CBC (complete blood count) and chest X-ray will be scheduled along with a **biopsy**.

Interpret William Shumaker's Chart Note

Directions: Access your *EduHub* subscription and listen to the recording of the physician reading William Shumaker's chart note. After listening to the recording, supply the medical term that matches each definition. You may encounter definitions and terms introduced in previous chapters.

Example: inflammation of the tonsils   *Answer:* tonsillitis

1. disease of the lymph glands   _____

2. Adam's apple   _____

3. blood pressure   _____

4. surgical removal of tissue for diagnostic examination   _____

5. malignant lymphoma characterized by painless and progressive enlargement of lymphoid tissue   _____

6. complete blood count   _____

SCORECARD: How Did You Do?

Number correct (_____), divided by 6 (_____), multiplied by 100 equals _____ (your score)

Working with Medical Records

In this activity, you will interpret the medical records (chart notes) of patients with health conditions related to the lymphatic and immune systems. These examples illustrate typical medical records prepared in a real-world healthcare environment. To interpret these chart notes, you will apply your knowledge of word elements (prefixes, combining forms, and suffixes), diseases and disorders, and procedures and treatments related to the lymphatic and immune systems.

Audio Activity: Sidney O'Brian's Chart Note

Directions: Access your *EduHub* subscription and listen to the recording of the physician reading Sidney O'Brian's chart note. Read along with the physician and pay attention to the pronunciation of each medical term.

CHART NOTE

Patient Name: O'Brian, Sidney
ID Number: SO4423
Examination Date: September 16, 20xx

SUBJECTIVE
Sidney is a 17-year-old patient who presents with a 7-day history of chills, sore throat, fatigue, fever, and headache. Over the weekend, her symptoms have worsened, and she is extremely tired. She states that she "shared a straw" with a friend when they were at the mall 2 weeks ago and now her friend is also sick.

OBJECTIVE
BP 120/76, temperature 102.4, respiratory rate 23, pulse 72. Lungs are clear. Lymph nodes are swollen. **Tonsils** are enlarged and have a whitish-yellow covering.

ASSESSMENT
Cervical **lymphadenopathy**. **Mononucleosis** test performed in the office is positive.

PLAN
The patient should drink plenty of fluids, gargle with warm salt water to ease sore throat pain, and get plenty of rest. She may take acetaminophen or ibuprofen for fever and discomfort.

Assessment 5.11

Interpret Sidney O'Brian's Chart Note

Directions: Access your *EduHub* subscription and listen to the recording of the physician reading Sidney O'Brian's chart note. After listening to the recording, supply the medical term that matches each definition.

Example: swelling of lymph   *Answer:* lymphedema

1. disease of the lymph glands   _____

2. viral infection characterized by enlarged lymph nodes, atypical lymphocytes, pharyngitis, fever, splenomegaly, and severe fatigue   _____

3. tissue structures that protect the body by trapping pathogens that enter through the mouth or nose   _____

SCORECARD: How Did You Do?

Number correct (_____), divided by 3 (_____), multiplied by 100 equals _____ (your score)

Audio Activity: Carter Rosari's Chart Note

Directions: Access your *EduHub* subscription and listen to the recording of the physician reading Carter Rosari's chart note. Read along with the physician and pay attention to the pronunciation of each medical term.

CHART NOTE

Patient Name: Rosari, Carter
ID Number: CR8062
Examination Date: November 21, 20xx

SUBJECTIVE

Carter presents with multiple raised, red, itchy welts on his left lower leg, thigh, and forearm after returning home from a camping trip with his Boy Scout troop. He states that it started about 3 days into the trip and that some of the welts seemed to get better, but then new ones began to erupt. "They seemed to move up my leg and onto my arm." He remembers something similar to this happening last year when he helped his father put up the Christmas tree.

OBJECTIVE

Wheals (welts or swellings) ranging in size from small spots on the left forearm to several large blotches about 1–2 cm in diameter on the lower leg and thigh. No fever. Vital signs are normal. History of pollen **allergy**.

ASSESSMENT

Urticaria (hives) of left leg and forearm. Allergic **contact dermatitis**.

PLAN

Apply hydrocortisone cream to the affected areas. Patient to return if condition does not improve or worsens.

Assessment 5.12

Interpret Carter Rosari's Chart Note

Directions: Access your *EduHub* subscription and listen to the recording of the physician reading Carter Rosari's chart note. After listening to the recording, supply the medical term that matches each definition. You may encounter definitions and terms introduced in previous chapters.

Example: softening of the spleen   *Answer:* splenomalacia

1. hives

   _____

2. edema and pruritic (itchy) skin as a result of contact with an allergen or irritant, causing edema and pruritic skin

   _____

3. welts or swellings

   _____

4. exaggerated response by the immune system to a substance that usually is recognized by the body as harmless

   _____

SCORECARD: How Did You Do?

Number correct (_____), divided by 4 (_____), multiplied by 100 equals _____ (your score)

Chapter Review

Word Elements Summary

Prefixes

Prefix	Meaning
auto-	self
hyper-	above; above normal
inter-	between
intra-	within

Combining Forms

Root Word/Combining Vowel	Meaning
aden/o	gland
adenoid/o	adenoids
angi/o	vessel
cyt/o	cell
immun/o	protection
leuk/o	white
lymph/o	lymph
path/o	disease
phag/o	eat; swallow; engulf
splen/o	spleen
thym/o	thymus
tonsill/o	tonsils

Suffixes

Suffix	Meaning
-ac	pertaining to
-ar	pertaining to
-atic	pertaining to
-cyte	cell
-ectomy	surgical removal; excision

(Continued)

Suffix	Meaning
-edema	swelling
-gen	producing; originating; causing
-ic	pertaining to
-itis	inflammation
-logist	specialist in the study and treatment of
-logy	study of
-malacia	softening
-megaly	enlargement
-oid	like; resembling
-oma	tumor; mass
-osis	abnormal condition
-pathy	disease
-pexy	surgical fixation
-rrhaphy	suture
-trophy	development

More Practice: Activities and Games

The following activities will help you reinforce your skills and check your mastery of the medical terminology you learned in this chapter. Access your *EduHub* subscription to complete more activities and vocabulary games for mastering the word parts and terms you have learned.

True or False

Directions: Indicate whether each statement is true or false.

True or False?

_____ 1. The prefix **inter-** means "through."

_____ 2. The root word **path** means "pathway to a disease."

_____ 3. The suffix **-cyte** means "cell."

_____ 4. The suffix **-pathy** means "pertaining to the study of pathology."

_____ 5. The term *adenoidectomy* contains one root word and one suffix.

_____ 6. The term *lymphadenitis* contains one root word and one suffix.

_____ 7. The term *autoimmune* contains a prefix and a suffix.

_____ 8. Pathogens are harmful invaders such as bacteria, viruses, parasites, and antibodies.

_____ 9. Nonspecific immunity is a protective mechanism that provides antibodies against a specific antigen.

_____ 10. An antigen is a specific substance that, when introduced into the body, stimulates the production of an antibody.

_____ 11. Tonsils help protect the body from infection by trapping pathogens that enter through the mouth or nose.

_____ 12. T lymphocytes are involved in a properly functioning immune system.

_____ 13. Hodgkin's disease is a disorder that causes the bronchi to narrow and swell and produce extra mucus.

_____ 14. An autoimmune disorder is a condition that occurs when the immune system attacks and destroys healthy body tissue.

_____ 15. There is only one type of autoimmune disorder.

_____ 16. Rheumatoid arthritis is a chronic, systemic disease that affects the joints.

_____ 17. Multiple sclerosis is caused by damage to the myelin sheaths that cover the nerves in the brain and spinal cord.

_____ 18. AIDS cannot be spread by contact with blood or bodily fluids.

_____ 19. An allergy is an exaggerated reaction of the immune system in response to a substance that the body ordinarily perceives as harmless.

_____ 20. _Tonsillectomy_ means "inflammation of the tonsils."

_____ 21. Sarcoidosis is an inflammatory disease that can affect almost any body part or system.

_____ 22. The Western blot test is a laboratory blood test to detect the presence of antibodies to specific antigens.

Dictionary Skills

Directions: Using a medical dictionary, such as _Taber's Cyclopedic Medical Dictionary_, look up the term **lymphocele**. For each medical term, indicate whether the term appears on the same page as **lymphocele** (_O_), before the page (_B_), or after the page (_A_). Then define each term.

Medical Term   **O, B, A**

1. lymphorrhea   _____

Definition: _____

_____

2. lymphology   _____

Definition: _____

_____

3. lymphocytosis   _____

Definition: _____

_____

4. lymphoblast   _____

Definition: _____

_____

5. lymphomatosis   _____

Definition: _____

_____

6. lymphogenous   _____

Definition: _____

_____

7. lymphangiography   _____

Definition: _____

_____

8. lymphocele   _____

Definition: _____

_____

9. lymphangiectomy   _____

Definition: _____

_____

10. lymphedema   _____

Definition: _____

_____

Break It Down

Directions: Dissect each medical term into its word parts (prefix, root word, combining vowel, and suffix) using one or more slashes. Then define each term.

Example:
Medical Term: lymphangiopathy
Dissection: lymph/angi/o/pathy
Definition: disease of the lymph vessels

Medical Term	Dissection
1. adenitis	a d e n i t i s

Definition: _____

_____

2. splenocyte	s p l e n o c y t e

Definition: _____

_____

3. immunogenic	i m m u n o g e n i c

Definition: _____

_____

4. tonsillopathy	t o n s i l l o p a t h y

Definition: _____

_____

5. adenoma	a d e n o m a

Definition: _____

_____

6. phagocytosis	p h a g o c y t o s i s

Definition: _____

_____

Medical Term	Dissection
7. pathogen	p a t h o g e n

Definition: _____

_____

| 8. lymphadenitis | l y m p h a d e n i t i s |

Definition: _____

_____

| 9. splenogenic | s p l e n o g e n i c |

Definition: _____

_____

| 10. adenolymphoma | a d e n o l y m p h o m a |

Definition: _____

_____

Spelling

Directions: For each medical term, indicate the correct spelling.

1.	lymphadenitis	lymphedenitis	lymphodenitis	lymphadynitis
2.	pathagenic	pathogenec	pathogenic	pathegenic
3.	splennopexy	splenopexxy	splaenopexy	splenopexy
4.	tonsilar	tonsillar	tonsiller	tonsillor
5.	anaphylaxis	anyphalaxis	anephylaxis	anaphalaxis
6.	reumatoid	rheumatoid	rhuematoid	rheumetoid
7.	antigen	antagen	antegen	antogen
8.	sarcoydosis	sarkoydosis	sarcoidossis	sarcoidosis
9.	splenorraphy	splenorhaphy	splenorrhaphy	splenoraphy
10.	lymphodema	lymphedema	lymphedemia	lymphadema
11.	tonsilitis	tonsillitis	tonsylitis	tonsolitis
12.	splenomelacia	splenomalacia	splenomalaysia	splenomalatia

Audio Activity: Kim Lee's Chart Note

Directions: Access your *EduHub* subscription and listen to the recording of the physician reading Kim Lee's chart note. Read along with the physician and pay attention to the pronunciation of each medical term.

CHART NOTE

Patient Name: Lee, Kim
ID Number: KL7214
Examination Date: May 14, 20xx

SUBJECTIVE

This 9-year-old patient presents with chronic nasal congestion, sore throat, and enlarged **tonsils**. Mother states that Kim always breathes through her mouth and snores at night. Also, mother said it is getting to the point where she is having difficulty understanding her since word formation is poor. Patient has a chronic history of strep throat.

OBJECTIVE

Temperature is 101. **Tympanic membranes** (eardrums) are clear. Exam of the **pharynx** reveals markedly enlarged tonsils, almost touching. **Erythema** is present. Nasal mucosa is edematous. Neck is supple without lymphadenopathy. Chest is clear.

ASSESSMENT

Tonsillitis and probable **hypertrophy** of the adenoids.

PLAN

Refer to **ENT** (ear, nose, and throat specialist) for possible **tonsillectomy** and **adenoidectomy**.

Interpret Kim Lee's Chart Note

Directions: Access your *EduHub* subscription and listen to the recording of the physician reading Kim Lee's chart note. After listening to the recording, supply the medical term that matches each definition. You may encounter definitions and terms introduced in previous chapters.

> *Example:* tumor of the lymph cells   *Answer:* lymphocytoma

1. excision of the tonsils

   _____

2. eardrums

   _____

3. excision of the adenoids

   _____

4. the throat

   _____

5. inflammation of the tonsils

   _____

6. tissue structures that protect the body from infection by trapping pathogens that enter through the mouth or nose

   _____

7. above-normal development

   _____

8. ear, nose, and throat specialist

   _____

9. redness

   _____

Chapter 6

Special Sensory Organs: Eye and Ear

ophthalm / o / logy = the study of the eye

ot / o / logy = the study of the ear

Chapter Organization

- Intern Experience
- Overview of Anatomy and Physiology of the Eye and Ear
- Word Elements
- Breaking Down and Building Terms Related to the Eye and Ear
- Diseases and Disorders
- Procedures and Treatments
- Analyzing the Intern Experience
- Working with Medical Records
- Chapter Review

Chapter Objectives

After completing this chapter, you will be able to

1. label anatomical diagrams of the eye and the ear;
2. dissect and define common medical terminology related to the special sensory organs of vision and hearing;
3. build terms used to describe diseases and disorders of the eye and ear, as well as diagnostic procedures and therapeutic treatments;
4. pronounce and spell common medical terminology related to the special sensory organs of vision and hearing;
5. understand that the process of building and dissecting a medical term based on its prefix, root word, and suffix enables you to analyze an extremely large number of medical terms beyond those presented in this chapter;
6. interpret the meaning of abbreviations associated with the special sensory organs of vision and hearing; and
7. interpret medical records containing terminology and abbreviations related to these special sensory organs.

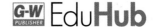

Your *EduHub* subscription that accompanies this text provides access to online assessments, assignments, activities, and resources. Throughout this chapter, access *EduHub* to

- use e-flash cards to review the medical terminology and word parts you learn;
- listen to the correct pronunciations of medical terms; and
- complete medical terminology activities and assignments.

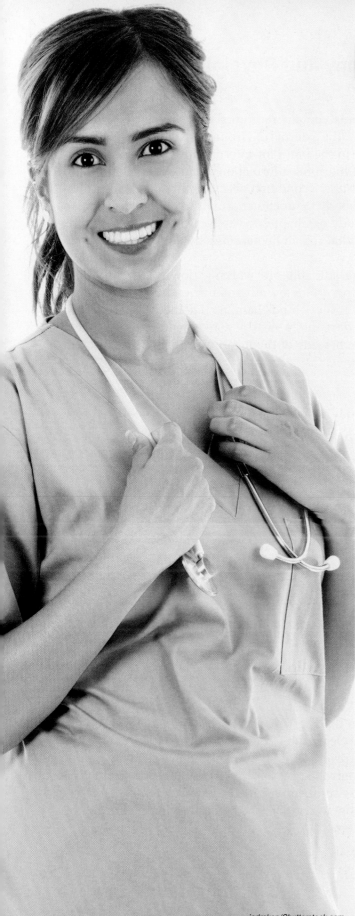

Intern Experience

Debra is in the second week of her internship with University Eye and Ear Specialists, Inc. Sofia Rodriguez called the office as soon as it opened, expressing concern for her four-year-old son, Juan. At the designated appointment time, Debra greets Mrs. Rodriguez and her son in the waiting room and escorts them to an exam room.

Mrs. Rodriguez appears fatigued. She states that she was awakened early that morning by her son's anguished screams. She informs Debra that Juan's face felt hot to the touch, and he was tugging at his left ear. Because Juan has had recurrent ear infections, Mrs. Rodriguez is worried about possible hearing loss. Debra notes the mother's concerns in Juan's chart, obtains Juan's vital signs, and, using her laptop computer, electronically signals to the physician that the patient is ready to be seen.

To help you understand Juan's health condition, this chapter will present word elements (combining forms, prefixes, and suffixes) that make up medical terminology related to the ear, the sensory organ that controls hearing and equilibrium (balance). You will also learn word elements and medical terminology related to the eye, the sensory organ of sight.

Let's begin our study with a brief anatomical and physiological overview of both the eye and the ear. We will cover major structures of these special sensory organs, along with their primary functions. Later in the chapter, you will learn about some common pathological conditions of the eye and ear, tests and procedures used to diagnose those conditions, and common treatment methods.

Overview of Anatomy and Physiology of the Eye and Ear

The special sensory organs contain receptors that receive information about stimuli outside the body (the external environment) and transmit neural impulses about these stimuli to the brain for interpretation. The special sensory organs also process and interpret information about external stimuli to help maintain internal *homeostasis*, a condition of stable physiological equilibrium (balance) that allows the body to function normally. (You will learn more about homeostasis in your study of Chapter 7: The Nervous System.) Organs of the sensory system play a vital role in homeostasis by alerting the body to potential danger.

For example, two college students are walking down a dark, windy street late at night after seeing a movie with some friends. They hear the muffled crunching of stones from behind them, as if someone is following them. The students quickly dart into a nearby convenience store and text their roommates, asking whether one of them can give them a ride back to their dormitory.

In this scenario, both the ears and the eyes—two of the special sensory organs—play a crucial role in alerting the body to potential danger.

Sensory systems of the body include the five commonly recognized sensory organs:

Organ	Function(s)
Eye	Sight (visual)
Ear	Hearing (auditory); equilibrium, or balance (vestibular)
Nose	Smell (olfactory)
Tongue	Taste (gustatory)
Skin	Touch (tactile or somatic)

For the purposes of this chapter, we will limit our discussion of special sensory organs to the eye and the ear.

The Eye

The eye operates much like a camera. Incoming light passes through the **cornea**, similar in function to the aperture (adjustable opening) of a camera (Figure 6.1). The cornea is the clear, outer layer of the eye that covers the iris and pupil; it allows light to travel to the interior of the eye. The amount of light that enters the eye is controlled by the **iris**, the colored portion of the anterior eye. Within the iris is an opening called the **pupil**, which contracts (narrows) and dilates (expands) to regulate the amount of light entering the eye, much like a camera shutter.

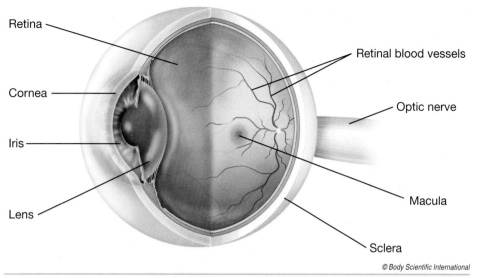

Retina

Cornea

Iris

Lens

Retinal blood vessels

Optic nerve

Macula

Sclera

© Body Scientific International

Figure 6.1 Major structures of the eye

The **lens**, located behind the pupil, focuses the light onto the retina. The **retina** (RĔT-ĭ-nă), the innermost layer of the eye, receives images formed by the lens. It contains light-sensing cells responsible for color vision and fine detail. The retina acts much like camera film—or, in today's technology, the memory card inside a cell phone that carries information about the subscriber's identity. The retina sends information via the **optic nerve** to the brain for interpretation. The **sclera** (SKLĒ-ră) is the white, outer protective layer of the eye.

The Ear

The ear has three main parts: the **external** (outer) **ear**, the **middle ear**, and the **internal** (inner) **ear** (Figure 6.2 on the next page). Sound waves enter the external ear, or **external auditory meatus** (mē-ĂT-ŭs), and pass through the middle ear to the **tympanic** (tĭm-PĂN-ĭk) **membrane** (eardrum), causing it to vibrate. Vibrations in the eardrum are transmitted to the internal ear by three very small bones called **ossicles**. The vibrations are detected by sensory receptors in the inner ear, where the information is transmitted by nerve impulses to the brain. The brain interprets these neural impulses as sound.

Besides the function of hearing, the ear is responsible for your sense of equilibrium, or balance. Fluid in the **semicircular canals**, tiny channels within the inner ear, control orientation and balance. They help you maintain steadiness while standing or walking.

Anatomy and Physiology Vocabulary

Now that you have been introduced to the basic anatomy and physiology of the eye and the ear, we will explore in more detail the key terms presented in the introduction (see table on the next page).

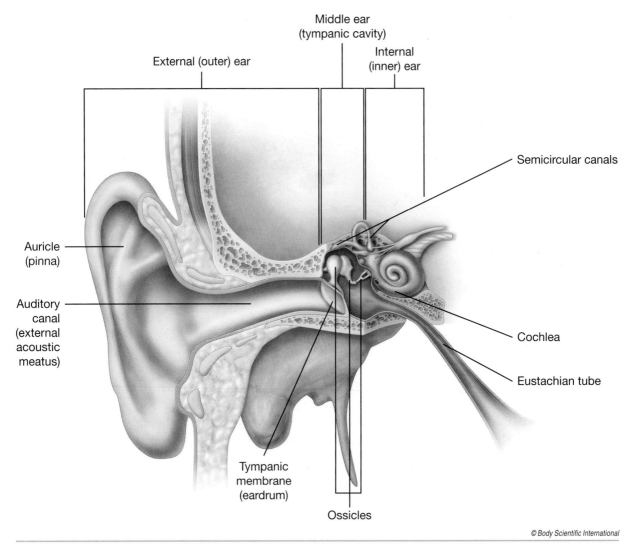

Figure 6.2 Major structures of the ear

© Body Scientific International

Key Term	Definition
cornea	transparent outer layer of the eye that covers the iris and pupil and allows light to enter
external auditory meatus	external (outer) ear
internal ear	inner ear
iris	colored portion of the anterior eye
lens	structure of the eye that focuses light onto the retina
middle ear	central cavity of the ear
optic nerve	nerve that carries impulses for the sense of sight from the retina to the brain

(Continued)

Key Term	Definition
ossicles	three small bones of the ear that transmit vibrations from the eardrum to the internal ear
pupil	opening in the iris that contracts and dilates, regulating the amount of light that enters the eye
retina	innermost layer of the eye that receives images formed by the lens
sclera	white, outer protective layer of the eye
semicircular canals	tiny channels in the inner ear that control balance
tympanic membrane	eardrum

E-Flash Card Activity: Anatomy and Physiology Vocabulary

Directions: After you have reviewed the anatomy and physiology vocabulary related to the sensory organs of sight and hearing, access your *EduHub* subscription and practice with the e-flash cards until you are comfortable with the spelling and definition of each term.

Assessment 6.1

Identifying Major Structures of the Eye

Directions: Label the anatomical diagram of the eye. You can also complete this activity online using *EduHub*.

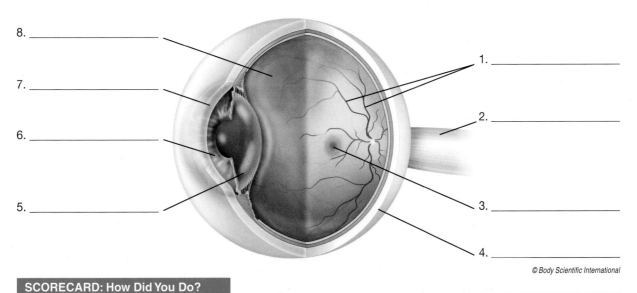

8. _____

7. _____

6. _____

5. _____

1. _____

2. _____

3. _____

4. _____

© Body Scientific International

SCORECARD: How Did You Do?

Number correct (_____), divided by 8 (_____), multiplied by 100 equals _____ (your score)

Identifying Major Structures of the Ear

Directions: Label the anatomical diagram of the ear. You can also complete this activity online using *EduHub*.

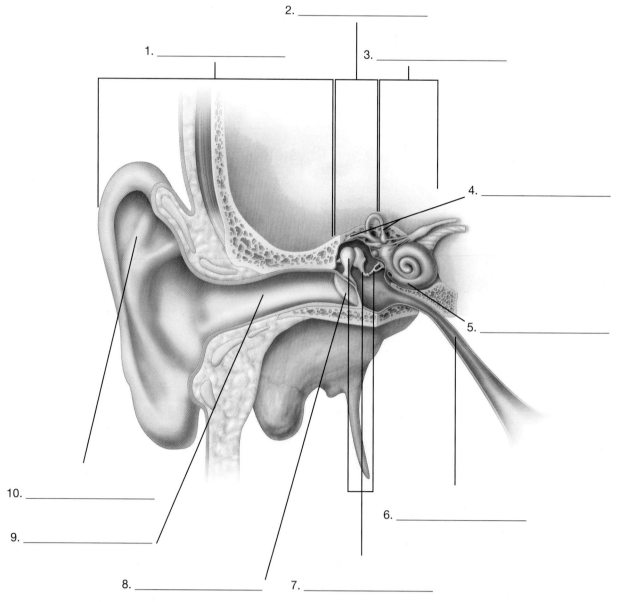

2. _____

1. _____

3. _____

4. _____

5. _____

10. _____

9. _____

6. _____

8. _____

7. _____

© Body Scientific International

Matching Anatomy and Physiology Vocabulary

Directions: Choose the correct vocabulary term for each meaning. You can also complete this activity online using *EduHub*.

_____ 1. colored portion of the anterior eye

_____ 2. nerve that carries impulses for the sense of sight from the retina to the brain

_____ 3. external (outer) ear

_____ 4. three small bones of the ear that transmit vibrations from the eardrum to the internal ear

_____ 5. innermost layer of the eye that receives images formed by the lens

_____ 6. structure of the eye that focuses light onto the retina

_____ 7. inner ear

_____ 8. white, outer protective layer of the eye

_____ 9. eardrum

_____ 10. central cavity of the ear

_____ 11. tiny channels in the inner ear that control balance

_____ 12. opening in the iris that contracts and dilates, regulating the amount of light that enters the eye

_____ 13. transparent outer layer of the eye that covers the iris and pupil and allows light to enter

A. internal ear

B. lens

C. middle ear

D. optic nerve

E. retina

F. tympanic membrane

G. cornea

H. semicircular canals

I. pupil

J. sclera

K. ossicles

L. iris

M. external auditory meatus

SCORECARD: How Did You Do?

Number correct (_____), divided by 13 (_____), multiplied by 100 equals _____ (your score)

Word Elements

In this section, you will learn word elements—prefixes, combining forms, and suffixes—that are common to the special senses. By learning these word elements and understanding how they are combined to build medical terms, you will be able to analyze Juan's health problem (described in the Intern Experience at the beginning of this chapter) and identify a large number of terms associated with the special senses.

E-Flash Card Activity: Word Elements

Directions: Review the word elements in the tables that follow. Then, access your *EduHub* subscription and practice with the e-flash cards until you are able to quickly recognize the different word parts (prefixes, combining forms, and suffixes) and their meanings. The e-flash cards are grouped together by prefixes, combining forms, and suffixes, followed by a cumulative review of all the word elements you are learning in this chapter.

Prefixes

This chapter presents terms that contain the prefixes listed below.

Prefix	Meaning
an-	not; without
extra-	outside
hemi-	half
intra-	inside; within
para-	near; beside
peri-	around

Combining Forms

Listed below are common combining forms used in medical terms pertaining to the sensory organs of vision and hearing.

Root Word/Combining Vowel	Meaning
audi/o	hearing
blephar/o	eyelid
ir/o	iris
irid/o	iris
kerat/o	cornea
myc/o	fungus
myring/o	tympanic membrane; eardrum
ocul/o	eye
ophthalm/o	eye
opt/o	eye; vision
optic/o	eye; vision
ot/o	ear
pleg/o	paralysis
presby/o	old age
retin/o	retina
scler/o	sclera (white of the eye)
tympan/o	tympanic membrane; eardrum

Suffixes

Listed below are suffixes used in medical terms related to the special sensory organs. You have already learned many of these suffixes.

Suffix	Meaning
-al	pertaining to
-algia	pain
-ar	pertaining to
-ectomy	surgical removal; excision
-gram	record; image
-ia	condition
-ic	pertaining to
-itis	inflammation
-logist	specialist in the study and treatment of
-logy	study of
-meter	instrument used to measure
-metry	measurement
-opia	vision
-osis	abnormal condition
-pexy	surgical fixation
-plasty	surgical repair
-ptosis	drooping; downward displacement
-rrhea	discharge; flow
-rrhexis	rupture
-scope	instrument used to observe
-scopy	process of observing
-spasm	involuntary muscle contraction
-stomy	new opening
-tomy	incision; cut into

Matching Prefixes, Combining Forms, and Suffixes

Directions: Choose the correct meaning for each word element. Some meanings may be used more than once. You can also complete this activity online using *EduHub*.

Prefixes

_____ 1. extra-	A.	inside; within
_____ 2. para-	B.	not; without
_____ 3. an-	C.	half
_____ 4. peri-	D.	outside
_____ 5. hemi-	E.	near; beside
_____ 6. intra-	F.	around

Combining Forms

_____ 1. retin/o	A.	iris
_____ 2. ir/o	B.	eye
_____ 3. myring/o	C.	ear
_____ 4. kerat/o	D.	sclera
_____ 5. tympan/o	E.	hearing
_____ 6. audi/o	F.	cornea
_____ 7. opt/o	G.	vision
_____ 8. blephar/o	H.	eyelid
_____ 9. myc/o	I.	fungus
_____ 10. scler/o	J.	tympanic membrane; eardrum
_____ 11. ot/o	K.	retina
_____ 12. irid/o	L.	paralysis
_____ 13. ophthalm/o	M.	old age
_____ 14. ocul/o		
_____ 15. pleg/o		
_____ 16. presby/o		

Suffixes

_____	1. -stomy	A.	pertaining to
_____	2. -metry	B.	pain
_____	3. -ia	C.	discharge; flow
_____	4. -tomy	D.	surgical removal; excision
_____	5. -al	E.	record; image
_____	6. -osis	F.	process of observing
_____	7. -ectomy	G.	inflammation
_____	8. -rrhea	H.	specialist in the study and treatment of
_____	9. -algia	I.	study of
_____	10. -scopy	J.	instrument used to measure
_____	11. -ar	K.	measurement
_____	12. -plasty	L.	vision
_____	13. -ic	M.	incision; cut into
_____	14. -scope	N.	abnormal condition
_____	15. -logist	O.	surgical fixation
_____	16. -meter	P.	surgical repair
_____	17. -spasm	Q.	condition
_____	18. -gram	R.	drooping; downward displacement
_____	19. -rrhexis	S.	involuntary muscle contraction
_____	20. -itis	T.	rupture
_____	21. -ptosis	U.	instrument used to observe
_____	22. -logy	V.	new opening
_____	23. -pexy		
_____	24. -opia		

SCORECARD: How Did You Do?

Number correct (_____), divided by 46 (_____), multiplied by 100 equals _____ (your score)

Breaking Down and Building Terms Related to the Eye and Ear

Now that you have mastered the prefixes, combining forms, and suffixes for medical terminology used to describe the special sensory organs of sight and hearing, you have the ability to dissect and build a large number of terms related to these special sensory systems.

Below is a list of common medical terms related to the study and treatment of the eye and the ear. For each term, a dissection has been provided, along with the meaning of each word element and the definition of the term as a whole.

Term	Dissection	Word Part/Meaning	Term Meaning
Note: *For simplification, combining vowels have been omitted from the Word Part/Meaning column.*			
1. **audiogram** (AW-dē-ō-grăm)	audi/o/gram	**audi** = hearing **gram** = record; image	record of hearing
2. **audiologist** (AW-dē-ŎL-ō-jĭst)	audi/o/logist	**audi** = hearing **logist** = specialist in the study and treatment of	specialist in the study and treatment of hearing
3. **audiology** (AW-dē-ŎL-ō-jē)	audi/o/logy	**audi** = hearing **logy** = study of	study of hearing
4. **audiometer** (AW-dē-ŎM-ě-ter)	audi/o/meter	**audi** = hearing **meter** = instrument used to measure	instrument used to measure hearing
5. **audiometry** (AW-dē-ŎM-ě-trē)	audi/o/metry	**audi** = hearing **metry** = measurement	measurement of hearing
6. **blepharitis** (BLĔF-ă-RĪ-tĭs)	blephar/itis	**blephar** = eyelid **itis** = inflammation	inflammation of the eyelid
7. **blepharoplasty** (BLĔF-ă-rō-PLĂS-tē)	blephar/o/plasty	**blephar** = eyelid **plasty** = surgical repair	surgical repair of the eyelid
8. **blepharoplegia** (BLĔF-ă-rō-PLĒ-jē-ă)	blephar/o/pleg/ia	**blephar** = eyelid **pleg** = paralysis **ia** = condition	condition of eyelid paralysis
9. **blepharoptosis** (BLĔF-ă-rŏp-TŌ-sĭs)	blephar/o/ptosis	**blephar** = eyelid **ptosis** = drooping; downward displacement	drooping of the eyelid
10. **blepharospasm** (BLĔF-ă-rō-SPĂZM)	blephar/o/spasm	**blephar** = eyelid **spasm** = involuntary muscle contraction	involuntary muscle contraction of the eyelid
11. **extraocular** (ĔKS-tră-ŎK-yū-lăr)	extra/ocul/ar	**extra** = outside **ocul** = eye **ar** = pertaining to	pertaining to the outside of the eye

Prefixes = Green   Root Words = Red   Suffixes = Blue

Term	Dissection	Word Part/Meaning	Term Meaning
12. **iridectomy** (ĬR-ĭ-DĔK-tō-mē)	irid/ectomy	**irid** = iris **ectomy** = surgical removal; excision	excision of the iris
13. **iridopexy** (ĬR-ĭd-ō-PĔK-sē)	irid/o/pexy	**irid** = iris **pexy** = surgical fixation	surgical fixation of the iris
14. **iridoplasty** (ĬR-ĭd-ō-PLĂS-tē)	irid/o/plasty	**irid** = iris **plasty** = surgical repair	surgical repair of the iris
15. **iridoplegia** (ĬR-ĭd-ō-PLĒ-jē-ă)	irid/o/pleg/ia	**irid** = iris **pleg** = paralysis **ia** = condition	condition of iris paralysis
16. **iritis** (ĭr-Ī-tĭs)	ir/itis	**ir** = iris **itis** = inflammation	inflammation of the iris
17. **keratometer** (kĕr-ă-TŎM-ĕ-ter)	kerat/o/meter	**kerat** = cornea **meter** = instrument used to measure	instrument used to measure the cornea
18. **keratometry** (kĕr-ă-TŎM-ĕ-trē)	kerat/o/metry	**kerat** = cornea **metry** = measurement	measurement of the cornea
19. **myringectomy** (mĭr-ĭn-JĔK-tō-mē)	myring/ectomy	**myring** = tympanic membrane; eardrum **ectomy** = surgical removal; excision	excision of the eardrum
20. **myringitis** (mĭr-ĭn-JĪ-tĭs)	myring/itis	**myring** = tympanic membrane; eardrum **itis** = inflammation	inflammation of the eardrum
21. **myringoplasty** (mĭr-ĬNG-gō-plăst-ē)	myring/o/plasty	**myring** = tympanic membrane; eardrum **plasty** = surgical repair	surgical repair of the eardrum
22. **myringotomy** (mĭr-ĭng-GŎT-ō-mē)	myring/o/tomy	**myring** = tympanic membrane; eardrum **tomy** = incision; cut into	incision to the eardrum
23. **ocular** (ŎK-yū-lăr)	ocul/ar	**ocul** = eye **ar** = pertaining to	pertaining to the eye
24. **oculomycosis** (ŎK-yū-lō-mī-KŌ-sĭs)	ocul/o/myc/osis	**ocul** = eye **myc** = fungus **osis** = abnormal condition	abnormal condition of fungus in the eye
25. **ophthalmic** (ŏf-THĂL-mĭk)	ophthalm/ic	**ophthalm** = eye **ic** = pertaining to	pertaining to the eye

Prefixes = Green   Root Words = Red   Suffixes = Blue

Term	Dissection	Word Part/Meaning	Term Meaning
26. **ophthalmologist** (ŎF-thăl-MŎL-ō-jĭst)	ophthalm/o/logist	**ophthalm** = eye **logist** = specialist in the study and treatment of	specialist in the study and treatment of the eye
27. **ophthalmology** (ŎF-thăl-MŎL-ō-jē)	ophthalm/o/logy	**ophthalm** = eye **logy** = study of	study of the eye
28. **ophthalmoscope** (ŏf-THĂL-mō-skōp)	ophthalm/o/scope	**ophthalm** = eye **scope** = instrument used to observe	instrument used to observe the eye
29. **optic** (ŎP-tĭk)	opt/ic	**opt** = eye; vision **ic** = pertaining to	pertaining to the eye or vision
30. **otalgia** (ō-TĂL-jē-ă)	ot/algia	**ot** = ear **algia** = pain	pain in the ear
31. **otitis** (ō-TĪ-tĭs)	ot/itis	**ot** = ear **itis** = inflammation	inflammation of the ear
32. **otologist** (ō-TŎL-ō-jĭst)	ot/o/logist	**ot** = ear **logist** = specialist in the study and treatment of	specialist in the study and treatment of the ear
33. **otology** (ō-TŎL-ō-jē)	ot/o/logy	**ot** = ear **logy** = study of	study of the ear
34. **otomycosis** (Ō-tō-mī-KŌ-sĭs)	ot/o/myc/osis	**ot** = ear **myc** = fungus **osis** = abnormal condition	abnormal condition of fungus in the ear
35. **otoplasty** (Ō-tō-PLĂS-tē)	ot/o/plasty	**ot** = ear **plasty** = surgical repair	surgical repair of the ear
36. **otorrhea** (ō-tō-RĒ-ă)	ot/o/rrhea	**ot** = ear **rrhea** = discharge; flow	discharge from the ear
37. **otoscope** (Ō-tō-skōp)	ot/o/scope	**ot** = ear **scope** = instrument used to observe	instrument used to observe the ear
38. **otoscopy** (ō-TŎS-kō-pē)	ot/o/scopy	**ot** = ear **scopy** = process of observing	process of observing the ear
39. **paraocular** (PĂR-ă-ŎK-yū-lăr)	para/ocul/ar	**para** = near; beside **ocul** = eye **ar** = pertaining to	pertaining to near the eye
40. **periocular** (PĔR-ē-ŎK-yū-lăr)	peri/ocul/ar	**peri** = around **ocul** = eye **ar** = pertaining to	pertaining to around the eye

Prefixes = Green   Root Words = **Red**   Suffixes = Blue

Term	Dissection	Word Part/Meaning	Term Meaning
41. **retinal** (RĔT-ĭ-năl)	retin/al	**retin** = retina **al** = pertaining to	pertaining to the retina
42. **retinitis** (RĔT-ĭ-NĪ-tĭs)	retin/itis	**retin** = retina **itis** = inflammation	inflammation of the retina
43. **scleral** (SKLĔR-ăl)	scler/al	**scler** = sclera **al** = pertaining to	pertaining to the sclera
44. **scleritis** (sklĕ-RĪ-tĭs)	scler/itis	**scler** = sclera **itis** = inflammation	inflammation of the sclera
45. **sclerotomy** (sklĕ-RŎT-ō-mē)	scler/o/tomy	**scler** = sclera **tomy** = incision; cut into	incision to the sclera
46. **tympanectomy** (tĭm-păn-ĔK-tō-mē)	tympan/ectomy	**tympan** = tympanic membrane; eardrum **ectomy** = excision; surgical removal	excision of the eardrum
47. **tympanic** (tĭm-PĂN-ĭk)	tympan/ic	**tympan** = tympanic membrane; eardrum **ic** = pertaining to	pertaining to the eardrum
48. **tympanometer** (TĬM-pă-NŎM-ĕ-tĕr)	tympan/o/meter	**tympan** = tympanic membrane; eardrum **meter** = instrument used to measure	instrument used to measure the eardrum
49. **tympanometry** (TĬM-pă-NŎM-ĕ-trē)	tympan/o/metry	**tympan** = tympanic membrane; eardrum **metry** = measurement	measurement of the eardrum
50. **tympanoplasty** (TĬM-păn-ō-PLĂS-tē)	tympan/o/plasty	**tympan** = tympanic membrane; eardrum **plasty** = surgical repair	surgical repair of the eardrum
51. **tympanorrhexis** (TĬM-păn-ŏr-RĔKS-ĭs)	tympan/o/rrhexis	**tympan** = tympanic membrane; eardrum **rrhexis** = rupture	rupture of the eardrum
52. **tympanostomy** (TĬM-păn-ŎS-tō-mē)	tympan/o/stomy	**tympan** = tympanic membrane; eardrum **stomy** = new opening	new opening in the eardrum

Prefixes = Green   Root Words = Red   Suffixes = Blue

Using the pronunciation guide from the Break It Down chart above, practice saying each medical term aloud. To hear the pronunciation of each term, complete the Pronounce It activity on the next page.

Audio Activity: Pronounce It

Directions: Access your *EduHub* subscription and listen to the correct pronunciations of the following medical terms. Practice pronouncing the terms until you are comfortable saying them aloud.

audiogram
(AW-dē-ō-grăm)

audiologist
(AW-dē-ŎL-ō-jĭst)

audiology
(AW-dē-ŎL-ō-jē)

audiometer
(AW-dē-ŎM-ĕ-ter)

audiometry
(AW-dē-ŎM-ĕ-trē)

blepharitis
(BLĔF-ă-RĪ-tĭs)

blepharoplasty
(BLĔF-ă-rō-PLĂS-tē)

blepharoplegia
(BLĔF-ă-rō-PLĒ-jē-ă)

blepharoptosis
(BLĔF-ă-rŏp-TŌ-sĭs)

blepharospasm
(BLĔF-ă-rō-SPĂZM)

extraocular
(ĔKS-tră-ŎK-yū-lăr)

iridectomy
(ĬR-ĭ-DĔK-tō-mē)

iridopexy
(ĬR-ĭd-ō-PĔK-sē)

iridoplasty
(ĬR-ĭd-ō-PLĂS-tē)

iridoplegia
(ĬR-ĭd-ō-PLĒ-jē-ă)

iritis
(ĭr-Ī-tĭs)

keratometer
(kĕr-ă-TŎM-ĕ-ter)

keratometry
(kĕr-ă-TŎM-ĕ-trē)

myringectomy
(mĭr-ĭn-JĔK-tō-mē)

myringitis
(mĭr-ĭn-JĪ-tĭs)

myringoplasty
(mĭr-ĬNG-gō-plăst-ē)

myringotomy
(mĭr-ĭng-GŎT-ō-mē)

ocular
(ŎK-yū-lăr)

oculomycosis
(ŎK-yū-lō-mī-KŌ-sĭs)

ophthalmic
(ŏf-THĂL-mĭk)

ophthalmologist
(ŎF-thăl-MŎL-ō-jĭst)

ophthalmology
(ŎF-thăl-MŎL-ō-jē)

ophthalmoscope
(ŏf-THĂL-mō-skōp)

optic
(ŎP-tĭk)

otalgia
(ō-TĂL-jē-ă)

otitis
(ō-TĪ-tĭs)

otologist
(ō-TŎL-ō-jĭst)

otology
(ō-TŎL-ō-jē)

otomycosis
(Ō-tō-mī-KŌ-sĭs)

otoplasty
(Ō-tō-PLĂS-tē)

otorrhea
(ō-tō-RĒ-ă)

otoscope
(Ō-tō-skōp)

otoscopy
(ō-TŎS-kō-pē)

paraocular
(PĂR-ă-ŎK-yū-lăr)

periocular
(PĔR-ē-ŎK-yū-lăr)

retinal
(RĔT-ĭ-năl)

retinitis
(RĔT-ĭ-NĪ-tĭs)

scleral
(SKLĔR-ăl)

scleritis
(sklĕ-RĪ-tĭs)

sclerotomy
(sklĕ-RŎT-ō-mē)

tympanectomy
(tĭm-păn-ĔK-tō-mē)

tympanic
(tĭm-PĂN-ĭk)

tympanometer
(TĬM-pă-NŎM-ĕ-tĕr)

tympanometry
(TĬM-pă-NŎM-ĕ-trē)

tympanoplasty
(TĬM-păn-ō-PLĂS-tē)

tympanorrhexis
(TĬM-păn-ŏr-RĔKS-ĭs)

tympanostomy
(TĬM-păn-ŎS-tō-mē)

Audio Activity: Spell It

Directions: Access your *EduHub* subscription and listen to the pronunciation for each number. As you hear each term, write its correct spelling.

1. _____
2. _____
3. _____
4. _____
5. _____
6. _____
7. _____
8. _____
9. _____
10. _____
11. _____
12. _____
13. _____
14. _____
15. _____
16. _____
17. _____
18. _____
19. _____
20. _____
21. _____
22. _____
23. _____
24. _____
25. _____
26. _____

27. _____
28. _____
29. _____
30. _____
31. _____
32. _____
33. _____
34. _____
35. _____
36. _____
37. _____
38. _____
39. _____
40. _____
41. _____
42. _____
43. _____
44. _____
45. _____
46. _____
47. _____
48. _____
49. _____
50. _____
51. _____
52. _____

SCORECARD: How Did You Do?

Number correct (_____), divided by 52 (_____), multiplied by 100 equals _____ (your score)

Break It Down

Directions: Dissect each medical term into its word parts (prefix, root word, combining vowel, and suffix) using one or more slashes. Then define each term. You can also complete this activity online using *EduHub*.

Example:

Medical Term: oculomycosis

Dissection: ocul/o/myc/osis

Definition: abnormal condition of fungus in the eye

Medical Term	Dissection
1. blepharoptosis	b l e p h a r o p t o s i s

Definition: _____

_____

| 2. scleritis | s c l e r i t i s |

Definition: _____

_____

| 3. opthalmoscope | o p t h a l m o s c o p e |

Definition: _____

_____

| 4. tympanic | t y m p a n i c |

Definition: _____

_____

| 5. audiometry | a u d i o m e t r y |

Definition: _____

_____

| 6. iridoplasty | i r i d o p l a s t y |

Definition: _____

_____

Medical Term	Dissection
7. paraocular	p a r a o c u l a r

Definition: _____

_____

8. myringectomy   m y r i n g e c t o m y

Definition: _____

_____

9. optic   o p t i c

Definition: _____

_____

10. otorrhea   o t o r r h e a

Definition: _____

_____

11. extraocular   e x t r a o c u l a r

Definition: _____

_____

12. iridectomy   i r i d e c t o m y

Definition: _____

_____

13. retinal   r e t i n a l

Definition: _____

_____

14. periocular   p e r i o c u l a r

Definition: _____

_____

Medical Term	Dissection
15. tympanorrhexis	t y m p a n o r r h e x i s

Definition: _____

_____

16. blepharoplegia   b l e p h a r o p l e g i a

Definition: _____

_____

17. iridopexy   i r i d o p e x y

Definition: _____

_____

18. keratometry   k e r a t o m e t r y

Definition: _____

_____

19. otitis   o t i t i s

Definition: _____

_____

20. otoscope   o t o s c o p e

Definition: _____

_____

SCORECARD: How Did You Do?

Number correct (_____), divided by 20 (_____), multiplied by 100 equals _____ (your score)

Build It

Directions: Build the medical term that matches each definition by supplying the correct word parts. You can also complete this activity online using *EduHub*.

P (Prefixes) = Green
RW (Root Words) = Red
S (Suffixes) = Blue
CV (Combining Vowel) = Purple

1. record of hearing

   _____ _____ _____
         RW   CV   S

2. excision of the eardrum **(two possible answers)**

   _____ _____
         RW   S

   _____ _____
         RW   S

3. instrument used to measure hearing

   _____ _____ _____
         RW   CV   S

4. rupture of the eardrum

   _____ _____ _____
         RW   CV   S

5. surgical repair of the eyelid

   _____ _____ _____
         RW   CV   S

6. excision of the iris

   _____ _____
         RW   S

7. study of the eye

   _____ _____ _____
         RW   CV   S

8. inflammation of the iris

_____ _____
RW   S

9. new opening in the eardrum

_____ _____ _____
RW   CV   S

10. instrument used to measure the cornea

_____ _____ _____
RW   CV   S

11. involuntary muscle contraction of the eyelid

_____ _____ _____
RW   CV   S

12. inflammation of the eardrum

_____ _____
RW   S

13. condition of eyelid paralysis

_____ _____ _____ _____
RW   CV   RW   S

14. pain in the ear

_____ _____
RW   S

15. specialist in the study and treatment of the ear

_____ _____ _____
RW   CV   S

SCORECARD: How Did You Do?

Number correct (_____), divided by 15 (_____), multiplied by 100 equals _____ (your score)

Diseases and Disorders

Diseases and disorders of the special sensory organs range from the mild to the severe and have a wide variety of causes. We will briefly examine some problems that commonly affect the eye and the ear.

The Eye

The eyes are among the most delicate organs of the body. Some eye conditions, such as minor infections, are short lived. Others require corrective treatment such as eyeglasses, contact lenses, or surgery. Left untreated, serious eye conditions—especially those linked with systemic pathology (for example, diabetic retinopathy)—can result in permanent loss of vision.

Astigmatism and Refractive Errors

Astigmatism (ă-STĬG-mă-tĭzm) is a common condition that causes blurred vision due to an irregularly shaped cornea or curvature of the lens (Figure 6.3). An irregular-shaped cornea or lens prevents light from properly focusing on the retina. As a result, vision becomes distorted or blurred at any distance, causing eye discomfort and headaches.

Astigmatism is often present at birth and may occur in conjunction with myopia or hyperopia (Figure 6.4 on the next page). **Myopia** (mī-ŌP-ē-ă), more commonly known as *nearsightedness*, is a condition in which close objects are seen clearly, but objects farther away appear blurred. **Hyperopia** (HĪ-pĕr-ŌP-ē-ă), or *farsightedness*, is a condition in which distant objects are usually seen clearly, but close ones do not come into proper focus. Together, myopia and hyperopia are referred to as *refractive errors* because they affect how the eyes *refract*, or bend, light. The specific cause of astigmatism is unknown.

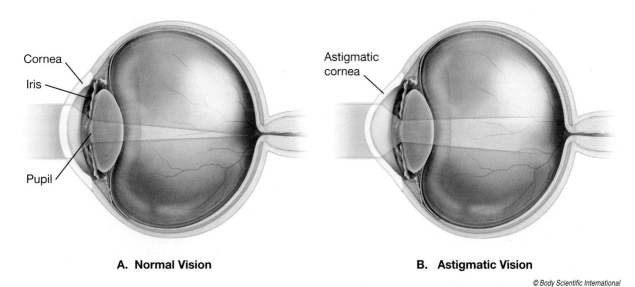

A. Normal Vision

B. Astigmatic Vision

© *Body Scientific International*

Figure 6.3 Astigmatism, the result of an irregularly shaped cornea or curvature of the lens, prevents light rays from properly focusing on the retina, causing blurred or distorted vision.

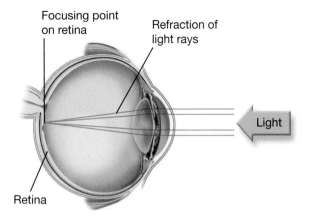

A. **Normal vision:**
Light rays focus on the retina.

Cataract

A **cataract** (KĂT-ă-răct) is a clouding of the lens of the eye (Figure 6.5). The lens of the eye is normally clear. It functions like the lens of a camera, focusing light that travels to the retina at the back of the eye. Normally, the shape of the lens is able to change, allowing the eye to focus on an object close or far away. With age, the lens begins to break down and becomes cloudy. As a result, vision may become blurred.

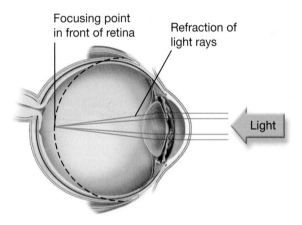

B. **Myopia (nearsightedness):**
Light rays focus in front of the retina.

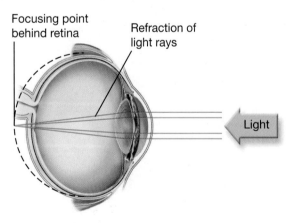

C. **Hyperopia (farsightedness):**
Light rays focus beyond the retina.

© Body Scientific International

Figure 6.4 Myopia and hyperopia

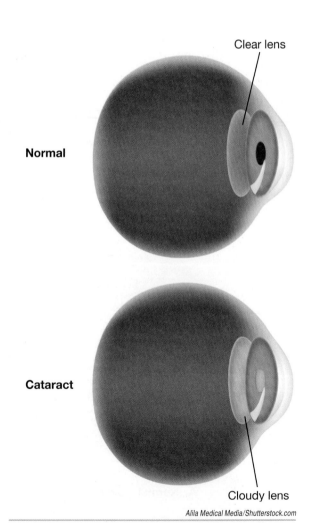

Alila Medical Media/Shutterstock.com

Figure 6.5 A cataract is a clouding of the lens of the eye. Cataracts are typically associated with aging.

Diabetic Retinopathy

Diabetic retinopathy (RĔT-ĭ-NŎP-ă-thē) is a serious complication of diabetes marked by progressive damage to the blood vessels of the retina. It is a chronic condition that can develop in patients with uncontrolled diabetes. In the early stages of diabetic retinopathy, patients are often asymptomatic (without symptoms). As the condition progresses, it may result in blurred or fluctuating vision (sight that "comes and goes"), floaters (small spots or specks that float around in the field of vision), dark or empty areas in the vision, or difficulty with color perception. Typically, diabetic retinopathy affects both eyes.

Glaucoma

Glaucoma (glaw-KŌ-mă) is a group of eye conditions that cause optic nerve damage, which may lead to loss of vision. The optic nerve carries visual information from the eye to the brain. In most cases, damage to this nerve is the result of abnormally high *intraocular pressure (IOP)*, or pressure within the eye. Because glaucoma damage is gradual, the patient may not notice any loss of vision until the disease has reached an advanced stage. Glaucoma is a major cause of blindness in the United States.

Macular Degeneration

Macular degeneration is a leading cause of vision loss among Americans 60 years of age and older. In macular degeneration, the central portion of the retina, called the *macular area*, degenerates over time, resulting in loss of central vision (Figure 6.6). Varying degrees of peripheral vision remain, but those afflicted with macular degeneration are often unable to read or drive, and other activities of daily living are severely restricted due to the loss of full, clear vision.

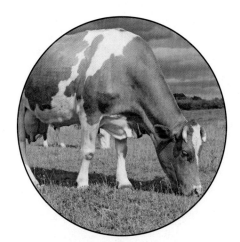 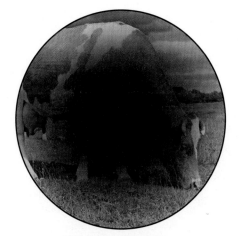

How a scene appears with normal vision

How a scene appears with vision affected by macular degeneration

Photo credit: smereka/Shutterstock.com. Concept adapted from Lighthouse International;
http://lighthouse.org/about-low-vision-blindness/vision-disorders/age-related-macular-degeneration-amd/

Figure 6.6 Macular degeneration

Presbyopia

Presbyopia (PRĔZ-bē-ŌP-ē-ă) is a condition in which the lens of the eye gradually loses its elasticity, or the ability to change its shape, causing difficulty seeing objects up close. Presbyopia occurs naturally with age; thus, it is often called the "aging eye condition." As the lens of the eye becomes less flexible, it no longer can change shape to focus on images at close range. As a result, objects appear out of focus.

The Ear

Infection or disease of the ear can affect hearing, balance, or both. Certain conditions of the ear can cause hearing disorders or deafness. We will take a brief look at some of the more common conditions.

Ménière's Disease

Ménière's (mĕn-YĔRZ) **disease** is a chronic inner-ear disorder that affects balance and hearing (Figure 6.7). The inner ear contains semicircular canals, or small fluid-filled tubes that help your body maintain its position and balance. Every time you move your head, the fluid within the canals stimulates tiny hairs lining each canal. These hairs interpret the movement of the fluid and transmit neural impulses to the brain. The cause of Ménière's disease is unknown. Symptoms include dizziness or a sensation of spinning called **vertigo** (VĔR-tĭ-gō or vĕr-TĒ-gō); **tinnitus** (TĬN-ĭ-tŭs or tĭ-NĪ-tŭs), commonly known as "ringing in the ears"; pressure within the ear; and hearing loss.

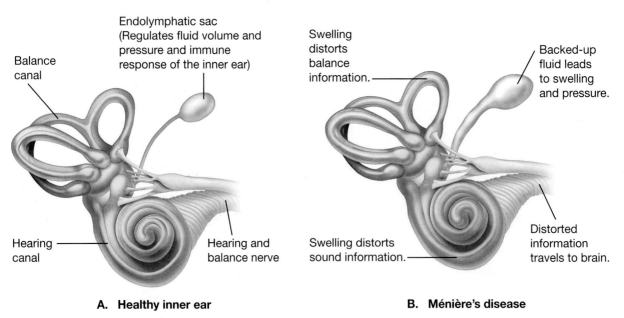

A. **Healthy inner ear**

Balance canal

Endolymphatic sac (Regulates fluid volume and pressure and immune response of the inner ear)

Hearing canal

Hearing and balance nerve

B. **Ménière's disease**

Swelling distorts balance information.

Backed-up fluid leads to swelling and pressure.

Swelling distorts sound information.

Distorted information travels to brain.

Figure 6.7 Ménière's disease

Otitis Media

Otitis media (ō-TĪ-tĭs MĒ-dē-ă) is a bacterial or viral infection of the middle ear (Figure 6.8). It is more common in children than in adults. The *otalgia* (ō-TĂL-jē-ă), or ear pain, that accompanies otitis media is due to inflammation and buildup of fluid in the middle ear. Persistent ear infections can cause hearing problems and other serious complications.

Presbycusis

Presbycusis (PRĔZ-bē-KŪ-sĭs) is the gradual loss of hearing that occurs as people age. Although there is no single known cause for presbycusis, it is most commonly associated with degenerative changes to the inner ear. One of the hallmarks of presbycusis is difficulty hearing high-frequency sound, such as that produced by someone talking, particularly amid background noise. Genetic factors as well as repeated or prolonged exposure to loud noises can contribute to age-related hearing loss.

Procedures and Treatments

We will now briefly review common diagnostic tests and procedures used to help identify disorders and diseases of the eyes and ears, as well as some common therapeutic treatments.

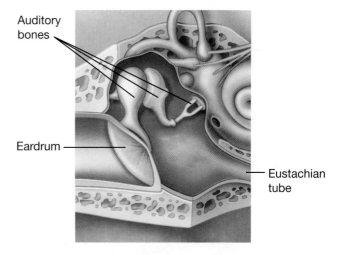

A. Normal middle ear

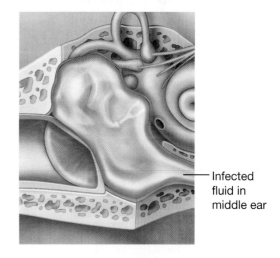

B. Otitis media

© *Body Scientific International*

Figure 6.8 Middle ear infection

The Eye

A variety of procedures are used to test visual acuity and help diagnose diseases and disorders of the eye, and rapidly developing technologies have brought about cutting-edge treatments. For the purpose of this brief overview, we will present a few common procedures and treatments.

Visual Acuity Test

The **visual acuity** (ă-KYŪ-ĭ-tē) **test** is a routine part of an eye examination. The Snellen chart, a standardized eye chart, is used to assess eyesight clarity and detect problems with vision (Figure 6.9).

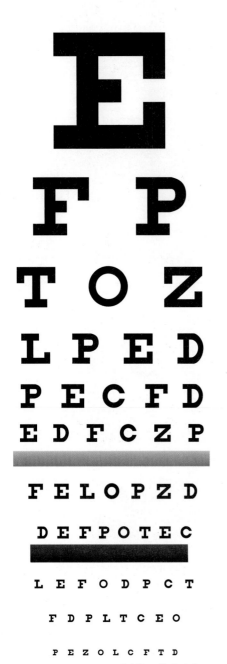

Radu Bercan/Shutterstock.com

Figure 6.9 The Snellen chart is used to test visual acuity.

During an eye exam, the patient covers one eye at a time and reads aloud the smallest line of letters that he or she can see on the Snellen chart. Visual acuity is expressed as a fraction. The top number refers to the distance from which the patient reads the chart, typically 20 feet. The bottom number indicates the distance from which a person with normal vision can read the line. Vision of 20/20 is considered normal. A reading of 20/30 indicates that the line read by the patient reading at a distance of 20 feet away can be read by a person with normal vision at a distance of 30 feet away.

Abnormal results of a visual acuity test may indicate a need for glasses or contact lenses due to an eye condition (such as astigmatism, myopia, or hyperopia) that needs further evaluation by an ophthalmologist. Besides attempting to read the smallest line of type on the Snellen chart, the patient may be asked to read letters or numbers from a card held 14 inches from the face in a test of near vision. For very young children or patients who cannot read, visual acuity is tested with pictures instead of letters.

Blepharoplasty

Blepharoplasty (BLĔF-ă-rō-PLĂS-tē) is the surgical repair of drooping eyelids (Figure 6.10). It can be both a functional (necessary) and a cosmetic surgery. During the procedure, excess skin and fat are removed or repositioned, and surrounding muscles and tendons may be reinforced.

With age, the eyelids stretch and muscular support weakens, resulting in excess fat above and below the eyelids. This causes sagging eyebrows, drooping upper lids, and puffy "bags" under the eyes. Severely sagging skin around the eyes can impair peripheral (side) vision. Blepharoplasty can reduce or eliminate impaired vision and improve appearance.

Fluorescein Angiography

Fluorescein (flor-ĔS-ē-ĭn) **angiography** (ĂN-jē-ŎG-ră-fē) is a photographic method of imaging the retina. A fluorescein dye (an orange fluorescent dye) is injected into a vein in the patient's arm. As the dye circulates throughout the body, multiple photographs are taken of the blood vessels in the eye. Fluorescein angiography is used to diagnose and document eye disease and to monitor response to therapy. It aids the physician in diagnosing retinal and vascular disease, diabetes, macular degeneration, intraocular tumors, and other conditions.

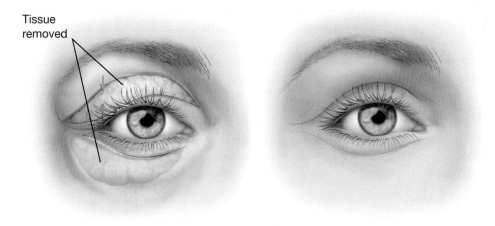

Tissue removed

© Body Scientific International

Figure 6.10 Blepharoplasty is the surgical repair of drooping eyelids.

LASIK

LASIK is an acronym for **laser-assisted in situ (SĪ-tū) keratomileusis** (KĔR-ă-tō-mī-LŪ-sĭs), a type of refractive surgery performed to correct myopia, hyperopia, or astigmatism (Figure 6.11). Other common names for LASIK include *laser eye surgery* and *laser vision correction*. The procedure changes the shape of the cornea so that light rays entering the eye focus more precisely on the retina rather than at some point before or beyond the retina. LASIK eliminates or reduces the need for eyeglasses or contact lenses.

Tonometry

Tonometry (tō-NŎM-ĕ-trē) is a test for measuring pressure within the eyes. It is used to screen for glaucoma. There are several tonometric methods of glaucoma testing. In one method, the surface of the eye is numbed with eyedrops to prevent discomfort. Then an orange or yellow fluorescein dye is applied to the eye with drops or a special strip of paper. A low-power microscope called a *slit lamp* is moved toward the

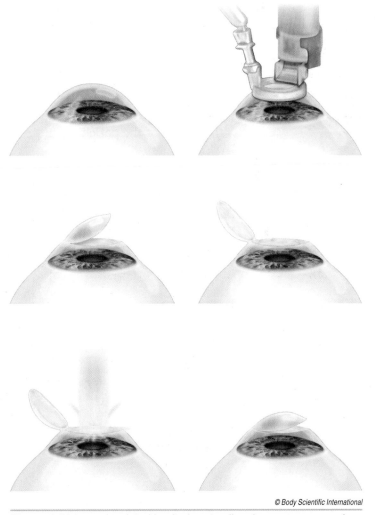

© Body Scientific International

Figure 6.11 Laser-assisted in situ keratomileusis, more commonly known as LASIK surgery

eye until it makes very light contact with the cornea, where it records a pressure reading. Another form of tonometric testing is a noncontact method that uses a puff of air to record eye pressure. A tiny device barely touches the outside of the eye and instantly records eye pressure by analyzing how the light reflections change as the air strikes the eye.

The Ear

In this section, you will learn about some common diagnostic technologies and treatment methods related to the special sensory organ of hearing and balance.

Audiometry

An **audiometry** exam is a hearing test that measures a person's ability to hear different sounds, pitches, and frequencies (Figure 6.12). Sounds vary based on their *intensity* (loudness) and *tone* (the speed of sound-wave vibrations). Hearing occurs when sound waves stimulate the nerves of the inner ear and then travel along neural pathways to the brain, where they are interpreted.

During an audiometry test, the patient wears headphones that cover both ears to eliminate outside noise. The headphones are connected to an **audiometer** (AW-dē-ŎM-ĕ-ter) that produces a series of tones at different frequencies (high or low pitches) and varying intensities (loud or soft). The patient presses a button or raises a hand to indicate when a tone is heard. Audiometry measures the ability of the patient to discriminate between different sound intensities,

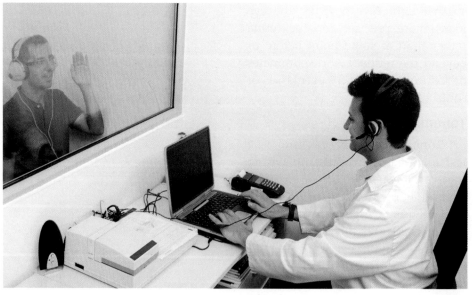

iStock.com/Maica

Figure 6.12 Audiometry

recognize different pitches, and distinguish speech from background noise. The test evaluates hearing loss and aids the physician in determining whether a patient needs a hearing aid.

Myringotomy

A **myringotomy** (mĭr-ĭng-GŎT-ō-mē), also called a **tympanostomy** (TĬM-păn-ŎS-tō-mē), is a surgical procedure in which a small incision is made in the *tympanic membrane* (eardrum) to relieve pressure and inflammation caused by fluid accumulation in the middle ear (Figure 6.13). Tympanostomy tubes, or small tubes that are open at both ends, are inserted into the surgically created opening. The procedure allows drainage of fluid or pus (*effusion*) and provides ventilation to the middle ear in patients suffering from otitis media. The tubes are left in place until they fall out by themselves or are removed by a physician.

Myringoplasty

Myringoplasty (mĭr-ĬNG-gō-plăst-ē), also known as **tympanoplasty** (TĬM-păn-ō-PLĂS-tē), is the surgical repair of a perforated tympanic membrane (hole in the eardrum). A perforated eardrum is usually caused by an infection in the middle ear that bursts through the eardrum, but it may also result from trauma. A perforated tympanic membrane may lead to repeated ear infections and hearing loss. Surgery can prevent recurring ear infection and sometimes improve hearing.

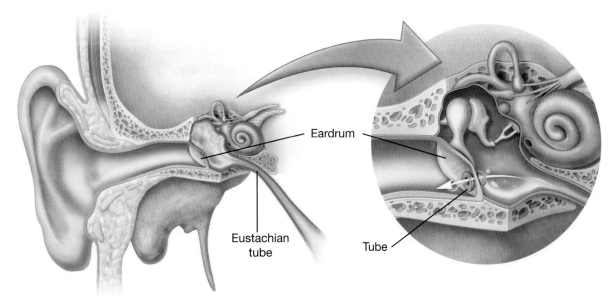

Eardrum

Eustachian tube

Tube

Figure 6.13 Myringotomy

Multiple Choice: Diseases and Disorders

Directions: Choose the disease or disorder that matches each definition. You can also complete this activity online using *EduHub*.

_____ 1. nearsightedness
    a. tinnitus   c. hyperopia
    b. myopia   d. vertigo

_____ 2. bacterial or viral infection of the middle ear
    a. presbycusis
    b. otitis media
    c. presbyopia
    d. Ménière's disease

_____ 3. ringing in the ears
    a. tinnitus   c. hyperopia
    b. myopia   d. vertigo

_____ 4. complication of diabetes that affects the eyes
    a. cataract
    b. glaucoma
    c. astigmatism
    d. diabetic retinopathy

_____ 5. chronic inner ear disorder that affects balance and hearing
    a. presbycusis
    b. otitis media
    c. presbyopia
    d. Ménière's disease

_____ 6. dizziness or sensation of spinning
    a. tinnitus   c. hyperopia
    b. myopia   d. vertigo

_____ 7. ear pain due to inflammation and buildup of fluid in the middle ear
    a. otalgia
    b. otitis media
    c. presbyopia
    d. Ménière's disease

_____ 8. farsightedness
    a. tinnitus   c. hyperopia
    b. myopia   d. vertigo

_____ 9. a group of eye conditions that cause optic nerve damage, which may lead to loss of vision
    a. cataract
    b. glaucoma
    c. astigmatism
    d. diabetic retinopathy

_____ 10. gradual loss of hearing that occurs as people age
    a. presbycusis
    b. otitis media
    c. presbyopia
    d. Ménière's disease

_____ 11. clouding of the lens of the eye
    a. cataract
    b. glaucoma
    c. astigmatism
    d. diabetic retinopathy

_____ 12. condition in which the lens of the eye naturally loses its elasticity or its ability to change its shape, making it difficult to see objects up close
    a. presbycusis
    b. otitis media
    c. presbyopia
    d. Ménière's disease

_____ 13. a common condition that causes blurred vision due to an irregularly shaped cornea or curvature of the lens
    a. cataract
    b. glaucoma
    c. astigmatism
    d. diabetic retinopathy

SCORECARD: How Did You Do?

Number correct (_____), divided by 13 (_____), multiplied by 100 equals _____ (your score)

Multiple Choice: Procedures and Treatments

Directions: Choose the procedure or treatment that matches each definition. You can also complete this activity online using *EduHub*.

_____ 1. laser eye surgery
   a. blepharoplasty
   b. LASIK
   c. myringotomy
   d. myringoplasty

_____ 2. surgical repair of drooping eyelids
   a. blepharoplasty
   b. LASIK
   c. myringotomy
   d. myringoplasty

_____ 3. surgical procedure in which a small incision is made in the tympanic membrane to relieve pressure and inflammation caused by accumulation of fluid in the middle ear
   a. blepharoplasty
   b. LASIK
   c. myringotomy
   d. myringoplasty

_____ 4. glaucoma screening test that measures pressure within the eyes
   a. audiometry
   b. tonometry
   c. visual acuity testing
   d. fluorescein angiography

_____ 5. hearing test that measures a person's ability to hear different sounds, pitches, and frequencies
   a. audiometry
   b. tonometry
   c. visual acuity testing
   d. fluorescein angiography

_____ 6. surgical repair of a perforated tympanic membrane
   a. blepharoplasty
   b. LASIK
   c. myringotomy
   d. myringoplasty

_____ 7. a routine part of an eye exam to detect vision problems
   a. audiometry
   b. tonometry
   c. visual acuity testing
   d. fluorescein angiography

_____ 8. photographic technique for imaging the retina
   a. audiometry
   b. tonometry
   c. visual acuity testing
   d. fluorescein angiography

SCORECARD: How Did You Do?

Number correct (_____), divided by 8 (_____), multiplied by 100 equals _____ (your score)

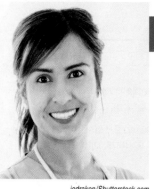

Analyzing the Intern Experience

In the Intern Experience described at the beginning of this chapter, we met Debra, an intern with University Eye and Ear Specialists. Debra met Mrs. Rodriguez and her four-year-old son, Juan, when the young boy was brought to the doctor's office because of severe otalgia (ear pain).

A physician examined Juan and obtained his personal and family health history from Mrs. Rodriguez. The doctor then made a medical diagnosis and provided Juan's mother with a treatment plan. Later, the physician made a dictated recording of the patient's health information, which was subsequently transcribed into a chart note.

We will now learn more about Juan's condition from a clinical perspective, interpreting the medical terms in his chart note as we analyze the scenario presented in the Intern Experience.

Audio Activity: Juan Rodriguez's Chart Note

Directions: Access your *EduHub* subscription and listen to the recording of the physician reading Juan Rodriguez's chart note. Read along with the physician and pay attention to the pronunciation of each medical term.

CHART NOTE

Patient Name: Rodriguez, Juan
ID Number: JR4239
Examination Date: February 6, 20xx

SUBJECTIVE
This 4-year-old male patient was brought in by his mother, who states he had a cold last week. He woke up this morning screaming, felt hot, and was tugging on his left ear. This is the third episode this year. Mother concerned with potential hearing loss.

OBJECTIVE
Temperature is 102.5° F and pulse is 100. Left **tympanic** membrane is dull, red, and bulging. Eyes are clear. Nose and throat clear. Neck is supple without adenopathy (disease of gland tissue). Lungs are clear.

ASSESSMENT
Left acute **otitis media**.

PLAN
Augmentin® (penicillin) 250 mg t.i.d. (three times a day) x 10 days. Recheck at end of treatment. Due to her concern with hearing loss, I discussed a **tympanometry** evaluation and/or referral to an **otorhinolaryngologist (ENT)**, an ear, nose, and throat specialist.

Interpret Juan Rodriguez's Chart Note

Directions: Access your *EduHub* subscription and listen to the recording of the physician reading Juan Rodriguez's chart note. After listening to the recording, supply the medical term that matches each definition.

> *Example*: discharge from the ear   *Answer*: otorrhea

1. specialist in the study of the ears, nose, and throat   _____

2. pertaining to the eardrum   _____

3. measurement of the eardrum   _____

4. bacterial or viral infection of the middle ear   _____

SCORECARD: How Did You Do?

Number correct (_____), divided by 4 (_____), multiplied by 100 equals _____ (your score)

Working with Medical Records

In this activity, you will interpret the medical records (chart notes) of patients with health conditions related to the special senses system. These examples illustrate typical medical records prepared in a real-world healthcare environment. To interpret these chart notes, you will apply your knowledge of word elements (prefixes, combining forms, and suffixes), diseases and disorders, and procedures and treatments related to the special sensory organs.

Audio Activity: Maria Jacobowitz's Chart Note

Directions: Access your *EduHub* subscription and listen to the recording of the physician reading Maria Jacobowitz's chart note. Read along with the physician and pay attention to the pronunciation of each medical term.

CHART NOTE

Patient Name: Jacobowitz, Maria
ID Number: MJ3321
Examination Date: August 12, 20xx

SUBJECTIVE
This 32-year-old female was struck in the left eye by the slats of a mini-blind, lacerating (scratching or tearing) the **sclera**. Mild pain was noted but no immediate visual problems, no **photophobia** (extreme sensitivity to light), and no blurred vision.

OBJECTIVE
There appears to be an abrasion of the left sclera with surrounding **subconjunctival** (below the membrane that lines the eyelids) hematoma. Pupils are equal, regular, and reactive to light. There does not appear to be any involvement of the **cornea**. Fluorescein stain shows some mild uptake over the injury site.

ASSESSEMENT
Scleral abrasion, left eye.

PLAN
Patient should apply Garamycin® **ophthalmic** solution (antibiotic medication), 1–2 drops to left eye every 4 hours for 3 days. Recheck if problem continues or symptoms worsen.

Assessment 6.11

Interpret Maria Jacobowitz's Chart Note

Directions: Access your *EduHub* subscription and listen to the recording of the physician reading Maria Jacobowitz's chart note. After listening to the recording, supply the medical term that matches each definition.

Example: inflammation of the retina   *Answer:* retinitis

1. clear, outer layer of the eye that covers the iris and pupil and admits light   _____

2. extreme sensitivity to light   _____

3. below the membrane that lines the eyelids   _____

4. white, outer protective layer of the eye   _____

5. pertaining to the eye   _____

SCORECARD: How Did You Do?

Number correct (_____), divided by 5 (_____), multiplied by 100 equals _____ (your score)

Chapter Review

Word Elements Summary

Prefixes

Prefix	Meaning
an-	not; without
extra-	outside
hemi-	half
intra-	inside; within
para-	near; beside
peri-	around

Combining Forms

Root Word/Combining Vowel	Meaning
audi/o	hearing
blephar/o	eyelid
ir/o	iris
irid/o	iris
kerat/o	cornea
myc/o	fungus
myring/o	tympanic membrane; eardrum
ocul/o	eye
ophthalm/o	eye
opt/o	eye; vision
optic/o	eye; vision
ot/o	ear
pleg/o	paralysis
presby/o	old age
retin/o	retina
scler/o	sclera (white of the eye)
tympan/o	tympanic membrane; eardrum

Suffixes

Suffix	Meaning
-al	pertaining to
-algia	pain
-ar	pertaining to
-ectomy	surgical removal; excision
-gram	record; image
-ia	condition
-ic	pertaining to
-itis	inflammation
-logist	specialist in the study and treatment of
-logy	study of
-meter	instrument used to measure
-metry	measurement
-opia	vision
-osis	abnormal condition
-pexy	surgical fixation
-plasty	surgical repair
-ptosis	drooping; downward displacement
-rrhea	discharge; flow
-rrhexis	rupture
-scope	instrument used to observe
-scopy	process of observing
-spasm	involuntary muscle contraction
-stomy	new opening
-tomy	incision; cut into

More Practice: Activities and Games

The following activities will help you reinforce your skills and check your mastery of the medical terminology you learned in this chapter. Access your *EduHub* subscription to complete more activities and vocabulary games for mastering the word parts and terms you have learned.

Break It Down

Directions: Dissect each medical term into its word parts (prefix, root word, combining vowel, and suffix) using one or more slashes. Then define each term.

Example:
Medical Term: blepharoptosis
Dissection: blephar/o/ptosis
Definition: drooping of the eyelid

Medical Term	Dissection
1. hemiplegia	h e m i p l e g i a

Definition: _____

_____

2. intraocular   i n t r a o c u l a r

Definition: _____

_____

3. intraretinal   i n t r a r e t i n a l

Definition: _____

_____

4. periophthalmic   p e r i o p h t h a l m i c

Definition: _____

_____

5. periotic   p e r i o t i c

Definition: _____

_____

6. blepharal   b l e p h a r a l

Definition: _____

_____

Medical Term	Dissection
7. blepharectomy	b l e p h a r e c t o m y

Definition: _____

_____

| 8. iridorrhexis | i r i d o r r h e x i s |

Definition: _____

_____

| 9. iridotomy | i r i d o t o m y |

Definition: _____

_____

| 10. keratitis | k e r a t i t i s |

Definition: _____

_____

Spelling

Directions: For each medical term that is misspelled, provide the correct spelling.

1. otomychosis _____
2. iridiplexy _____
3. presbycosis _____
4. miryngitis _____
5. occular _____
6. otagia _____
7. otorhea _____
8. blepharplegea _____
9. perocular _____
10. ophtaloscope _____
11. sclarotomy _____
12. optomology _____

Audio Activity: Phuong Tao's Chart Note

Directions: Access your *EduHub* subscription and listen to the recording of the physician reading Phuong Tao's chart note. Read along with the physician and pay attention to the pronunciation of each medical term.

CHART NOTE

Patient Name: Tao, Phuong
ID Number: TP9231
Examination Date: January 7, 20xx

SUBJECTIVE
This 58-year-old female patient presents with declining vision. She states that she failed her driver's license eye exam two weeks ago. She wants a "solution" because she drives herself and her mother to the grocery store and to doctor appointments on a monthly basis.

OBJECTIVE
Vision is **20/50** in the right eye and 20/70 in the left eye.

ASSESSMENT
Senile cataracts.

PLAN
Slight improvement in left eye can be obtained by increasing the prescription. Copy of prescription for left eye **lens** change was given to the patient. Driver's license form completed. Patient instructed to drive only during the daytime. I informed the patient that **cataract** surgery is warranted in the near future. I discussed the need for the procedure and its risks and benefits. She was given a pamphlet explaining the procedure and will follow up.

Assessment

Interpret Phuong Tao's Chart Note

Directions: Access your *EduHub* subscription and listen to the recording of the physician reading Phuong Tao's chart note. After listening to the recording, supply the medical term that matches each definition.

Example: pertaining to near the eye   *Answer*: paraocular

1. clouding of the lens of the eye   _____

2. fractional number that represents visual acuity (In this case, the line read by the patient reading from a distance of 20 feet can be read by a person with normal vision from a distance of 50 feet.)   _____

3. structure of the eye that focuses light onto the retina   _____

Chapter 7

The Nervous System

neur / o / logy: the study of the nervous system

Chapter Organization

- Intern Experience
- Overview of Nervous System Anatomy and Physiology
- Word Elements
- Breaking Down and Building Nervous System Terms
- Diseases and Disorders
- Procedures and Treatments
- Analyzing the Intern Experience
- Working with Medical Records
- Chapter Review

Chapter Objectives

After completing this chapter, you will be able to

1. label an anatomical diagram of the nervous system;
2. dissect and define common medical terminology related to the nervous system;
3. build terms used to describe nervous system diseases and disorders, diagnostic procedures, and therapeutic treatments;
4. pronounce and spell common medical terminology related to the nervous system;
5. understand that the process of building and dissecting a medical term based on its prefix, root word, and suffix enables you to analyze an extremely large number of medical terms beyond those presented in this chapter;
6. interpret the meaning of abbreviations associated with the nervous system; and
7. interpret medical records containing terminology and abbreviations related to the nervous system.

Your *EduHub* subscription that accompanies this text provides access to online assessments, assignments, activities, and resources. Throughout this chapter, access *EduHub* to

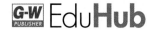

- use e-flash cards to review the medical terminology and word parts you learn;
- listen to the correct pronunciations of medical terms; and
- complete medical terminology activities and assignments.

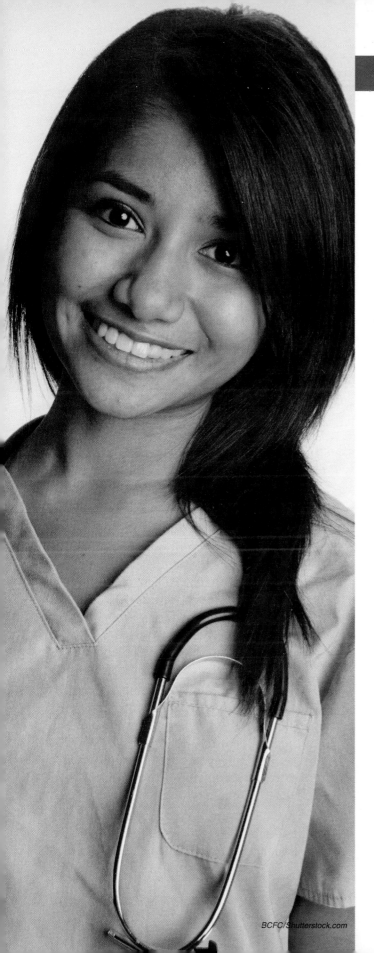

Intern Experience

Today is Nancy Chang's second day as an intern with Egan Immediate Care Center. Nancy has been assigned to "shadow" Beth, a medical assistant who works with Dr. Gangliola. Nancy and Beth escort their first patient, Steven Rutter, to the examination room. Mr. Rutter, 84 years of age, lives with his daughter, who brought him to the immediate care center. Mr. Rutter is agitated, angry, and frightened. His daughter explains that he left a pot of soup cooking on the stove while he went to get the mail, and he "almost burned down the house." Mr. Rutter found himself wandering along the street and did not know how he got there.

Steven Rutter is suffering from a disorder that has affected his nervous system, a complex network of nerve fibers and organs that carry messages to and from the brain, coordinating voluntary and involuntary muscular action, thought, sensation, and emotion. To help you understand what is happening to Mr. Rutter, this chapter will present word elements (combining forms, prefixes, and suffixes) that make up medical terms related to the nervous system.

By now, you know that many of the same medical word elements appear in terms used to describe different body systems. This systematic use of combining forms, prefixes, and suffixes helps make the study of medical terminology logical, consistent, and predictable.

We will begin our study of the nervous system with a brief overview of its anatomy and physiology. Later in the chapter, you will learn about some common pathological conditions of the nervous system, tests and procedures used to diagnose these conditions, and common treatment methods.

Overview of Nervous System Anatomy and Physiology

The **nervous system** consists of the brain, spinal cord, and nerves (Figure 7.1). As the body's "command" center, the nervous system sends, receives, and interprets messages both from the body (internal stimuli) and from the environment (external stimuli).

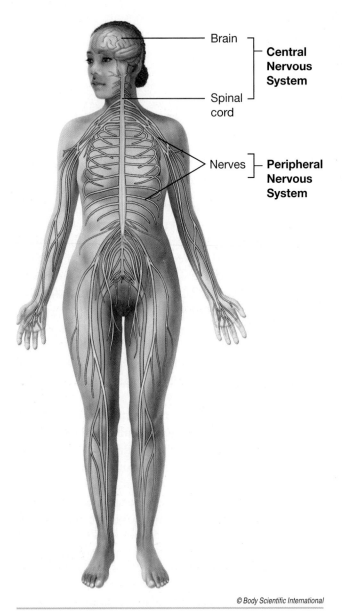

© Body Scientific International

Figure 7.1 The nervous system is divided into two branches: the central nervous system, consisting of the brain and spinal cord, and the peripheral nervous system, which includes all nerve tissue outside the brain and spinal cord.

Brain — Central Nervous System

Spinal cord

Nerves — Peripheral Nervous System

The nervous system is divided into two branches: the **central nervous system (CNS)**, which consists of the brain and spinal cord, and the **peripheral nervous system (PNS)**, which is made up of all nerve tissue outside the brain and spinal cord. The peripheral nervous system transmits sensory and motor information to and from the central nervous system. The central nervous system receives, processes, and interprets this information.

Major Functions and Structures of the Nervous System

The primary functions of the nervous system include

- coordinating the body's responses to internal and external stimuli; and

- regulating body systems to maintain *homeostasis*, a condition of stable internal balance that allows the body to function normally. To achieve homeostasis, your body is constantly working to keep physiological processes such as heart rate, blood pressure, body temperature, glucose levels, and hormonal activity within normal limits.

The human brain is a complex, multifaceted organ composed of multiple regions and subregions with interrelated functions. For the purposes of this overview, we will discuss four major parts of the brain: the cerebrum, cerebellum, brain stem, and diencephalon (Figure 7.2 on the next page).

- The **cerebrum** is the largest part of the brain, located in the anterior (upper) part of the skull. It controls

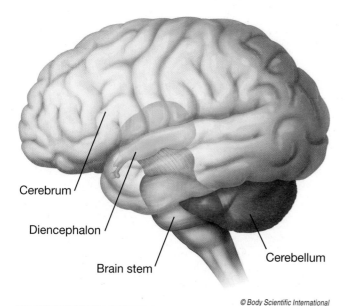

Cerebrum

Diencephalon

Brain stem

Cerebellum

© Body Scientific International

Figure 7.2 Four major parts of the brain

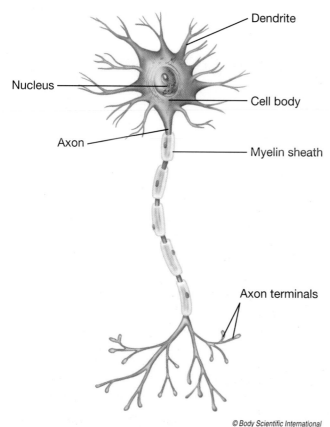

Dendrite

Nucleus

Cell body

Axon

Myelin sheath

Axon terminals

© Body Scientific International

Figure 7.3 Simplified anatomy of a neuron, the basic functional cell of the nervous system

voluntary movement and is the "seat" of higher-level mental processes, such as thinking, speaking, imagining, remembering, and planning.

- The **cerebellum** (Latin for "little brain") is located posterior to the cerebrum, behind the brain stem. It coordinates voluntary muscle activity, including fine-motor movement and equilibrium (balance).

- The **brain stem**, situated in the most inferior part of the brain, connects the brain to the spinal cord. It is composed of the *midbrain, pons,* and *medulla oblongata.* The brain stem controls life-sustaining cardiovascular and respiratory activities, such as heart rate, blood pressure, and breathing. It also relays sensory and motor information to and from the cerebellum.

- The **diencephalon** is located superior and anterior to the midbrain. It serves as a "relay station" by directing nerve impulses to and from the cerebrum.

The diencephalon contains three glands: the thalamus, hypothalamus, and pineal gland. The *thalamus* routes sensory input to the correct areas of the brain. The *hypothalamus* controls involuntary homeostatic functions such as heart rate; blood pressure; temperature; hormone production; and the senses of sight, hearing, smell, taste, and touch. The *pineal gland* produces the hormone melatonin, which regulates sleep.

The brain and spinal cord are protected by the *cranium, vertebral column,* and three membranous layers collectively called the *meninges.*

Neurons are the basic functional cells of the nervous system (Figure 7.3). They conduct electrical impulses that carry critical information between the CNS and the body. Neurons do not touch each other; instead, a gap called a *synaptic cleft* exists between them (Figure 7.4). Chemical messengers called **neurotransmitters** carry electrical impulses across this gap.

Neurology is the study of the nervous system. A **neurologist** is a physician who specializes in the study and treatment of nervous system diseases and disorders. Neurologists may also treat patients with muscular conditions caused by a nervous system disorder.

Anatomy and Physiology Vocabulary

Now that you have been introduced to the basic structure and functions of the nervous system, we will explore in more detail the key terms presented in the introduction.

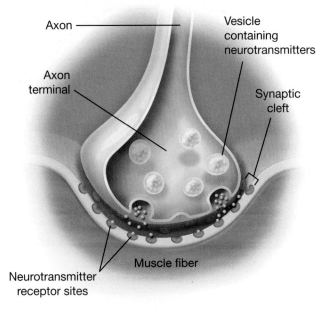

Axon

Axon terminal

Vesicle containing neurotransmitters

Synaptic cleft

Muscle fiber

Neurotransmitter receptor sites

© Body Scientific International

Figure 7.4 Neurotransmitters transport electrical impulses across the synaptic cleft between neurons.

Key Term	Definition
brain stem	structure that connects the brain to the spinal cord; relays sensory and motor information to and from the cerebellum; also controls life-sustaining, involuntary functions such as heart rate, blood pressure, and breathing
central nervous system (CNS)	the part of the nervous system consisting of the brain and spinal cord
cerebellum	the part of the brain that coordinates voluntary muscle activity and equilibrium (balance)
cerebrum	the largest part of the brain; controls higher-level mental processes and voluntary movement
diencephalon	"relay station" of the brain, which directs nerve impulses to and from the cerebrum and also controls involuntary homeostatic activity
nervous system	the system of the body that transmits nerve impulses between parts of the body and regulates the body's responses to internal and external stimuli
neurologist	physician who specializes in the study and treatment of nervous system diseases and disorders
neurology	the study of the nervous system
neuron	the basic functional cell of the nervous system; responsible for sending and receiving nerve impulses between parts of the body and the brain
peripheral nervous system (PNS)	the part of the nervous system made up of all nerve tissue outside the brain and spinal cord

E-Flash Card Activity: Anatomy and Physiology Vocabulary

Directions: After you have reviewed the anatomy and physiology vocabulary related to the nervous system, access your *EduHub* subscription and practice with the e-flash cards until you are comfortable with the spelling and definition of each term.

Assessment 7.1

Identifying Major Structures of the Nervous System

Directions: Label the diagram of the nervous system. You can also complete this activity online using *EduHub*.

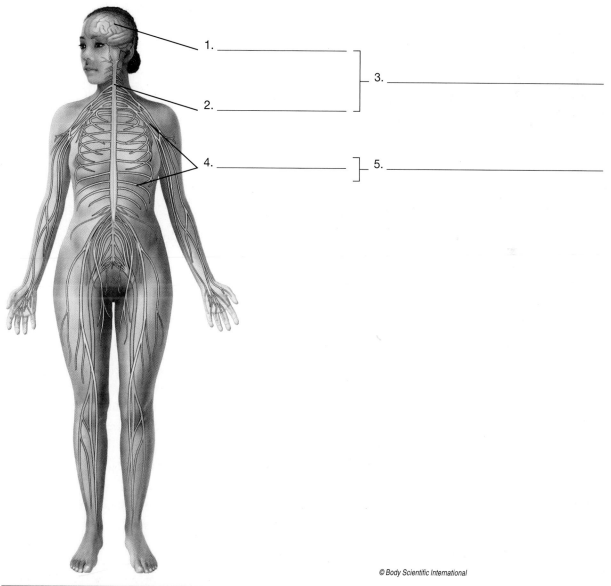

1. _____

2. _____

3. _____

4. _____

5. _____

© Body Scientific International

SCORECARD: How Did You Do?

Number correct (_____), divided by 5 (_____), multiplied by 100 equals _____ (your score)

Identifying Major Parts of the Brain

Directions: Label the four major parts of the brain. You can also complete this activity online using *EduHub*.

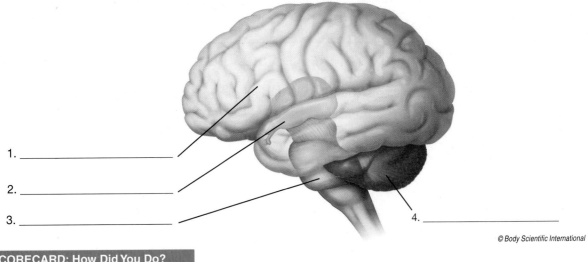

1. _____

2. _____

3. _____

4. _____

© Body Scientific International

SCORECARD: How Did You Do?

Number correct (_____), divided by 4 (_____), multiplied by 100 equals _____ (your score)

Matching Anatomy and Physiology Vocabulary

Directions: Choose the correct vocabulary term for each meaning. You can also complete this activity online using *EduHub*.

_____ 1. connects the brain and spinal cord

_____ 2. contains all nerve tissue outside the brain and spinal cord

_____ 3. controls muscle activity and balance

_____ 4. physician who specializes in the study and treatment of the nervous system

_____ 5. directs nerve impulses to and from the cerebrum

_____ 6. part of the nervous system made up of the brain and spinal cord

_____ 7. basic functional cell of the nervous system

_____ 8. largest part of the brain; controls mental processes and voluntary movement

_____ 9. the study of the nervous system

_____ 10. transmits nerve impulses and controls responses to stimuli

A. nervous system
B. neurology
C. diencephalon
D. brain stem
E. cerebellum
F. cerebrum
G. neuron
H. neurologist
I. central nervous system
J. peripheral nervous system

SCORECARD: How Did You Do?

Number correct (_____), divided by 10 (_____), multiplied by 100 equals _____ (your score)

Word Elements

In this section, you will learn word elements—prefixes, combining forms, and suffixes—that are common to the study of the nervous system. By learning these word elements and understanding how they are combined to build medical terms, you will be able to analyze Mr. Rutter's health condition (described in the Intern Experience at the beginning of this chapter) and identify a large number of terms associated with the nervous system.

E-Flash Card Activity: Word Elements

Directions: Review the word elements in the tables that follow. Then, access your *EduHub* subscription and practice with the e-flash cards until you are able to quickly recognize the different word parts (prefixes, combining forms, and suffixes) and their meanings. The e-flash cards are grouped together by prefixes, combining forms, and suffixes, followed by a cumulative review of all the word elements you are learning in this chapter.

Prefixes

Let's start our study of word elements by looking at the prefixes listed in the table below. As you know by now, these prefixes appear not only in medical terms related to the nervous system, but also in many terms used to describe other body systems.

Prefix	Meaning
a-	not; without
an-	not; without
dys-	painful; difficult
hemi-	half
hyper-	above; above normal
poly-	many; much
quadri-	four

Combining Forms

Listed below are combining forms that appear in medical terms used to describe the anatomy and physiology of the nervous system, as well as pathological conditions, diagnostic procedures, and therapeutic treatments related to this body system. Some of these combining forms also appear in medical terms related to other body systems.

Root Word/Combining Vowel	Meaning
angi/o	vessel
cephal/o	head
cerebr/o	cerebrum
cerebell/o	cerebellum

(Continued)

Root Word/Combining Vowel	Meaning
cran/o, crani/o	skull; cranium
encephal/o	brain
hydr/o	water
mening/o, meningi/o	meninges (membranes covering the brain and spinal cord)
myel/o	spinal cord
neur/o	nerve
path/o	disease
pleg/o	paralysis
psych/o	mind
radicul/o	nerve root
spin/o	spine; backbone
vascul/o	blood vessel

Suffixes

Listed below are suffixes that appear in medical terms used to describe the nervous system. You are already familiar with these suffixes, which were introduced in previous chapters.

Suffix	Meaning
-al	pertaining to
-algia	pain
-ar	pertaining to
-ary	pertaining to
-asthenia	weakness
-cele	hernia; swelling; protrusion
-eal	pertaining to
-esthesia	sensation; feeling
-gram	record; image
-graphy	process of recording an image
-ia	condition
-ic	pertaining to
-ical	pertaining to
-itis	inflammation
-logist	specialist in the study and treatment of
-logy	study of
-malacia	softening
-metry	process of measuring

(Continued)

Suffix	Meaning
-oma	tumor; mass
-osis	abnormal condition
-pathy	disease
-phasia	speech
-plasty	surgical repair
-rrhaphy	suture
-sclerosis	hardening
-tomy	incision; cut into
-us	structure; thing

Matching Prefixes, Combining Forms, and Suffixes

Directions: Choose the correct meaning for each word element. Some meanings may be used more than once. You can also complete this activity online using *EduHub*.

Prefixes

_____ 1. poly-

_____ 2. hemi-

_____ 3. quadri-

_____ 4. a-

_____ 5. dys-

_____ 6. an-

_____ 7. hyper-

A. not; without

B. four

C. many; much

D. above; above normal

E. painful; difficult

F. half

Combining Forms

_____ 1. neur/o

_____ 2. encephal/o

_____ 3. radicul/o

_____ 4. cerebr/o

_____ 5. myel/o

_____ 6. angi/o

_____ 7. mening/o, meningi/o

_____ 8. cephal/o

_____ 9. psych/o

_____ 10. cerebell/o

A. water

B. brain

C. meninges

D. nerve root

E. spine; backbone

F. nerve

G. head

H. cerebellum

I. vessel

J. disease

_____ 11. vascul/o   K. cerebrum

_____ 12. cran/o, crani/o   L. spinal cord

_____ 13. path/o   M. skull; cranium

_____ 14. hydr/o   N. mind

_____ 15. spin/o   O. paralysis

_____ 16. pleg/o   P. blood vessel

Suffixes

_____ 1. -sclerosis   A. pertaining to

_____ 2. -ical   B. process of measuring

_____ 3. -esthesia   C. structure; thing

_____ 4. -pathy   D. tumor; mass

_____ 5. -us   E. abnormal condition

_____ 6. -al   F. hernia; swelling; protrusion

_____ 7. -metry   G. condition

_____ 8. -rrhaphy   H. disease

_____ 9. -ary   I. sensation; feeling

_____ 10. -osis   J. weakness

_____ 11. -tomy   K. study of

_____ 12. -cele   L. surgical repair

_____ 13. -algia   M. suture

_____ 14. -ar   N. process of recording an image

_____ 15. -ia   O. record; image

_____ 16. -asthenia   P. pain

_____ 17. -ic   Q. incision; cut into

_____ 18. -eal   R. hardening

_____ 19. -logy

_____ 20. -graphy

_____ 21. -oma

_____ 22. -plasty

_____ 23. -gram

SCORECARD: How Did You Do?

Number correct (_____), divided by 46 (_____), multiplied by 100 equals _____ (your score)

Breaking Down and Building Nervous System Terms

Now that you have mastered the prefixes, combining forms, and suffixes for medical terminology used to describe the nervous system, you have the ability to dissect and build a large number of terms related to this body system.

Below is a list of common medical terms related to the study and treatment of the nervous system. For each term, a dissection has been provided, along with the meaning of each word element and the definition of the term as a whole.

Term	Dissection	Word Part/Meaning	Term Definition
Note: *For simplification, combining vowels have been omitted from the Word Part/Meaning column.*			
1. **anesthesia** (ĂN-ĕs-THĒ-zē-ă)	an/esthesia	an = not; without esthesia = sensation; feeling	without sensation or feeling
2. **aphasia** (ă-FĀ-zē-ă)	a/phasia	a = not; without phasia = speech	condition of without speech
3. **cephalalgia** (SĔF-ă-LĂL-jē-ă)	cephal/algia	cephal = head algia = pain	pain in the head (headache)
4. **cephalic** (sĕ-FĂL-ĭk)	cephal/ic	cephal = head ic = pertaining to	pertaining to the head
5. **cerebral** (SĔR-ĕ-brăl) (sĕ-RĒ-brăl)	cerebr/al	cerebr = cerebrum al = pertaining to	pertaining to the cerebrum
6. **cerebrospinal** (SĔR-ĕ-brō-SPĪ-năl)	cerebr/o/spin/al	cerebr = cerebrum spin = spine; backbone al = pertaining to	pertaining to the cerebrum and spine
7. **cerebrovascular** (SĔR-ĕ-brō-VĂS-kū-lăr)	cerebr/o/vascul/ar	cerebr = cerebrum vascul = blood vessel ar = pertaining to	pertaining to the blood vessels in the cerebrum
8. **cranial** (KRĀ-nē-ăl)	crani/al	crani = skull; cranium al = pertaining to	pertaining to the skull/cranium
9. **craniotomy** (KRĀ-nē-ŎT-ō-mē)	crani/o/tomy	crani = skull; cranium tomy= incision; cut into	incision to the skull/cranium
10. **dysphasia** (dĭs-FĀ-zē-ă)	dys/phasia	dys = painful; difficult phasia = speech	condition of difficult speech
11. **encephalitis** (ĕn-SĔF-ă-LĪ-tĭs)	encephal/itis	encephal = brain itis = inflammation	inflammation of the brain
12. **encephalomyelopathy** (ĕn-SĔF-ă-lō-MĪ-ĕ-LŎP-ă-thē)	encephal/o/myel/o/pathy	encephal = brain myel = spinal cord pathy = disease	disease of the brain and spinal cord
Prefixes = Green Root Words = Red Suffixes = Blue			

Term	Dissection	Word Part/Meaning	Term Definition
13. **hemiplegia** (HĔM-ē-PLĒ-jē-ă)	hemi/pleg/ia	**hemi** = half **pleg** = paralysis **ia** = condition	condition of half paralysis (paralysis of two extremities)
14. **hydrocephalus** (HĪ-drō-SĔF-ă-lŭs)	hydr/o/cephal/us	**hydr** = water **cephal** = head **us** = structure; thing	pertaining to water in the head*
15. **meningeal** (mě-NĬN-jē-ăl)	mening/eal	**mening** = meninges **eal** = pertaining to	pertaining to the meninges
16. **meningitis** (MĔN-ĭn-JĪ-tĭs)	mening/itis	**mening** = meninges **itis** = inflammation	inflammation of the meninges
17. **myelogram** (MĪ-ě-lō-grăm)	myel/o/gram	**myel** = spinal cord **gram** = record; image	record or image of the spinal cord
18. **neural** (NŪ-răl)	neur/al	**neur** = nerve **al** = pertaining to	pertaining to the nerves
19. **neuralgia** (nū-RĂL-jē-ă)	neur/algia	**neur** = nerve **algia** = pain	pain in the nerve (nerve pain)
20. **neurologist** (nū-RŎL-ō-jĭst)	neur/o/logist	**neur** = nerve **logist** = specialist in the study and treatment of	specialist in the study and treatment of the nerves
21. **neurology** (nū-RŎL-ō-jē)	neur/o/logy	**neur** = nerve **logy** = study of	study of the nerves
22. **neuropathy** (nū-RŎP-ă-thē)	neur/o/pathy	**neur** = nerve **pathy** = disease	disease of the nerves
23. **psychology** (sī-KŎL-ō-jē)	psych/o/logy	**psych** = mind **logy** = study of	study of the mind
24. **quadriplegia** (KWAH-drĭ-PLĒ-jē-ă)	quadri/pleg/ia	**quadri** = four **pleg** = paralysis **ia** = condition	condition of paralysis of four (paralysis of all four extremities)
25. **radiculitis** (ră-DĬK-ū-LĪ-tĭs)	radicul/itis	**radicul** = nerve root **itis** = inflammation	inflammation of the nerve root

Prefixes = **Green**   Root Words = **Red**   Suffixes = **Blue**

*__Hydrocephalus__ comes from two Greek words: *hydros*, which means "water," and *cephalus*, which means "head."
The suffix **-us** is a Latin noun form that means "structure or thing." In this case, **-us** refers to an anatomical structure.

Using the pronunciation guide in the Breaking Down and Building chart, practice saying each medical term aloud. To hear the pronunciation of each term, complete the Pronounce It activity on the next page.

Audio Activity: Pronounce It

Directions: Access your *EduHub* subscription and listen to the correct pronunciations of the following medical terms. Practice pronouncing the terms until you are comfortable saying them aloud.

anesthesia
(ĂN-ĕs-THĒ-zē-ă)

aphasia
(ă-FĀ-zē-ă)

cephalalgia
(SĔF-ă-LĂL-jē-ă)

cephalic
(sĕ-FĂL-ĭk)

cerebral
(SĔR-ĕ-brăl)
(sĕ-RĒ-brăl)

cerebrospinal
(SĔR-ĕ-brō-SPĪ-năl)

cerebrovascular
(SĔR-ĕ-brō-VĂS-kū-lăr)

cranial
(KRĀ-nē-ăl)

craniotomy
(KRĀ-nē-ŎT-ō-mē)

dysphasia
(dĭs-FĀ-zē-ă)

encephalitis
(ĕn-SĔF-ă-LĪ-tĭs)

encephalomyelopathy
(ĕn-SĔF-ă-lō-MĪ-ĕ-LŎP-ă-thē)

hemiplegia
(HĔM-ē-PLĒ-jē-ă)

hydrocephalus
(HĪ-drō-SĔF-ă-lŭs)

meningeal
(mĕ-NĬN-jē-ăl)

meningitis
(MĔN-ĭn-JĪ-tĭs)

myelogram
(MĪ-ĕ-lō-grăm)

neural
(NŪ-răl)

neuralgia
(nū-RĂL-jē-ă)

neurologist
(nū-RŎL-ō-jĭst)

neurology
(nū-RŎL-ō-jē)

neuropathy
(nū-RŎP-ă-thē)

psychology
(sī-KŎL-ō-jē)

quadriplegia
(KWAH-drĭ-PLĒ-jē-ă)

radiculitis
(ră-DĬK-ū-LĪ-tĭs)

Audio Activity: Spell It

Directions: Access your *EduHub* subscription and listen to the pronunciation for each number. As you hear each term, write its correct spelling.

1. _____
2. _____
3. _____
4. _____
5. _____
6. _____
7. _____
8. _____
9. _____
10. _____
11. _____
12. _____
13. _____
14. _____
15. _____
16. _____
17. _____
18. _____
19. _____
20. _____
21. _____
22. _____
23. _____
24. _____
25. _____

SCORECARD: How Did You Do?

Number correct (_____), divided by 25 (_____), multiplied by 100 equals _____ (your score)

Break It Down

Directions: Dissect each medical term into its word parts (prefix, root word, combining vowel, and suffix) using one or more slashes. Then define each term. You can also complete this activity online using *EduHub*.

Example:

Medical Term: meningitis
Dissection: mening/itis
Definition: inflammation of the meninges

Medical Term	Dissection
1. anesthesia	a n e s t h e s i a

Definition: _____

_____

2. radiculitis   r a d i c u l i t i s

Definition: _____

_____

3. quadriplegia   q u a d r i p l e g i a

Definition: _____

_____

4. cerebrospinal   c e r e b r o s p i n a l

Definition: _____

_____

5. encephalitis   e n c e p h a l i t i s

Definition: _____

_____

6. myelogram   m y e l o g r a m

Definition: _____

_____

Medical Term	Dissection
7. psychology	p s y c h o l o g y

Definition: _____

_____

8. hydrocephalus   h y d r o c e p h a l u s

Definition: _____

_____

9. cranial   c r a n i a l

Definition: _____

_____

10. hemiplegia   h e m i p l e g i a

Definition: _____

_____

11. meningeal   m e n i n g e a l

Definition: _____

_____

12. dysphasia   d y s p h a s i a

Definition: _____

_____

13. craniotomy   c r a n i o t o m y

Definition: _____

_____

14. neuralgia   n e u r a l g i a

Definition: _____

_____

SCORECARD: How Did You Do?

Number correct (_____), divided by 14 (_____), multiplied by 100 equals _____ (your score)

Build It

Directions: Build the medical term that matches each definition by supplying the correct word elements. You can also complete this activity online using *EduHub*.

P (Prefixes) = Green
RW (Root Words) = Red
S (Suffixes) = Blue
CV (Combining Vowel) = Purple

1. pertaining to the head

   _____ _____
         RW   S

2. condition of without speech

   _____ _____
     P   S

3. study of the nerves

   _____ _____ _____
         RW   CV   S

4. specialist in the study and treatment of the nerves

   _____ _____ _____
         RW   CV   S

5. without sensation or feeling

   _____ _____
     P   S

6. record or image of the spinal cord

   _____ _____ _____
         RW   CV   S

7. pertaining to water in the head

   _____ _____ _____ _____
    RW   CV   RW   S

8. pertaining to the skull/cranium

   _____ _____
         RW   S

9. pertaining to the blood vessels in the cerebrum

   _____ _____ _____ _____
         RW   CV   RW   S

10. pertaining to the nerves

    _____ _____
          RW   S

11. pertaining to the meninges

   _____ _____
            RW   S

12. condition of paralysis of four (paralysis of all four extremities)

   _____ _____ _____
      P   RW   S

13. pertaining to the cerebrum

   _____ _____
            RW   S

14. pain in the head

   _____ _____
            RW   S

15. incision to the skull/cranium

   _____ _____ _____
            RW   CV   S

16. inflammation of the meninges

   _____ _____
            RW   S

17. inflammation of the nerve root

   _____ _____
            RW   S

18. condition of difficult speech

   _____ _____
      P   S

19. condition of half paralysis (paralysis of two extremities)

   _____ _____ _____
      P   RW   S

20. disease of the nerves

   _____ _____ _____
            RW   CV   S

21. inflammation of the brain

   _____ _____
            RW   S

22. disease of the brain and spinal cord

   _____ _____ _____ _____ _____
            RW   CV   RW   CV   S

SCORECARD: How Did You Do?

Number correct (_____), divided by 22 (_____), multiplied by 100 equals _____ (your score)

Diseases and Disorders

Diseases and disorders of the nervous system run the spectrum from the mild to the severe in nature and etiology (cause). In this section, we will briefly explore some common pathological conditions of this body system.

Cerebral Aneurysm

A **cerebral aneurysm** is a bulge or ballooning of an artery in the brain due to thinning and weakening of the arterial wall (Figure 7.5). Aneurysms can appear anywhere in the brain, but they are more common in arteries at the base of the brain. A cerebral aneurysm can leak or rupture, causing bleeding into the brain. A sudden, extremely severe headache is the key symptom of a ruptured aneurysm. Patients often describe this event as "the worst headache they have ever had." However, a cerebral aneurysm that is small and intact may produce no symptoms.

Cerebral Embolism

Cerebral embolism is the sudden blockage of an artery in the brain due to a thrombus or other foreign matter (Figure 7.6). A stationary blood clot is called a *thrombus*. When the thrombus breaks away from the site at which it was lodged, it becomes an *embolism*.

Emboli (plural of *embolus*) can move through the bloodstream from their original location to another part of the body, where they can obstruct arterial blood flow. An embolism can develop anywhere within the cardiovascular (circulatory) system. When an embolism obstructs a cerebral artery, it is called a **cerebral embolism**.

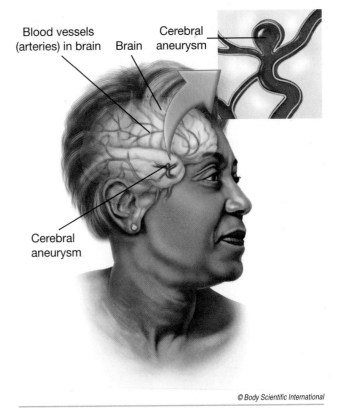

© Body Scientific International

Figure 7.5 Cerebral aneurysm. Note the ballooning of the weakened artery.

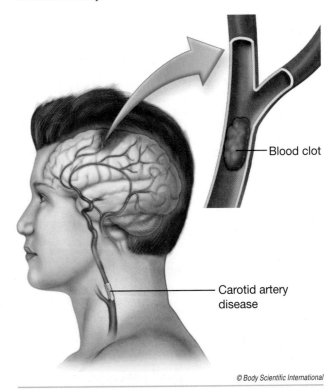

© Body Scientific International

Figure 7.6 Cerebral embolism

Cerebral Palsy

Cerebral palsy (CP) is a group of neurological disorders caused by damage to the brain and nervous system during embryonic development or soon after birth. CP impairs muscle movement and is associated with intellectual disabilities, vision and hearing problems, and in some cases, seizures. The effect of cerebral palsy on functional abilities varies greatly from one patient to the next. It is not yet known what triggers the abnormality in brain development that leads to CP.

Cerebral Vascular Attack

A **cerebral vascular attack (CVA)** is a sudden interruption in blood flow to a part of the brain (Figure 7.7). An embolism travels from another part of the body and lodges within an artery in the brain. The blocked artery deprives the brain of oxygen, damaging the surrounding brain tissue. If blood flow is cut off for longer than a few seconds, the brain cannot receive blood and oxygen. Brain cells die, causing permanent damage to brain function. A cerebral vascular attack is more commonly known as a "brain attack" or "stroke."

Concussion

A **concussion** is a *traumatic brain injury (TBI)* caused by a severe blow or jolt to the head. The force of impact causes the brain to slide back and forth inside the skull (Figure 7.8). The result is a brief or prolonged loss of consciousness that affects normal brain function.

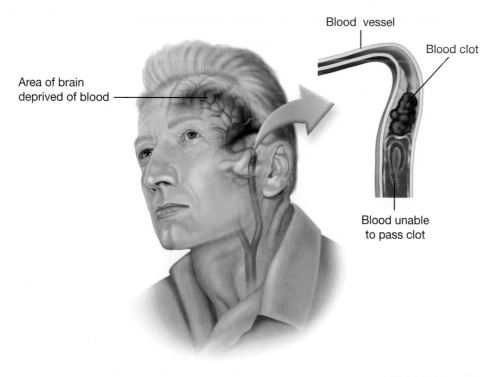

Blood vessel

Blood clot

Area of brain deprived of blood

Blood unable to pass clot

© Body Scientific International

Figure 7.7 Cerebral vascular attack

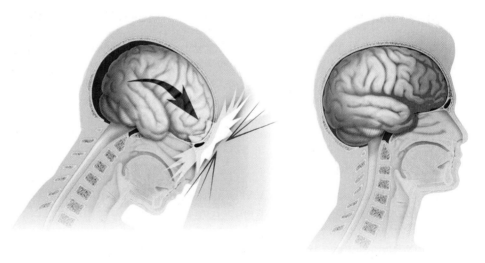

Figure 7.8 A concussion is a traumatic brain injury caused by a severe blow or jolt to the head.

Concussions are often caused by head trauma sustained during car accidents, contact sports, or falls. According to the Centers for Disease Control and Prevention (CDC), concussions are also a leading cause of child abuse deaths due to Shaken Baby Syndrome in the United States. The head trauma associated with Shaken Baby Syndrome is the result of an infant being violently shaken by the shoulders, arms, or legs.

Because some head injuries produce no loss of consciousness, some patients who experience a concussion may not be aware of it. Aftermath of concussion may include problems with headache, concentration, memory, judgment, balance, or coordination. The person must be closely watched for signs of disorientation, sleepiness, irritability, and impaired speech or muscle coordination. The patient must get sufficient rest so that the injured brain can heal.

Dementia

Dementia is a broad term for a group of cognitive disorders caused by the slow, progressive death of cerebral neurons and deteriorating mental function. It is attributed to brain trauma, substance abuse, or any of a number of neuro-degenerative diseases. Common signs of dementia include impaired memory, motor activity, and language processing skills. **Alzheimer's disease** is the most common form of dementia. It is a hereditary dementia associated with certain inherited chromosomal mutations.

Encephalitis

Encephalitis is inflammation of the brain due to a bacterial or viral infection. Abrupt fever, severe headache, muscle weakness, restlessness, and lethargy are typical symptoms. Blood tests can identify the causative bacterium or virus.

Encephalitis may also be diagnosed through an electroencephalogram (EEG), a lumbar puncture to evaluate the cerebrospinal fluid (CSF) for infection, and brain imaging tests such as computerized tomography (CT) or magnetic resonance imaging (MRI). CT and MRI technologies were discussed in Chapter 4: The Musculoskeletal System.

Epilepsy

Epilepsy is a disorder in which nerve cells in the brain send out abnormal signals, producing seizures. In milder cases of epilepsy, seizures may take the form of staring spells or strange sensations. More severe cases are marked by convulsions (seizures), violent muscle spasms, and loss of consciousness. Repeated seizures can result in long-term memory loss and personality changes. Prior to a seizure, some patients experience an *aura*, a strange sensation such as a tingling or buzzing sound, an unusual odor, or a flashing light, which signals the impending seizure.

The type of epileptic seizure that a patient experiences depends on the cause of the epilepsy and the part of the brain that is affected. Common causes include illness, brain injury, or abnormal brain development. In many cases, though, epilepsy's cause is *idiopathic* (unknown). Electroencephalograms (EEGs) and brain scans are used to diagnose epilepsy.

Meningitis

Meningitis is inflammation of the meninges, the three-layer membrane that surrounds and protects the brain and spinal cord. Meningitis may be caused by a virus, bacterium, or other microorganism such as a fungus or parasite.

Because of the proximity of the meninges to the brain and spinal cord, this disease is often considered a medical emergency. The swelling associated with meningitis produces symptoms of high fever, stiff neck, severe headache, nausea, and vomiting. A lumbar puncture may be performed to diagnose or exclude meningitis. Treatment involves immediate administration of antibiotics, corticosteroids (inflammation-reducing steroid drugs), and in some cases, antiviral drugs. Some forms of meningitis may be prevented by immunization.

Migraine Headache

A **migraine headache** (commonly called a **migraine**) is a recurring episode of moderate or severe throbbing pain, typically on one side of the head. The pain is accompanied by sensitivity to light and sound, as well as nausea and vomiting in some cases. Migraines can be triggered by any of a number of factors, including stress, anxiety, hunger, sleep deprivation, and in women, hormonal changes. Before the onset of a migraine, some patients experience an aura that produces visual disturbances. This aura serves as a warning sign that a severe headache is imminent. Medications can help prevent migraines or relieve symptoms when they occur.

Parkinson's Disease

Parkinson's disease is a chronic, degenerative neurological disorder marked by muscle tremor and rigidity (Figure 7.9). Bradykinesia (slow movement) is common, along with stiff posture and gait. Patients often have speech problems and display an immobile, mask-like face that shows little or no expression.

Parkinson's disease develops when neural cells in the brain fail to produce enough dopamine, a neurotransmitter involved in regulating bodily movement. While it may be genetic or environmental, the etiology (cause) of Parkinson's disease is unknown, and symptoms worsen over time.

Transient Ischemic Attack

A **transient ischemic attack (TIA)** occurs when blood flow to a section of the brain is briefly interrupted. A TIA, or "mini stroke," produces signs and symptoms similar to those of a stroke; however, a TIA usually lasts only a few minutes and causes no permanent damage. A TIA is a warning sign that a stroke might occur and provides an opportunity for preventive measures.

Procedures and Treatments

We will now take a brief look at some diagnostic tests and procedures used to help identify disorders and diseases of the nervous system, as well as common therapeutic methods for treating some of these conditions.

Babinski Reflex

A *reflex* is a predictable, involuntary response to a stimulus. A *stimulus* is an action that produces a reaction from a muscle, nerve, or other body tissue.

The **Babinski reflex** (also called **Babinski's sign**) is a reflex that happens in infants. It is evoked during a physical examination by a healthcare specialist.

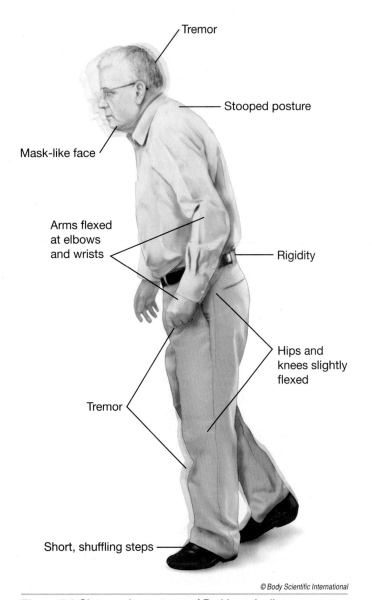

Tremor

Stooped posture

Mask-like face

Arms flexed at elbows and wrists

Rigidity

Hips and knees slightly flexed

Tremor

Short, shuffling steps

© Body Scientific International

Figure 7.9 Signs and symptoms of Parkinson's disease

The doctor or other medical specialist stimulates the heel of the foot with a small object and then moves the object along the outer edge of the sole, to the base of the toes. The great (big) toe moves toward the top surface of the foot, and the other toes fan out after the sole of the foot has been firmly stroked (Figure 7.10).

The Babinski reflex is normal between infancy and two years of age. The presence of this reflex in children older than two years or in adults indicates damage to the nerve pathways that connect the brain and spinal cord. The Babinski reflex may be a sign of tumor, defect, or injury to the brain or spinal cord, multiple sclerosis, or another neurological disorder.

Cerebral Angiography

Cerebral angiography is a diagnostic procedure that uses a contrast agent ("dye") and X-rays to evaluate the vessels that supply blood to the brain. A thin, flexible catheter (tube) is inserted into the femoral artery in the groin. The physician threads the catheter past the heart into an artery of the brain. Then the contrast agent is injected into the catheter, through which it travels to selected cerebral arteries. Cerebral angiography can identify or confirm cerebral vascular abnormalities or pathologies that may indicate an aneurysm, brain tumor, or stenosis (abnormal narrowing of blood vessels).

Computerized Tomography

Computerized tomography (CT), also called *computed tomography*, is a diagnostic imaging procedure that uses X-rays and a computer to scan and display cross-sectional images of internal body structures in multiple planes. A radiopaque (RĀ-dē-ō-PĀK) contrast agent (a dye that sharpens X-ray detail) is sometimes injected into the patient to enhance anatomical imagery during the scanning process.

Because of its ability to "image" body structures in multiple planes, CT technology can detect tumors, masses, and diseases that otherwise could go undetected if they were visualized in only one plane, as is the case with radiographs. A more detailed explanation of computerized tomography is presented in chapter 4.

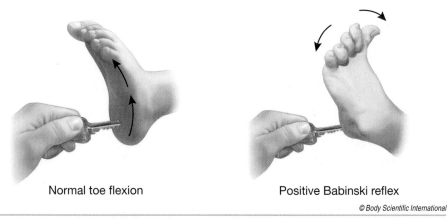

Normal toe flexion

Positive Babinski reflex

© Body Scientific International

Figure 7.10 In a positive Babinski reflex, the great toe moves toward the top surface of the foot, and the other toes fan out.

Electroencephalogram

An **electroencephalogram (EEG)** is a test that measures the electrical activity of the brain. A series of flat, metal disks called *electrodes* are affixed to the scalp. The electrodes are held in place with a sticky substance and are connected by wires to a recording device (Figures 7.11A and 7.11B). The device translates electrical signals from the brain into waveforms (wavy patterns), which are interpreted by a neurologist (Figure 7.11C).

The EEG test is used to confirm an epilepsy diagnosis. It is also used to diagnose sleep disorders, dementia, and other brain disorders.

Finger-to-Nose Test

The **finger-to-nose test** is a neurological test used to evaluate physical coordination. The patient is asked to close his or her eyes, extend the arms outward, and then slowly touch the nose with an index finger. Inability to do so may indicate cerebellar dysfunction.

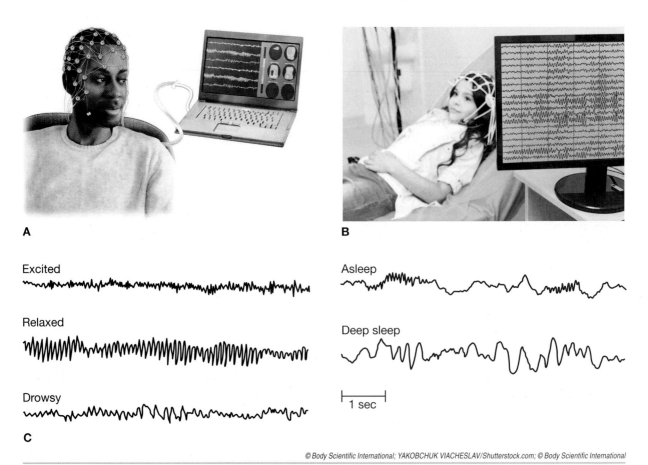

Figure 7.11 An electroencephalogram measures the electrical activity of the brain. A—Electrodes are placed on the scalp and connected by wires to a recording device. B—The device translates electrical signals from the brain into waveforms. C—Waveforms, which signify different types of brain activity, are interpreted by a neurologist.

Kernig's Sign

Kernig's sign (also called **Kernig sign**) is a test that facilitates the diagnosis of meningitis. The maneuver is usually performed with the patient in a supine position (lying face upward) with the hips and knees flexed to 90 degrees (Figure 7.12). Inability to extend the legs beyond 135 degrees without experiencing pain, stiffness, and involuntary contraction of the hamstrings (the group of muscles in the back of the thigh) constitutes a positive test for Kernig's sign. A positive Kernig's sign indicates meningeal inflammation.

Lumbar Puncture

A **lumbar puncture (LP)**, sometimes called a *spinal tap*, is a diagnostic or therapeutic procedure that involves inserting a needle into the lumbar region (lower back) to extract cerebrospinal fluid (Figure 7.13). Cerebrospinal fluid (CSF) is the protective fluid that surrounds and cushions the brain and spinal column. The CSF obtained from a lumbar puncture is analyzed for the presence of infection, injury, or another pathological condition of the brain or spinal cord.

Magnetic Resonance Angiogram

A **magnetic resonance angiogram (MRA)** is a type of magnetic resonance imaging (MRI) scan. MRA provides critical information about the condition and function of blood vessels that cannot be obtained from X-rays, ultrasound tests, or CT scans. It can detect an aneurysm (blood-filled bulge in an artery), vascular stenosis (narrowing of a blood vessel), and other disorders and diseases of the blood vessels. (For more detailed information on MRI technology, see the Procedures and Treatments section of chapter 4.)

Romberg's Sign

Romberg's sign (also called **Romberg sign** or **Romberg test**) is a measure of *sensory ataxia*, defective muscle coordination resulting from loss of input from the senses of sight and equilibrium (balance). The patient is asked to stand erect with the eyes closed and the feet close together. If the patient sways and falls when the eyes are closed, the Romberg's sign is positive, indicating sensory ataxia.

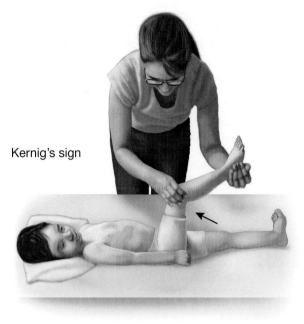

Kernig's sign

© Body Scientific International

Figure 7.12 Kernig's sign helps diagnose meningitis.

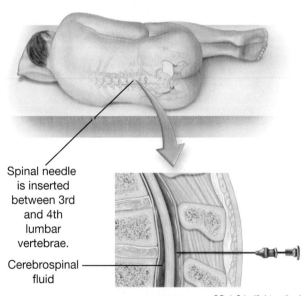

Spinal needle is inserted between 3rd and 4th lumbar vertebrae.

Cerebrospinal fluid

© Body Scientific International

Figure 7.13 Cerebrospinal fluid extracted during a lumbar puncture helps detect infection, injury, or disease of the brain or spinal cord.

Multiple Choice: Diseases and Disorders

Directions: Choose the disease or disorder that matches each definition. You can also complete this activity online using *EduHub*.

_____ 1. a bulge or ballooning of an artery in the brain due to thinning and weakening of the arterial wall
    a. cerebral aneurysm
    b. cerebral embolism
    c. cerebral vascular attack
    d. cerebral palsy

_____ 2. the sudden blockage of an artery in the brain due to a thrombus or other foreign matter
    a. cerebral palsy
    b. cerebral embolism
    c. cerebral aneurysm
    d. cerebral vascular attack

_____ 3. a sudden interruption in blood flow to a part of the brain; caused by an embolism that lodges in an artery of the brain after traveling from another part of the body
    a. cerebral vascular attack
    b. cerebral aneurysm
    c. cerebral palsy
    d. cerebral embolism

_____ 4. a disorder in which nerve cells in the brain send out abnormal signals, producing seizures
    a. epilepsy
    b. dementia
    c. transient ischemic attack
    d. encephalitis

_____ 5. a group of neurological disorders caused by damage to the brain and nervous system during embryonic development or soon after birth; characterized in part by impaired muscle movement and intellectual disabilities
    a. cerebral vascular attack
    b. cerebral embolism
    c. cerebral aneurysm
    d. cerebral palsy

_____ 6. broad term for a group of cognitive disorders caused by the slow, progressive death of cerebral neurons and marked by deteriorating mental function
    a. epilepsy
    b. dementia
    c. transient ischemic attack
    d. encephalitis

_____ 7. inflammation of the brain due to a bacterial or viral infection
    a. encephalitis
    b. dementia
    c. transient ischemic attack
    d. epilepsy

_____ 8. a traumatic brain injury (TBI) caused by a severe blow or jolt to the head, resulting in brief or prolonged loss of consciousness
    a. migraine headache   c. epilepsy
    b. concussion   d. dementia

_____ 9. a symptom of an aneurysm is
    a. sudden, extremely severe headache
    b. repeated seizures
    c. muscle tremor
    d. mini stroke

_____ 10. a recurring headache characterized by moderate or severe pain, usually on one side of the head
    a. concussion   c. meningitis
    b. migraine headache d. encephalitis

_____ 11. an interruption in blood flow to the brain that lasts only a few minutes and causes no permanent damage; mini stroke
    a. cerebral embolism
    b. cerebral aneurysm
    c. migraine headache
    d. transient ischemic attack

SCORECARD: How Did You Do?

Number correct (_____), divided by 11 (_____), multiplied by 100 equals _____ (your score)

Multiple Choice: Procedures and Treatments

Directions: Choose the procedure or treatment that matches each definition. You can also complete this activity online using *EduHub*.

_____ 1. a diagnostic or therapeutic procedure that involves inserting a needle into the lumbar region (lower back) to extract cerebrospinal fluid
   a. electroencephalogram
   b. lumbar puncture
   c. magnetic resonance angiography
   d. cerebral angiography

_____ 2. a test that measures the electrical activity of the brain by means of electrodes connected to a recording device that generates waveforms
   a. electroencephalogram
   b. magnetic resonance angiography
   c. cerebral angiography
   d. computerized tomography

_____ 3. a test that facilitates the diagnosis of meningitis
   a. Babinski reflex   c. Romberg's sign
   b. Kernig's sign   d. finger-to-nose test

_____ 4. a test in which the outer edge of the sole of the foot is firmly stroked
   a. Babinski reflex   c. Romberg's sign
   b. Kernig's sign   d. sole test

_____ 5. a neurological test used to evaluate physical coordination and test for cerebellar dysfunction
   a. Babinski reflex   c. Romberg's sign
   b. Kernig's sign   d. finger-to-nose test

_____ 6. measure of *sensory ataxia,* defective muscle coordination resulting from loss of input from the senses of sight and balance
   a. Babinski reflex   c. Romberg's sign
   b. Kernig's sign   d. finger-to-nose test

_____ 7. a form of MRI that can detect aneurysms, vascular stenosis, and other blood vessel diseases and disorders
   a. electroencephalogram
   b. lumbar puncture
   c. magnetic resonance angiography
   d. cerebral angiography

_____ 8. a diagnostic procedure that uses a contrast agent and X-rays to evaluate the vessels that supply blood to the brain
   a. electroencephalogram
   b. lumbar puncture
   c. magnetic resonance angiography
   d. cerebral angiography

_____ 9. a diagnostic procedure involving the use of X-rays and a computer to scan and display cross-sectional images of internal body structures in multiple planes
   a. electroencephalogram
   b. computerized tomography
   c. magnetic resonance angiogram
   d. lumbar puncture

SCORECARD: How Did You Do?

Number correct (_____), divided by 9 (_____), multiplied by 100 equals _____ (your score)

Identifying Abbreviations

Directions: Supply the correct abbreviation for each medical term. You can also complete this activity online using *EduHub*.

Medical Term	Abbreviation
1. central nervous system	_____
2. cerebral palsy	_____
3. cerebrospinal fluid	_____
4. cerebral vascular attack	_____
5. magnetic resonance imaging	_____
6. computerized tomography	_____
7. electroencephalogram	_____
8. lumbar puncture	_____
9. traumatic brain injury	_____
10. magnetic resonance angiography	_____
11. peripheral nervous system	_____
12. transient ischemic attack	_____

SCORECARD: How Did You Do?

Number correct (_____), divided by 12 (_____), multiplied by 100 equals _____ (your score)

Spelling

Directions: For each medical term that is misspelled, provide the correct spelling. You can also complete this activity online using *EduHub*.

1. cerabellum _____

2. diencepholon _____

3. nuerologist _____

4. encephylitis _____

5. neuralgea _____

6. hydracephalis _____

SCORECARD: How Did You Do?

Number correct (_____), divided by 6 (_____), multiplied by 100 equals _____ (your score)

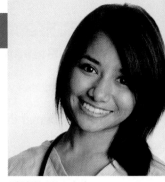

In the Intern Experience described at the beginning of this chapter, we met Nancy, an intern with the Egan Immediate Care Center. Nancy was assigned to shadow (follow and observe) Beth, medical assistant to Dr. Gangliola. Their first patient was Steven Rutter, an 84-year-old man brought to the clinic by his daughter, who explained that her father had nearly "burned down the house." He had left a pot of soup cooking on the stove while he walked outside to the mailbox. He found himself wandering along the street with no awareness of how he had gotten there. During his physical exam in the doctor's office, Mr. Rutter appeared agitated, angry, and frightened.

Dr. Gangliola examined Mr. Rutter and obtained his personal and family health history. He then made a medical diagnosis and provided Mr. Rutter and his daughter with a treatment plan. Later, Dr. Gangliola made a dictated recording of the patient's health information, which was subsequently transcribed into a chart note.

We will now learn more about Steven Rutter's condition from a clinical perspective, interpreting the medical terms in his chart note as we analyze the scenario presented in the Intern Experience.

Audio Activity: Steven Rutter's Chart Note

Directions: Access your *EduHub* subscription and listen to the recording of the physician reading Steven Rutter's chart note. Read along with the physician and pay attention to the pronunciation of each medical term.

CHART NOTE

Patient Name: Rutter, Steven
ID Number: 257RS
Examination Date: December 6, 20xx

SUBJECTIVE
Mr. Rutter is an anxious 84-year-old gentleman who appears older than his stated age. He states that he has been experiencing increasing episodes of memory loss.

OBJECTIVE
Physical exam reveals an agitated but depressed-appearing male who is underweight but in no acute distress. He denies any falls or head injuries. He has a history of **TIAs** and a **CVA** that occurred 3 years ago. Vital signs normal. **Cranial** nerves II through XII are intact in detail to visual fields and ophthalmoscopic (pertaining to an instrument used to visualize the eyes) examination. Motor and sensory exams and reflexes within normal limits.

ASSESSMENT
Patient has memory loss without objective findings relating to organic (causing a change in physical structure) **etiology**. Depression may be a key factor. Rule out **dementia**.

PLAN
I will order a **CT** scan of the brain. Pending results may necessitate a neurology consult.

Interpret Steven Rutter's Chart Note

Directions: Access your *EduHub* subscription and listen to the recording of the physician reading Steven Rutter's chart note. After listening to the recording, supply the medical term that matches each definition. You may encounter definitions and terms introduced in previous chapters.

Example: inflammation of the meninges   *Answer:* meningitis

1. sudden interruption in blood flow to a part of the brain

   _____

2. cause of a disorder or disease

   _____

3. diagnostic imaging procedure that uses X-rays and a computer to scan and display cross-sectional images of internal body structures in multiple planes; computerized tomography

   _____

4. brief interruptions in blood flow to a section of the brain; also called "mini strokes"

   _____

5. pertaining to the skull or cranium

   _____

6. term used to describe a group of cognitive disorders caused by the slow, progressive death of cerebral neurons and marked by deteriorating mental function

   _____

SCORECARD: How Did You Do?

Number correct (_____), divided by 6 (_____), multiplied by 100 equals _____ (your score)

Working with Medical Records

In this activity, you will interpret the medical records (chart notes) of patients with nervous system disorders. These examples illustrate typical medical records prepared in a real-world healthcare environment. To interpret these chart notes, you will apply your knowledge of word elements (prefixes, combining forms, and suffixes), diseases and disorders, and procedures and treatments related to the nervous system.

Audio Activity: Ellen Wyamback's Chart Note

Directions: Access your *EduHub* subscription and listen to the recording of the physician reading Ellen Wyamback's emergency department (ED) report. Read along with the physician and pay attention to the pronunciation of each medical term.

Emergency Department Report

Patient Name: Wyamback, Ellen
ID Number: 138EW
Examination Date: August 25, 20xx

SUBJECTIVE
16-year-old patient presents with a history of falling off her bike. While performing "tricks," she fell into a fence. She complains of head, neck, and left knee pain. A brief loss of consciousness was observed by a friend. She is slow to answer questions and repeats questions about the accident.

OBJECTIVE
Patient presents on a rigid backboard with a **C-collar** (cervical spine brace) in place. Pupils equal and reactive to light. No blood in the ears. There is tenderness over the mid-posterior **C-spine** (cervical spine) without obvious swelling or deformity. Heart and chest exam normal. Patient moves all 4 extremities well. Mild tenderness over the left patella (kneecap) but no instability or limited **ROM** (range of motion) noted. Cranial nerves II–VII intact. C-spine X-rays and **CT** scan of head are negative.

ASSESSMENT
Mild **concussion**.

PLAN
Patient sent home with treatment instructions. She should follow up with her physician in 1–2 days or return **PRN*** (as needed) or if any change in mental status.

*The abbreviation **PRN** comes from the Latin phrase *pro re nata* (prō-rā-NÄ-tä), which means "as the circumstances require" (as needed).

Assessment 7.13

Interpret Ellen Wyamback's Chart Note

Directions: Access your *EduHub* subscription and listen to the recording of the physician reading Ellen Wyamback's emergency department (ED) report. After listening to the recording, supply the medical term that matches each definition.

Example: pain in the head   *Answer:* cephalalgia

1. cervical spine   _____

2. procedure that uses X-rays and a computer to scan and display cross-sectional images   _____

3. neck brace worn to stabilize the cervical spine   _____

4. as needed   _____

5. range of motion   _____

6. traumatic brain injury caused by a severe blow or jolt to the head   _____

SCORECARD: How Did You Do?

Number correct (_____), divided by 6 (_____), multiplied by 100 equals _____ (your score)

Audio Activity: Lucy Carmel's Chart Note

Directions: Access your *EduHub* subscription and listen to the recording of the physician reading Lucy Carmel's chart note. Read along with the physician and pay attention to the pronunciation of each medical term.

Emergency Department Report

Patient Name: Carmel, Lucy
ID Number: 495LC
Examination Date: February 19, 20xx

CHIEF COMPLAINT
Nausea, vomiting, and headache.

HISTORY OF PRESENT ILLNESS
This is an 18-year-old female who was seen by her **PCP** (primary care physician) early this morning. She has a 5-day history of nausea, vomiting, headache, and elevated temperature with increasing lethargy. She was evaluated and sent to the emergency department for a **lumbar puncture** to rule out **meningitis**.

ALLERGIES
None known.

PHYSICAL EXAMINATION
Physical examination reveals a well-developed, well-nourished, somewhat lethargic young female. **BP** is 110/74, pulse 94, respirations 25, and temperature 101.2. Examination of the neck revealed marked stiffness with rigidity and positive **Babinski reflex** and **Kernig's sign**. Cardiac exam is regular in rate and rhythm with no murmurs (atypical, extra sounds heard while examining heartbeat). Lungs are clear bilaterally. During the course of the exam, the patient became profoundly lethargic and did not respond appropriately to pain stimuli.

LABORATORY DATA
Lumbar puncture revealed gram-negative cocci (type of bacteria). A **CBC** (complete blood count) is also consistent for a bacterial process.

IMPRESSION
Acute bacterial meningitis.

PLAN
Request **neurological** consult for probable acute bacterial meningitis.

Interpret Lucy Carmel's Chart Note

Directions: Access your *EduHub* subscription and listen to the recording of the physician reading Lucy Carmel's chart note. After listening to the recording, supply the medical term that matches each definition. You may encounter definitions and terms introduced in previous chapters.

Example: condition of difficult speech   *Answer:* dysphasia

1. test that facilitates the diagnosis of meningitis   _____

2. complete blood count   _____

3. pertaining to study of the nerves   _____

4. inflammation of the meninges   _____

5. diagnostic or therapeutic procedure that involves inserting a needle into the lumbar region (lower back) to extract cerebrospinal fluid; also called a *spinal tap*   _____

6. procedure that involves stimulating the heel of the foot with a small object and then moving the object along the outer edge of the sole, to the base of the toes   _____

7. blood pressure   _____

8. primary care physician   _____

SCORECARD: How Did You Do?

Number correct (_____), divided by 8 (_____), multiplied by 100 equals _____ (your score)

Chapter Review

Word Elements Summary

Prefixes

Prefix	Meaning
a-	not; without
an-	not; without
dys-	painful; difficult
hemi-	half
hyper-	above; above normal
poly-	many; much
quadri-	four

Combining Forms

Root Word/Combining Vowel	Meaning
angi/o	vessel
cephal/o	head
cerebr/o	cerebrum
cerebell/o	cerebellum
cran/o, crani/o	skull; cranium
encephal/o	brain
hydr/o	water
mening/o, meningi/o	meninges (membranes covering the brain and spinal cord)
myel/o	spinal cord
neur/o	nerve
path/o	disease
pleg/o	paralysis
psych/o	mind
radicul/o	nerve root
spin/o	spine; backbone
vascul/o	blood vessel

Suffixes

Suffix	Meaning
-al	pertaining to
-algia	pain
-ar	pertaining to
-ary	pertaining to
-asthenia	weakness
-cele	hernia; swelling; protrusion
-eal	pertaining to
-esthesia	sensation; feeling
-gram	record; image
-graphy	process of recording an image
-ia	condition
-ic	pertaining to
-ical	pertaining to
-itis	inflammation
-logist	specialist in the study and treatment of
-logy	study of
-malacia	softening
-metry	process of measuring
-oma	tumor; mass
-osis	abnormal condition
-pathy	disease
-phasia	speech
-plasty	surgical repair
-rrhaphy	suture
-sclerosis	hardening
-tomy	incision; cut into
-us	structure; thing

More Practice: Activities and Games

The following activities will help you reinforce your skills and check your mastery of the medical terminology you learned in this chapter. Access your *EduHub* subscription to complete more activities and vocabulary games for mastering the word parts and terms you have learned.

Audio Activity: Nigel Dixon's Chart Note

Directions: Access your *EduHub* subscription and listen to the recording of the physician reading Nigel Dixon's chart note. Read along with the physician and pay attention to the pronunciation of each medical term.

CHART NOTE

Patient Name: Dixon, Nigel
ID Number: 602DN
Examination Date: April 7, 20xx

SUBJECTIVE
Nigel is now 5 weeks post (after) completion of radiation therapy. He is alert, cooperative, and responsive to questions. He is often tired and sleepy.

OBJECTIVE
Neurological assessment reveals pupils equal, round, and reactive to light. Normal fundoscopic examination (of the inner part of the eye). Extraocular (pertaining to outside the eye) movements still show limitations on the right. The face is symmetric, including eye and lip closure. Nigel continues to have a mild right **hemiplegia** that is unchanged from his examination 5 weeks ago. Sensory exam is normal to touch, pinprick, and position. **Cerebellar** examination is normal with a negative **Romberg test** and a good **finger-to-nose test**.

ASSESSMENT
The repeated **MRA** study indicates a diminished brain stem lesion. Sustained clinical improvement over the course of his radiation therapy treatments.

PLAN
Patient will return in 6 weeks for follow-up.

Interpret Nigel Dixon's Chart Note

Directions: Access your *EduHub* subscription and listen to the recording of the physician reading Nigel Dixon's chart note. After listening to the recording, supply the medical term that matches each definition. You may encounter definitions and terms introduced in previous chapters.

Example: inflammation   *Answer:* radiculitis

1. condition of half paralysis (paralysis of two extremities)   _____

2. neurological test used to evaluate physical coordination   _____

3. type of magnetic resonance imaging test that provides information about the condition and function of blood vessels   _____

4. test used to measure sensory ataxia   _____

5. pertaining to the study of the nerves   _____

6. pertaining to the cerebellum   _____

True or False

Directions: Indicate whether each statement is true or false.

True or False?

_____ 1. The prefix **hemi-** means "full."

_____ 2. The prefix **quadri-** means "four."

_____ 3. The root word **cerebr** means "cerebellum."

_____ 4. The root word **neur** means "nervous."

_____ 5. The root word **pleg** means "paralysis."

_____ 6. The suffix **-ical** means "pertaining to."

_____ 7. A CVA is also called a *stroke*.

_____ 8. A positive Romberg's sign is a failure to maintain balance while sitting.

_____ 9. A stationary blood clot is called a *thrombus*.

_____ 10. A TIA causes permanent damage to the brain.

_____ 11. All patients who get migraine headaches have warning symptoms.

_____ 12. Alzheimer's disease is the most common form of dementia.

Break It Down

Directions: Dissect each medical term into its word parts (prefix, root word, combining vowel, and suffix) using one or more slashes. Then define each term.

Example:
Medical Term: polyneuritis
Dissection: poly/neur/itis
Definition: inflammation of many nerves

Medical Term	Dissection
1. encephalomalacia	e n c e p h a l o m a l a c i a

Definition: _____

_____

2. meningioma   m e n i n g i o m a

Definition: _____

_____

3. polyneuritis   p o l y n e u r i t i s

Definition: _____

_____

4. quadriplegic   q u a d r i p l e g i c

Definition: _____

_____

5. radiculopathy   r a d i c u l o p a t h y

Definition: _____

_____

6. hemicerebrum   h e m i c e r e b r u m

Definition: _____

_____

Medical Term	Dissection
7. neurorrhaphy	n e u r o r r h a p h y

Definition: _____

_____

8. neurasthenia   n e u r a s t h e n i a

Definition: _____

_____

9. meningocele   m e n i n g o c e l e

Definition: _____

_____

Spelling

Directions: For each medical term, indicate the correct spelling.

1.	aphasia	aphaesia	aphasea	aphazia
2.	craneal	cranial	craenial	chranial
3.	cerebovasular	cerebralvascolar	cerebrovascular	cerebrovascullar
4.	disphasia	dysphasia	disphasea	dysphasea
5.	polyneuritis	polynuritis	polynueritis	polineuritis
6.	hemipeglia	hemiplegia	hemaplegia	hemipledgia
7.	menyngitis	menangitis	meninghitis	meningitis
8.	meningocele	meningiocele	meningecele	meningacele
9.	nueral	nural	neural	neureal
10.	neurosthenia	neuresthenia	neuresthaenia	neurasthenia
11.	quodriplegia	quadroplegia	quadriplegia	quodreplegia
12.	ridiculopathy	radiculopathy	radicculopathy	rediculapathy

Cumulative Review

Chapters 5–7: Lymphatic and Immune Systems, Special Sensory Organs, and Nervous System

Directions: Check your mastery of word elements used in medical terminology related to the lymphatic and immune systems, special sensory organs (eyes and ears), and nervous system by defining the following prefixes, combining forms, and suffixes.

Prefixes

a- _____

an- _____

auto- _____

dys- _____

extra- _____

hemi- _____

hyper- _____

inter- _____

intra- _____

para- _____

peri- _____

poly- _____

quadri- _____

Combining Forms

aden/o _____

adenoid/o _____

angi/o _____

audi/o _____

blephar/o _____

cephal/o _____

cerebell/o _____

cerebr/o _____

cran/o, crani/o _____

cyt/o _____

encephal/o _____

hydr/o _____

immun/o _____

ir/o _____

irid/o _____

kerat/o _____

leuk/o _____

lymph/o _____

mening/o, meningi/o _____

myc/o _____

myel/o _____

myring/o _____

neur/o _____

ocul/o _____

ophthalm/o _____

opt/o _____

optic/o _____

ot/o _____

path/o _____

pleg/o _____

phag/o _____

psych/o _____

radicul/o _____

retin/o _____

scler/o _____

spin/o _____

splen/o _____

thym/o _____

tonsill/o _____

tympan/o _____

vascul/o _____

Suffixes

-ac _____

-al _____

-algia _____

-ar _____

-ary _____

-asthenia _____

-atic _____

-cele _____

-cyte _____

-eal _____

-ectomy _____

-edema _____

-esthesia _____

-gen _____

-gram _____

-graphy _____

-ia _____

-ic _____

-ical _____

-itis _____

-logist _____

-logy _____

-malacia _____

-megaly _____

-meter _____

-metry _____

-oid _____

-oma _____

-opia _____

-osis _____

-pathy _____

-pexy _____

-phasia _____

-plasty _____

-ptosis _____

-rrhaphy _____

-rrhea _____

-rrhexis _____

-sclerosis _____

-scope _____

-scopy _____

-spasm _____

-stomy _____

-tomy _____

-trophy _____

-us _____

Chapter 8

The Male and Female Reproductive Systems

gynec / o / logy: the study of the woman (female reproductive system)

ur / o / logy: the study of the urinary tract (male reproductive system)

Chapter Organization

- Intern Experience
- Overview of Reproductive System Anatomy and Physiology
- Word Elements
- Breaking Down and Building Reproductive System Terms
- Diseases and Disorders
- Procedures and Treatments
- Analyzing the Intern Experience
- Working with Medical Records
- Chapter Review

Chapter Objectives

After completing this chapter, you will be able to

1. label anatomical diagrams of the male and female reproductive systems;

2. dissect and define common medical terminology related to the male and female reproductive systems;

3. build terms used to describe reproductive system diseases and disorders, diagnostic procedures, and therapeutic treatments;

4. pronounce and spell common medical terminology related to the male and female reproductive systems;

5. understand that the process of building and dissecting a medical term based on its prefix, root word, and suffix enables you to analyze an extremely large number of medical terms beyond those presented in this chapter;

6. interpret the meaning of abbreviations associated with the reproductive systems; and

7. interpret medical records containing terminology and abbreviations related to the reproductive systems.

Your *EduHub* subscription that accompanies this text provides access to online assessments, assignments, activities, and resources. Throughout this chapter, access *EduHub* to

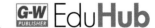

- use e-flash cards to review the medical terminology and word parts you learn;
- listen to the correct pronunciations of medical terms; and
- complete medical terminology activities and assignments.

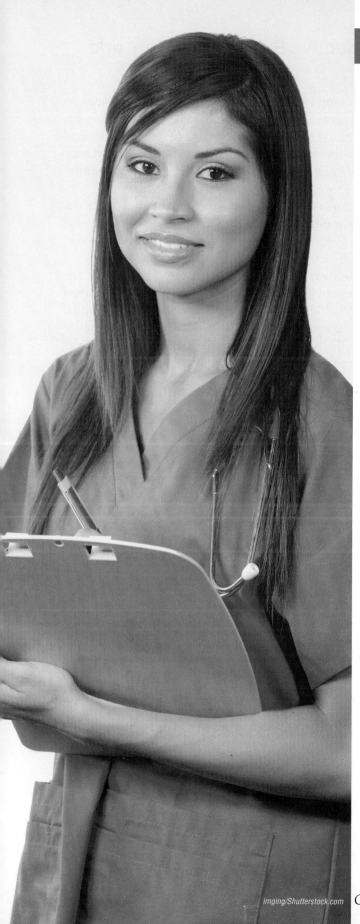

Emily is serving an internship with the Village Square Institute. She is delighted about the opportunity because the medical facility has an excellent reputation in the healthcare community. Emily has heard that the Institute has an opening for a medical assistant; she hopes that her internship experience will result in an employment offer.

On her first day, Emily reports to Pam Masters, RN. She escorts her first patient, Nancy Hopps, to the examination room. Mrs. Hopps is an older woman who recently discovered a lump in her right breast. Her primary care physician referred Mrs. Hopps to the Village Square Institute for further evaluation.

As you will learn later in this chapter, Nancy Hopps has a disorder that has affected one of the mammary organs of her reproductive system. She will be clinically evaluated for a possible cancerous tumor of the breast, and you will have the opportunity to interpret her chart note, the medical record dictated by her physician following Nancy's physical examination.

In this chapter, you will learn common word elements (prefixes, combining forms, and suffixes) used to form medical terms related to both the male and female reproductive systems. Mastery of these terms and the word parts from which they are constructed will enable you to understand the health conditions and diagnostic procedures summarized in the patient chart notes presented throughout this chapter.

Let's begin our study of the male and female reproductive systems with a brief overview of their anatomy and physiology. Afterward, you will learn about diseases and disorders, diagnostic tests and procedures, and therapeutic methods for treating common reproductive health conditions.

Overview of Reproductive System Anatomy and Physiology

As the name implies, the reproductive system enables human beings to reproduce, ensuring the survival of the species. **Gonads** are the primary organs of reproduction. Male gonads, called the **testes**, produce sperm and the hormone *testosterone* (tĕs-TŎS-tĕ-rōn). The testes, also called *testicles*, are suspended in a sac called the **scrotum**, situated behind the **penis** (Figure 8.1). Testosterone stimulates development of the male sex organs and production of sperm.

Sperm is produced in the testes and transported through genital ducts: the **epididymis** (ĕp-ĭ-DĬD-ĭ-mĭs), **vas deferens** (also called the *ductus deferens*), and **urethra**. The seminal vesicles, bulbourethral (BŬL-bō-yū-RĒ-thrăl) gland, and prostate gland contribute fluids along the way to produce semen.

Female gonads, called the **ovaries**, produce **ova** (eggs) and secrete the hormones *estrogen* and *progesterone* (prō-JĔS-tĕr-ōn). These hormones regulate the reproductive cycle and development of the **breasts** (**mammary glands**) and other female sexual characteristics. Fertilization of the ovum (singular form of *ova*) usually occurs in the **uterine tubes** (also called **fallopian tubes**). If fertilization occurs, the ovum implants in the **uterus**, where the female reproductive system continues to nurture and protect the developing fetus during pregnancy. During childbirth, the baby is expelled from the **vagina** (Figure 8.2 on the next page).

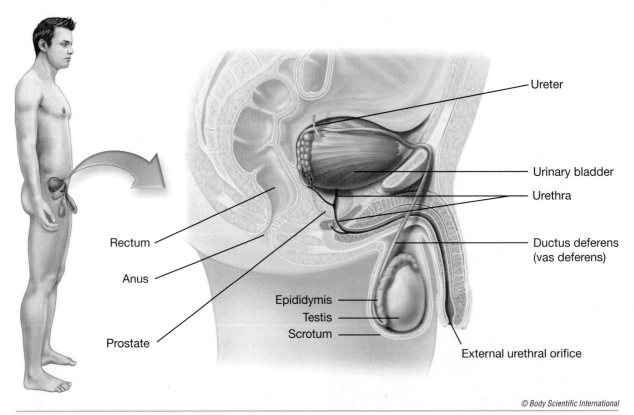

Rectum

Anus

Prostate

Epididymis

Testis

Scrotum

Ureter

Urinary bladder

Urethra

Ductus deferens (vas deferens)

External urethral orifice

© *Body Scientific International*

Figure 8.1 Major organs of the male reproductive system, sagittal view

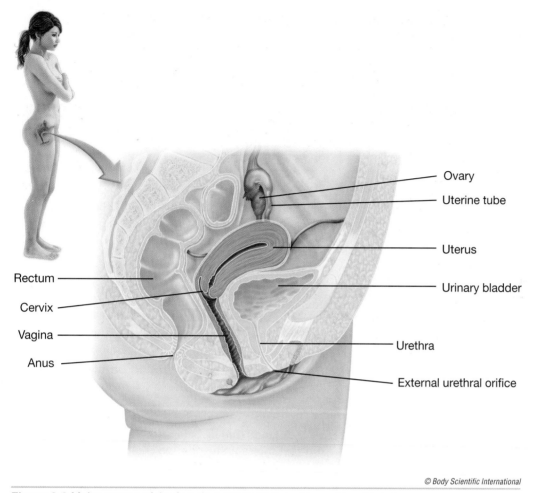

Rectum

Cervix

Vagina

Anus

Ovary

Uterine tube

Uterus

Urinary bladder

Urethra

External urethral orifice

Figure 8.2 Major organs of the female reproductive system, midsagittal view

In summary, the primary functions of the male and female reproductive systems are to

- produce ova (eggs) and sperm;
- secrete hormones; and
- facilitate conception (fertilization) and pregnancy.

The study of the male reproductive system is encompassed within the medical practice of **urology**, the study of the urinary tract. A **urologist** is a physician who specializes in the study, diagnosis, and treatment of diseases and disorders of the male reproductive system and urinary tract. **Gynecology** is the study of the female reproductive system. A specialist in the study, diagnosis, and treatment of female reproductive system disorders is called a **gynecologist**.

Anatomy and Physiology Vocabulary

Now that you have been introduced to the major organs and basic functions of the male and female reproductive systems, following are brief definitions of the key terms presented in the anatomy and physiology overview.

Key Term	Definition
breasts	mammary glands
bulbourethral gland	small gland on either side of the prostate gland; secretes fluid that lubricates the penis during sexual intercourse
epididymis	small, oblong body that rests upon and beside the posterior surface of the testes; stores and transports sperm from the testes
gonads	primary organs of reproduction (testes in the male, ovaries in the female)
ovaries	female gonads
penis	male organ of reproduction and urination
prostate gland	gland that surrounds the neck of the bladder and the urethra in the male; aids in production and ejaculation of semen
scrotum	pouch that contains the testes
seminal vesicles	sac-like glands that lie behind the male bladder; hold fluid that mixes with sperm to create semen
sperm	fluid produced in the testes that consists of sperm cells
testes	male gonads
urethra	canal through which urine is discharged from the bladder to the outside of the body
uterine tubes	fallopian tubes
uterus	organ that contains and nourishes the developing fetus
vagina	tube that leads from the cervix, the neck-like passage at the lower end of the uterus, to the vulva (external genitals)
vas deferens	excretory duct of the testis; *ductus deferens*

E-Flash Card Activity: Anatomy and Physiology Vocabulary

Directions: After you have reviewed the anatomy and physiology vocabulary related to the male and female reproductive systems, access your *EduHub* subscription and practice with the e-flash cards until you are comfortable with the spelling and definition of each term.

Identifying Major Organs of the Male Reproductive System

Directions: Label the diagram of the male reproductive system. You can also complete this activity online using *EduHub*.

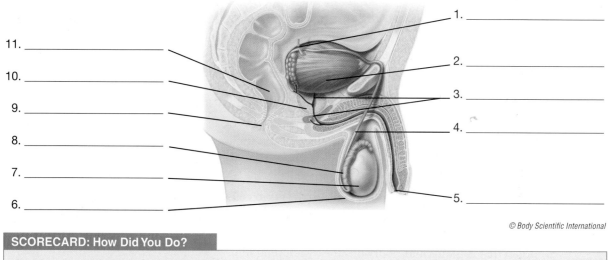

11. _____

10. _____

9. _____

8. _____

7. _____

6. _____

1. _____

2. _____

3. _____

4. _____

5. _____

© Body Scientific International

SCORECARD: How Did You Do?

Number correct (_____), divided by 11 (_____), multiplied by 100 equals _____ (your score)

Identifying Major Organs of the Female Reproductive System

Directions: Label the diagram of the female reproductive system. You can also complete this activity online using *EduHub*.

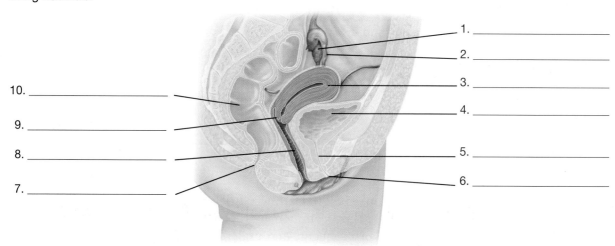

10. _____

9. _____

8. _____

7. _____

1. _____

2. _____

3. _____

4. _____

5. _____

6. _____

© Body Scientific International

SCORECARD: How Did You Do?

Number correct (_____), divided by 10 (_____), multiplied by 100 equals _____ (your score)

Matching Anatomy and Physiology Vocabulary

Directions: Choose the correct vocabulary term for each meaning. You can also complete this activity online using *EduHub*.

_____ 1. female gonads

_____ 2. fallopian tubes

_____ 3. tube that leads from the cervix, the neck-like passage at the lower end of the uterus, to the vulva (external genitals)

_____ 4. sac-like glands that lie behind the male bladder; hold fluid that mixes with sperm to create semen

_____ 5. gland that surrounds the neck of the bladder and the urethra in the male; aids in production and ejaculation of semen

_____ 6. pouch that contains the testes

_____ 7. fluid produced in the testes that consists of sperm cells

_____ 8. canal through which urine is discharged from the bladder to the outside of the body

_____ 9. organ that contains and nourishes the developing fetus

_____ 10. excretory duct of the testis; *ductus deferens*

_____ 11. primary organs of reproduction (testes in the male, ovaries in the female)

_____ 12. small gland on either side of the prostate gland; secretes fluid that lubricates the penis during sexual intercourse

_____ 13. small, oblong body that rests upon and beside the posterior surface of the testes; stores and transports sperm from the testes

_____ 14. male gonads

_____ 15. mammary glands

_____ 16. male organ of reproduction and urination

A. gonads
B. testes
C. sperm
D. ovaries
E. breasts
F. uterine tubes
G. uterus
H. vagina
I. scrotum
J. epididymis
K. vas deferens
L. urethra
M. prostate gland
N. penis
O. seminal vesicles
P. bulbourethral gland

SCORECARD: How Did You Do?

Number correct (_____), divided by 16 (_____), multiplied by 100 equals _____ (your score)

Word Elements

In this section, you will learn word elements—prefixes, combining forms, and suffixes—that are common to reproductive system terminology. By learning these word elements and understanding how they are combined to build medical terms, you will be able to analyze Mrs. Hopps's health condition (described in the Intern Experience at the beginning of this chapter) and identify a large number of terms associated with the reproductive systems.

E-Flash Card Activity: Word Elements

Directions: Review the word elements in the tables that follow. Then, access your *EduHub* subscription and practice with the e-flash cards until you are able to quickly recognize the different word parts (prefixes, combining forms, and suffixes) and their meanings. The e-flash cards are grouped together by prefixes, combining forms, and suffixes, followed by a cumulative review of all the word elements you are learning in this chapter.

Prefixes

Let's begin our study of medical word elements by looking at the prefixes listed in the table below. By now, you have mastered each of these prefixes and their meanings.

Prefix	Meaning
a-	not; without
dys-	painful; difficult
endo-	within
intra-	inside; within
trans-	across

Combining Forms

Following are combining forms that appear in medical terms used to describe reproductive system anatomy and physiology, pathological conditions, diagnostic procedures, and therapeutic treatments. A few of these combining forms appear in medical terms used to describe other body systems.

Root Word/Combining Vowel	Meaning
cervic/o	cervix; neck
colp/o	vagina
cyst/o	sac containing fluid; bladder
gynec/o	woman; female
hyster/o	uterus
lapar/o	abdomen
mamm/o	breast
mast/o	breast
men/o	menstruation
metr/o, metri/o	uterus

(Continued)

Root Word/Combining Vowel	Meaning
oophor/o	ovary
orchid/o	testes
prostat/o	prostate gland
salping/o	uterine tube; fallopian tube
scrot/o	scrotum
testicul/o	testes
ur/o	urine; urinary tract
vagin/o	vagina
vas/o	vessel; duct

Suffixes

Following are suffixes commonly encountered in medical terms pertaining to the male and female reproductive systems. From your studies of other body systems, you are already familiar with most of these suffixes.

Suffix	Meaning
-al	pertaining to
-algia	pain
-ectomy	surgical removal; excision
-gram	record; image
-graphy	process of recording an image
-ic	pertaining to
-itis	inflammation
-logist	specialist in the study and treatment of
-logy	study of
-osis	abnormal condition
-pexy	surgical fixation
-plasty	surgical repair
-rrhagia	bursting forth (of blood)
-rrhaphy	suture
-rrhea	discharge; flow
-rrhexis	rupture
-scope	instrument used to observe
-scopy	process of observing

Matching Prefixes, Combining Forms, and Suffixes

Directions: Choose the correct meaning for each word element. Some meanings may be used more than once. You can also complete this activity online using *EduHub*.

Prefixes

_____ 1. trans-	A. within
_____ 2. dys-	B. across
_____ 3. a-	C. not; without
_____ 4. intra-	D. painful; difficult
_____ 5. endo-	E. inside; within

Combining Forms

_____ 1. scrot/o

_____ 2. mast/o

_____ 3. colp/o

_____ 4. vas/o

_____ 5. hyster/o

_____ 6. oophor/o

_____ 7. cervic/o

_____ 8. testicul/o

_____ 9. mamm/o

_____ 10. prostat/o

_____ 11. cyst/o

_____ 12. vagin/o

_____ 13. men/o

_____ 14. ur/o

_____ 15. gynec/o

_____ 16. salping/o

_____ 17. metr/o, metri/o

_____ 18. orchid/o

_____ 19. lapar/o

A. woman; female

B. abdomen

C. cervix; neck

D. vagina

E. uterus

F. sac containing fluid; bladder

G. testes

H. uterine tube; fallopian tube

I. breast

J. menstruation

K. scrotum

L. prostate gland

M. urine; urinary tract

N. vessel; duct

O. ovary

Suffixes

_____ 1. -scope

_____ 2. -logist

_____ 3. -algia

_____ 4. -ic

_____ 5. -rrhaphy

_____ 6. -al

_____ 7. -ectomy

_____ 8. -rrhexis

_____ 9. -plasty

_____ 10. -gram

_____ 11. -scopy

_____ 12. -graphy

_____ 13. -logy

_____ 14. -rrhagia

_____ 15. -rrhea

_____ 16. -osis

_____ 17. -itis

_____ 18. -pexy

A. specialist in the study and treatment of

B. pertaining to

C. surgical fixation

D. suture

E. pain

F. process of observing

G. inflammation

H. instrument used to observe

I. surgical removal; excision

J. study of

K. record; image

L. process of recording an image

M. surgical repair

N. discharge; flow

O. bursting forth (of blood)

P. rupture

Q. abnormal condition

SCORECARD: How Did You Do?

Number correct (_____), divided by 42 (_____), multiplied by 100 equals _____ (your score)

Breaking Down and Building Reproductive System Terms

Now that you have mastered common word parts used in medical terminology related to the reproductive systems, you have the ability to dissect and build a large number of terms that apply to reproductive anatomy and physiology, pathology, diagnostics, and treatments.

Term	Dissection	Word Part/Meaning	Term Meaning
Note: *For simplification, combining vowels have been omitted from the Word Part/Meaning column.*			
1. **amenorrhea** (ă-MĔN-ō-RĒ-ă)	a/men/o/rrhea	**a** = not; without **men** = menstruation **rrhea** = discharge; flow	without flow of menstruation
2. **cervical** (SĔR-vĭ-kăl)	cervic/al	**cervic** = cervix; neck **al** = pertaining to	pertaining to the cervix/neck
3. **colposcopy** (kŏl-PŎS-kō-pē)	colp/o/scopy	**colp** = vagina **scopy** = process of observing	process of observing the vagina
4. **dysmenorrhea** (dĭs-MĔN-ō-RĒ-ă)	dys/men/o/rrhea	**dys** = painful; difficult **men** = menstruation **rrhea** = discharge; flow	painful and difficult flow of menstruation
5. **endometriosis** (ĔN-dō-mē-trē-Ō-sĭs)	endo/metri/osis	**endo** = within **metr** = uterus **osis** = abnormal condition	abnormal condition within the uterus
6. **gynecology** (gī-nĕ-KŎL-ō-jē)	gynec/o/logy	**gynec** = woman; female **logy** = study of	study of the woman/female
7. **gynecologist** (gī-nĕ-KŎL-ō-jĭst)	gynec/o/logist	**gynec** = woman; female **logist** = specialist in the study and treatment of	specialist in the study and treatment of the woman/female
8. **hysterectomy** (HĬS-tĕr-ĔK-tō-mē)	hyster/ectomy	**hyster** = uterus **ectomy** = surgical removal; excision	excision of the uterus
9. **hysterosalpingogram** (HĬS-tĕr-ō-săl-PĬNG-gō-grăm)	hyster/o/salping/o/gram	**hyster** = uterus **salping** = uterine tube; fallopian tube **gram** = record; image	record/image of the uterus and uterine/fallopian tube
10. **hysterosalpingo-oophorectomy** (HĬS-tĕr-ō-săl-PING-gō ō-ŏ-for-ĔK-tō-mē)	hyster/o/salping/o oophor/ectomy	**hyster** = uterus **salping** = uterine tube; fallopian tube **oophor** = ovary **ectomy** = surgical removal; excision	excision of the uterus, uterine/fallopian tube, and ovary
11. **laparoscopy** (LĂP-ă-RŎS-kō-pē)	lapar/o/scopy	**lapar** = abdomen **scopy** = process of observing	process of observing the abdomen
12. **mammography** (mă-MŎG-ră-fē)	mamm/o/graphy	**mamm** = breast **graphy** = process of recording an image	process of recording an image of the breast
13. **mastectomy** (măs-TĔK-tō-mē)	mast/ectomy	**mast** = breast **ectomy** = surgical removal; excision	excision of the breast
Prefixes = **Green** Root Words = **Red** Suffixes = **Blue**			

Term	Dissection	Word Part/Meaning	Term Meaning
14. **menorrhagia** (měn-ō-RĀ-jē-ă)	men/o/rrhagia	**men** = menstruation **rrhagia** = bursting forth (of blood)	bursting forth of menstruation
15. **menorrhea** (měn-ō-RĒ-ă)	men/o/rrhea	**men** = menstruation **rrhea** = discharge; flow	flow of menstruation
16. **oophorectomy** (ō-ŎF-ō-RĔK-tō-mē)	oophor/ectomy	**oophor** = ovary **ectomy** = surgical removal; excision	excision of the ovary
17. **orchidectomy** (or-kĭ-DĔK-tō-mē)	orchid/ectomy	**orchid** = testes **ectomy** = surgical removal; excision	excision of the testes
18. **prostatectomy** (PRŎS-tă-TĔK-tō-mē)	prostat/ectomy	**prostat** = prostate gland **ectomy** = surgical removal; excision	excision of the prostate gland
19. **prostatic** (prŏs-TĂT-ĭk)	prostat/ic	**prostat** = prostate gland **ic** = pertaining to	pertaining to the prostate gland
20. **prostatitis** (prŏs-tă-TĪ-tĭs)	prostat/itis	**prostat** = prostate gland **itis** = inflammation	inflammation of the prostate gland
21. **salpingitis** (săl-pĭn-JĪ-tĭs)	salping/itis	**salping** = uterine tube; fallopian tube **itis** = inflammation	inflammation of the uterine/fallopian tube
22. **urologist** (ū-RŎL-ō-jĭst)	ur/o/logist	**ur** = urine; urinary tract **logist** = specialist in the study and treatment of	specialist in the study and treatment of the urinary tract
23. **urology** (ū-RŎL-ō-jē)	ur/o/logy	**ur** = urine; urinary tract **logy** = study of	study of the urine/ urinary tract
24. **vaginitis** (VĂJ-ĭn-Ī-tĭs)	vagin/itis	**vagin** = vagina **itis** = inflammation	inflammation of the vagina
25. **vasectomy** (văs-ĔK-tō-mē)	vas/ectomy	**vas** = vessel; duct **ectomy** = surgical removal; excision	excision of a vessel/ duct

Prefixes = Green   Root Words = Red   Suffixes = Blue

Using the pronunciation guide in the Breaking Down and Building chart, practice saying each medical term aloud. To hear the pronunciation of each term, complete the Pronounce It activity on the next page.

Audio Activity: Pronounce It

Directions: Access your *EduHub* subscription and listen to the correct pronunciations of the following medical terms. Practice pronouncing the terms until you are comfortable saying them aloud.

amenorrhea
(ă-MĔN-ō-RĒ-ă)

cervical
(SĔR-vĭ-kăl)

colposcopy
(kŏl-PŎS-kō-pē)

dysmenorrhea
(dĭs-MĔN-ō-RĒ-ă)

endometriosis
(ĔN-dō-mē-trē-Ō-sĭs)

gynecology
(gī-nĕ-KŎL-ō-jē)

gynecologist
(gī-nĕ-KŎL-ō-jĭst)

hysterectomy
(HĬS-tĕr-ĔK-tō-mē)

hysterosalpingogram
(HĬS-tĕr-ō-săl-PĬNG-gō-grăm)

hysterosalpingo-
oophorectomy
(HĬS-tĕr-ō-săl-PING-gō
ō-ŏ-for-ĔK-tō-mē)

laparoscopy
(LĂP-ă-RŎS-kō-pē)

mammography
(mă-MŎG-ră-fē)

mastectomy
(măs-TĔK-tō-mē)

menorrhagia
(mĕn-ō-RĀ-jē-ă)

menorrhea
(mĕn-ō-RĒ-ă)

oophorectomy
(ō-ŎF-ō-RĔK-tō-mē)

orchidectomy
(or-kĭ-DĔK-tō-mē)

prostatectomy
(PRŎS-tă-TĔK-tō-mē)

prostatic
(prŏs-TĂT-ĭk)

prostatitis
(prŏs-tă-TĪ-tĭs)

salpingitis
(săl-pĭn-JĪ-tĭs)

urologist
(ū-RŎL-ō-jĭst)

urology
(ū-RŎL-ō-jē)

vaginitis
(VĂJ-ĭn-Ī-tĭs)

vasectomy
(văs-ĔK-tō-mē)

Assessment 8.5

Audio Activity: Spell It

Directions: Access your *EduHub* subscription and listen to the pronunciation for each number. As you hear each term, write its correct spelling.

1. _____
2. _____
3. _____
4. _____
5. _____
6. _____
7. _____
8. _____
9. _____
10. _____
11. _____
12. _____
13. _____
14. _____
15. _____
16. _____
17. _____
18. _____
19. _____
20. _____
21. _____
22. _____
23. _____
24. _____
25. _____

SCORECARD: How Did You Do?

Number correct (_____), divided by 25 (_____), multiplied by 100 equals _____ (your score)

Break It Down

Directions: Dissect each medical term into its word parts (prefix, root word, combining vowel, and suffix) using one or more slashes. Then define each term. You can also complete this activity online using *EduHub*.

Example:
Medical Term: salpingitis
Dissection: salping/itis
Definition: inflammation of the uterine (fallopian) tube

Medical Term	Dissection
1. prostatitis	p r o s t a t i t i s

Definition: _____

_____

2. oophorectomy — o o p h o r e c t o m y

Definition: _____

_____

3. mammography — m a m m o g r a p h y

Definition: _____

_____

4. hysterosalpingo-oophorectomy — h y s t e r o s a l p i n g o -

o o p h o r e c t o m y

Definition: _____

_____

5. endometriosis — e n d o m e t r i o s i s

Definition: _____

_____

Medical Term	Dissection
6. dysmenorrhea	d y s m e n o r r h e a

Definition: _____

_____

| 7. urologist | u r o l o g i s t |

Definition: _____

_____

| 8. salpingitis | s a l p i n g i t i s |

Definition: _____

_____

| 9. prostatectomy | p r o s t a t e c t o m y |

Definition: _____

_____

| 10. urology | u r o l o g y |

Definition: _____

_____

| 11. gynecologist | g y n e c o l o g i s t |

Definition: _____

_____

| 12. vasectomy | v a s e c t o m y |

Definition: _____

_____

| 13. amenorrhea | a m e n o r r h e a |

Definition: _____

_____

Medical Term	Dissection
14. vaginitis	v a g i n i t i s

Definition: _____

_____

15. gynecology   g y n e c o l o g y

Definition: _____

_____

16. menorrhagia   m e n o r r h a g i a

Definition: _____

_____

17. hysterosalpingogram   h y s t e r o s a l p i n g o g r a m

Definition: _____

_____

18. hysterectomy   h y s t e r e c t o m y

Definition: _____

_____

19. colposcopy   c o l p o s c o p y

Definition: _____

_____

20. cervical   c e r v i c a l

Definition: _____

_____

SCORECARD: How Did You Do?

Number correct (_____), divided by 20 (_____), multiplied by 100 equals _____ (your score)

Build It

Directions: Build the medical term that matches each definition by supplying the correct word parts. You can also complete this activity online using *EduHub*.

P (Prefixes) = Green
RW (Root Words) = Red
S (Suffixes) = Blue
CV (Combining Vowel) = Purple

1. excision of a vessel/duct

   _____ _____
   RW   S

2. specialist in the study and treatment of the woman/female

   _____ _____ _____
   RW   CV   S

3. process of recording an image of the breast

   _____ _____ _____
   RW   CV   S

4. record/image of the uterus and uterine/fallopian tube

   _____ _____ _____ _____ _____
   RW   CV   RW   CV   S

5. abnormal condition within the uterus

   _____ _____ _____
   P   RW   S

6. without flow of menstruation

   _____ _____ _____ _____
   P   RW   CV   S

7. inflammation of the uterine/fallopian tube

   _____ _____
   RW   S

8. process of observing the vagina

   _____ _____ _____
   RW   CV   S

9. process of observing the abdomen

   _____ _____ _____
   RW   CV   S

10. excision of the breast

——————————————— ————
RW   S

11. painful and difficult flow of menstruation

———— ——————————————— ———— ————
P   RW   CV   S

12. specialist in the study and treatment of the urinary tract

——————————————— ———— ————
RW   CV   S

13. flow of menstruation

——————————————— ———— ————
RW   CV   S

14. inflammation of the vagina

——————————————— ————
RW   S

15. study of the woman/female

——————————————— ———— ————
RW   CV   S

16. pertaining to the cervix

——————————————— ————
RW   S

17. study of the urine/urinary tract

——————————————— ———— ————
RW   CV   S

18. excision of the uterus

——————————————— ————
RW   S

19. excision of the prostate gland

——————————————— ————
RW   S

20. pertaining to the prostate

——————————————— ————
RW   S

SCORECARD: How Did You Do?

Number correct (_____), divided by 20 (_____), multiplied by 100 equals _____ (your score)

Identify the Medical Word Part

Directions: For each medical word part, identify the type of word part (prefix, root word, or suffix) and provide its meaning. You can also complete this activity online using *EduHub*.

1. **metr**   Prefix   Root Word   Suffix

Meaning: _____

2. **graphy**   Prefix   Root Word   Suffix

Meaning: _____

3. **dys**   Prefix   Root Word   Suffix

Meaning: _____

4. **salping**   Prefix   Root Word   Suffix

Meaning: _____

5. **cervic**   Prefix   Root Word   Suffix

Meaning: _____

6. **oophor**   Prefix   Root Word   Suffix

Meaning: _____

7. **rrhagia**   Prefix   Root Word   Suffix

Meaning: _____

8. **prostat**   Prefix   Root Word   Suffix

Meaning: _____

SCORECARD: How Did You Do?

Number correct (_____), divided by 8 (_____), multiplied by 100 equals _____ (your score)

Diseases and Disorders

Diseases and disorders of the male and female reproductive systems run the spectrum from the mild to the severe and have a number of different causes. In this section, we will briefly examine some common pathological conditions of these body systems.

Benign Prostatic Hypertrophy

Benign prostatic hypertrophy (prŏs-TĂT-ĭk hī-PĔR-trō-phē) (**BPH**) is a noncancerous enlargement of the prostate gland, or *prostate* (Figure 8.3). The prostate surrounds the urethra, a tube that carries urine from the bladder out of the body. As the prostate enlarges, it constricts (narrows) the urethra, impeding urine flow. Symptoms of BPH include *nocturia* (urinating often at night), *urinary retention* (inability to empty urine from the bladder), and *frequency* (urinating frequently). BPH occurs in many men as they age.

Breast Cancer

Breast cancer originates in the tissues of the breast (Figure 8.4 on the next page). It may be *invasive* or *noninvasive.* Breast cancer that is invasive has spread from the *lobule* (LŎB-yūl), or milk duct, to other tissue in the breast. Breast cancer that is noninvasive has not affected other tissue in the breast.

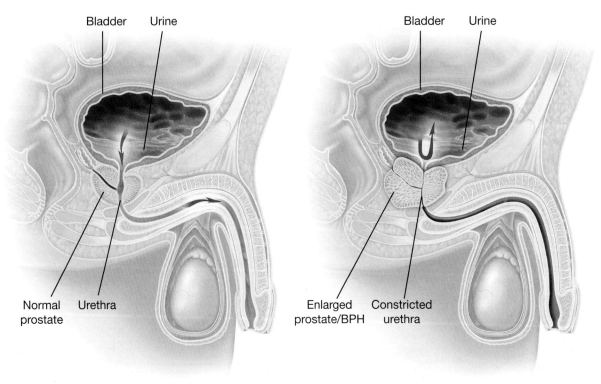

Bladder   Urine

Bladder   Urine

Normal prostate   Urethra

Enlarged prostate/BPH   Constricted urethra

© *Body Scientific International*

Figure 8.3 Benign prostatic hypertrophy is a noncancerous enlargement of the prostate gland.

Early-stage breast cancer usually does not cause symptoms. As the cancer grows, a woman may feel a painless lump in the breast or in the armpit. The lump is typically hard with uneven edges. There may be a change in the size, shape, or feel of the breast or nipple or a discharge from the nipple. Breast cancer is not limited to females. Men, too, can develop this type of cancer.

Different tests are used to diagnose breast cancer. A physician will perform a physical examination of both breasts, armpits, and the neck and chest area. **Mammography** (mă-MŎG-ră-fē) is used to screen for breast cancer. If a suspicious growth is detected in a mammogram, a breast ultrasound may be performed to determine whether the lump is solid (indicative of a tumor) or fluid-filled (characteristic of a cyst). Further testing may include a breast biopsy, computerized tomography (CT) scan, or magnetic resonance imaging (MRI) scan. These tests help the physician determine whether or not the cancer has spread. Use of a series of tests to establish the extent of cancerous growth—especially whether or not cancer has spread to other parts of the body—is called *staging*. Staging helps in guiding future treatment.

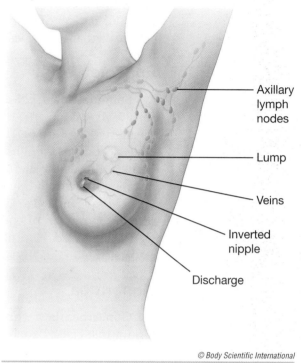

© Body Scientific International

Figure 8.4 Breast cancer may originate anywhere within the tissues of the breast.

Chlamydia

Chlamydia is a common sexually transmitted infection (STI) caused by a bacterium (Figure 8.5). Sexually active individuals and those with multiple partners are at highest risk of contracting the disease.

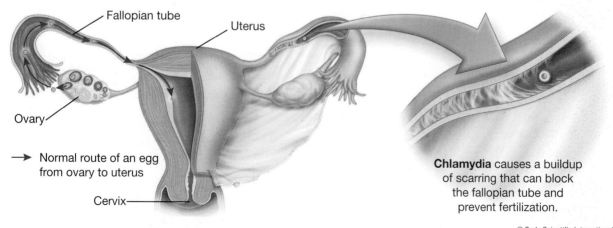

Chlamydia causes a buildup of scarring that can block the fallopian tube and prevent fertilization.

© Body Scientific International

Figure 8.5 Untreated chlamydia can lead to fallopian tube damage.

Chlamydia infections in women may lead to **cervicitis** (sĕr-vĭ-SĪ-tĭs), inflammation of the cervix. Left untreated, chlamydia can result in fallopian tube damage. In men, chlamydia can lead to **urethritis** (yū-rĕ-THRĪ-tĭs), inflammation of the urethra. Male patients may experience a burning sensation during urination and/or discharge from the penis or rectum. Some males also experience testicular tenderness. Chlamydia typically is treated with antibiotics.

Endometriosis

Endometriosis (ĔN-dō-mē-trē-Ō-sis) is a disorder in which the *endometrium* (ĕn-dō-MĒ-trē-ŭm), the tissue that lines the inside of the uterus, grows outside the uterus (Figure 8.6). The displaced endometrium continues to function normally. It thickens, sloughs off, and bleeds with each menstrual cycle. Because the tissue is outside the uterus, it has no way to exit the body. It is trapped, causing irritation to surrounding body tissues and eventually leading to the formation of scar tissue and *adhesions* (abnormal tissue that binds organs together). The primary symptom of endometriosis is pelvic pain, often associated with the menstrual period. Painful intercourse, painful defecation, and infertility can be associated with this disease. The cause of endometriosis is unknown.

Gonorrhea

Gonorrhea is a curable sexually transmitted infection (STI). The bacterium that causes gonorrhea can infect the genital tract, mouth, or anus. In men, gonorrhea can cause pain with urination and discharge from the penis. In women, it can cause bleeding between periods, pain with urination, and increased vaginal discharge. Gonorrhea does not always cause symptoms, so an infected person can unknowingly transmit the disease. Left untreated, the STI can lead to pelvic inflammatory disease (PID), which causes infertility or problems during pregnancy. Gonorrhea can pass from mother to baby during pregnancy. It is treated with antibiotics.

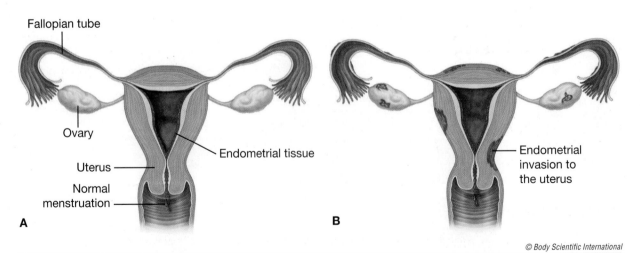

Fallopian tube

Ovary

Uterus

Normal menstruation

Endometrial tissue

A

Endometrial invasion to the uterus

B

© Body Scientific International

Figure 8.6 In endometriosis, the tissue that lines the inside of the uterus grows outside the uterus. The displaced tissue becomes trapped, causing irritation and eventually scar tissue and adhesions.

Genital Herpes

Genital herpes is a highly contagious sexually transmitted infection (STI) caused by the *herpes simplex virus* (*HSV*) (Figure 8.7). It is characterized by periodic outbreaks of painful, itchy, ulcer-like lesions of the genitals, skin, and mucous membranes. Some people infected with HSV are asymptomatic (without signs or symptoms). In fact, an infected person can still be contagious even if no sores are visible. Genital herpes cannot be cured, but it can be controlled with medication. Once a person has been infected, the virus lies dormant in the body and can reactivate several times a year. Use of condoms can help prevent transmission of the virus.

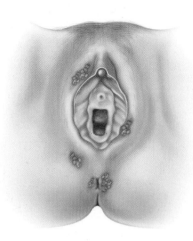

- Sexually transmitted virus
- Small, painful sores or blisters
- Usually heal in 1-3 weeks
- Can come back weeks, months, or years later

© Body Scientific International

Figure 8.7 Genital herpes is a highly contagious, incurable sexually transmitted infection.

Pelvic Inflammatory Disease

Pelvic inflammatory disease (PID) is an infection of the female reproductive organs (Figure 8.8). Symptoms may include fever, chills, malaise (general feeling of unwellness), backache, tender abdomen, and a foul-smelling vaginal discharge. The initial infection is usually caused by an STI. PID occurs when disease-causing microorganisms travel from the cervix to the upper genital tract. Untreated gonorrhea and chlamydia cause nearly all cases of PID. Antibiotic treatment is prescribed for PID.

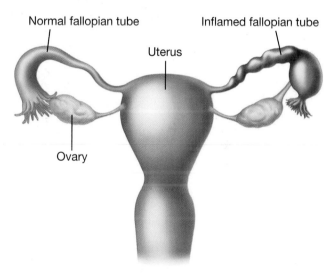

Normal fallopian tube

Inflamed fallopian tube

Uterus

Ovary

© Body Scientific International

Figure 8.8 Pelvic inflammatory disease is an infection of the female reproductive organs. It is usually caused by a sexually transmitted infection.

Premenstrual Syndrome

Premenstrual syndrome (PMS) is a group of symptoms linked to the menstrual cycle. Its cause is unclear. PMS is characterized by a variety of symptoms, including tender breasts, mood swings, irritability, depression, fatigue, and food cravings. These problems tend to peak in women in their late 20s and early 30s. There are no specific physical or laboratory tests for the positive diagnosis of premenstrual syndrome.

Prostate Cancer

Prostate cancer originates in the prostate gland, a small, walnut-sized gland that surrounds the neck of the male bladder and urethra (Figure 8.9 on the next page). The prostate secretes an alkaline substance that

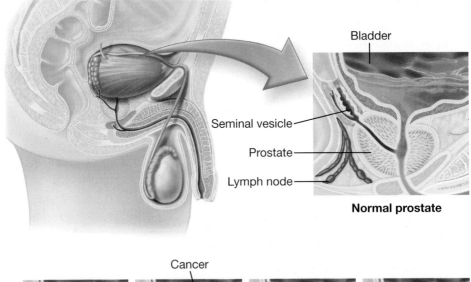

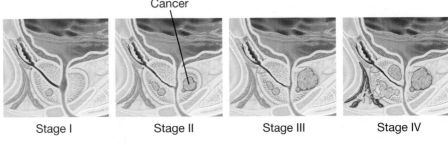

Bladder

Seminal vesicle

Prostate

Lymph node

Normal prostate

Cancer

Stage I   Stage II   Stage III   Stage IV

© *Body Scientific International*

Figure 8.9 Stages of prostate cancer, from early to advanced stage. The cancer originates in the prostate gland, which surrounds the neck of the male bladder and urethra.

is a component of semen. Symptoms of prostate cancer are similar to those of benign prostatic hypertrophy (BPH): slow or weak urine stream, incontinence (leakage), inability to fully empty the bladder, and nocturia. A biopsy may be performed if a rectal exam reveals that the prostate is enlarged or has a hard, uneven surface. During the biopsy, a sample of tissue is removed from the prostate and sent to a lab for analysis.

Syphilis

Syphilis (SĬF-ĭ-lĭs) is a sexually transmitted infection (STI) caused by a bacterium. It infects the genital area, lips, mouth, or anus by producing red, elevated areas on the skin that erode into small ulcers called *chancres* (SHĂNG-kĕrs). Syphilis is transmitted by direct sexual contact with an infected person. A pregnant woman infected with syphilis can pass the disease to her fetus. The disease is treated with antibiotics. Without treatment, syphilis can be life-threatening, severely damaging the heart, brain, or other vital organs.

Procedures and Treatments

In this section, you will learn about tests and procedures used to help diagnose pathological conditions of the male and female reproductive systems, as well as therapeutic methods commonly used to treat certain conditions.

Circumcision

Circumcision (sĕr-kŭm-SĬZH-ŭn) is the surgical removal of the foreskin, the skin that covers the tip of the penis (Figure 8.10). The procedure is performed soon after birth. There are medical benefits and risks to circumcision. Benefits include a lower risk of urinary tract infections (UTIs), penile cancer, and STIs. Risks include bleeding, pain, and infection after the procedure. Parents of a male newborn decide whether or not they want circumcision to be performed based on their religious, cultural, and personal beliefs.

Colposcopy

Colposcopy (kŏl-PŎS-kō-pē) is a diagnostic procedure used to examine the cervix, vagina, and vulva (external genitalia) (Figure 8.11 on the next page). It is performed using a *colposcope* (KŎL-pō-skōp), a surgical instrument that provides an enlarged view of the tissues in these areas. This enhanced view enables the physician to visually distinguish between normal and abnormal-appearing tissue and to take biopsies for pathological examination. Colposcopy is often performed if a pelvic exam or Pap test (discussed on the next pages) reveals abnormalities. The main goal of colposcopy is to prevent cervical cancer by detecting precancerous lesions and treating them before they become cancerous.

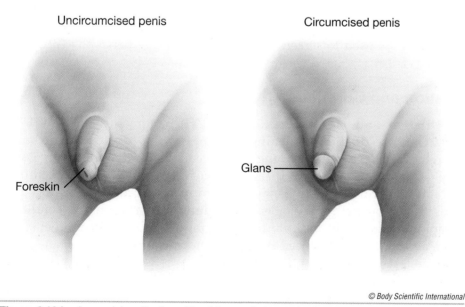

Uncircumcised penis

Circumcised penis

Glans

Foreskin

© Body Scientific International

Figure 8.10 In circumcision, the foreskin of the penis is surgically removed shortly after birth.

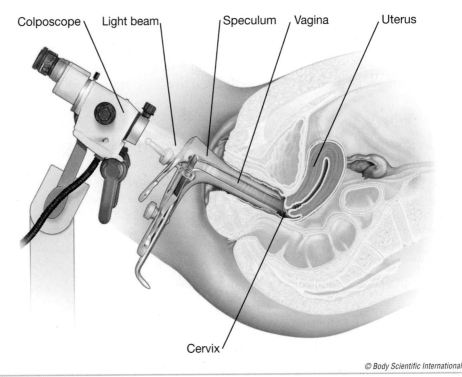

Colposcope   Light beam   Speculum   Vagina   Uterus

Cervix

© Body Scientific International

Figure 8.11 Colposcopy is the diagnostic examination of the cervix, vagina, and vulva using a colposcope.

Digital Rectal Exam

A **digital rectal exam** is performed to evaluate the size and shape of the prostate gland. A physician inserts a finger into the rectum to *palpate* (lightly press with the fingers) the prostate through the wall of the rectum. A digital rectal exam is used to screen for benign prostatic hypertrophy (BPH) and prostate cancer.

Dilation and Curettage

Dilation and curettage (kū-rĕ-TĀHZH), commonly referred to as a **D&C**, is the dilation (widening/opening) of the cervix and the surgical removal of part of the lining and/or contents of the uterus by curettage (scraping and scooping). Tissue removed during a D&C is sent to a laboratory for analysis. D&C may be performed as a diagnostic procedure or as a therapeutic gynecological procedure to treat a uterine condition. Symptoms that might indicate the need for a D&C are severe menstrual pain, abnormal uterine bleeding, postmenopausal bleeding, or an abnormal Pap test (discussed on the next page).

Laparoscopic Hysterectomy

Laparoscopic hysterectomy (LĂP-ă-rō-SKŎP-ĭk HĬS-tĕr-ĔK-tō-mē) is a minimally invasive surgical technique that allows the uterus to be removed without a large incision (Figure 8.12). The surgeon makes multiple, small incisions to insert instruments and uses a tiny camera to visualize the surgical site. The laparoscopic approach to hysterectomy is safer than open surgery because less tissue is cut, resulting in a lower risk of infection and faster healing time.

Pap Test

A **Pap test**, or **Pap smear**, is the microscopic examination of cells from the cervix (Figure 8.13). It is used as a screening tool for cervical cancer. During a Pap test, the physician inserts an instrument called a *speculum* into the vagina to open it slightly. Then cells are gently scraped from the opening of the cervix and sent to a lab for analysis.

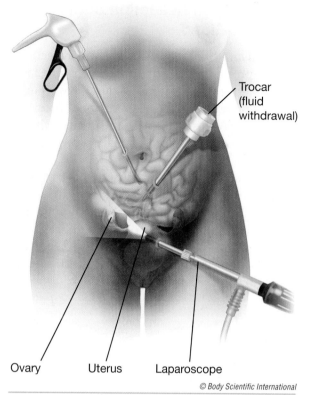

Trocar (fluid withdrawal)

Ovary   Uterus   Laparoscope

© Body Scientific International

Figure 8.12 Laparoscopic hysterectomy is a safer alternative than open surgery for removal of the uterus.

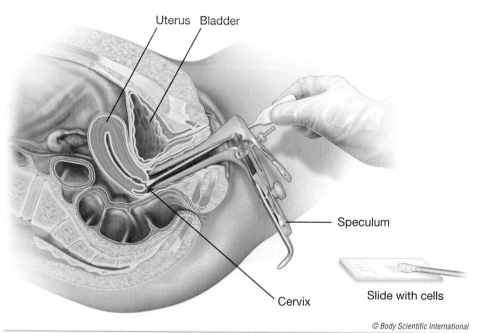

Uterus Bladder

Speculum

Cervix

Slide with cells

© Body Scientific International

Figure 8.13 A Pap test, or Pap smear, is a common screening tool for cervical cancer.

Transurethral Resection of the Prostate Gland

Transurethral (trăns-yū-RĒ-thrăl) **resection of the prostate (TURP)** is a type of prostate surgery done to relieve moderate to severe urinary symptoms caused by an enlarged prostate (Figure 8.14). As you learned earlier, another term for an enlarged prostate is *benign prostatic hypertrophy* (BPH).

During the TURP procedure, an instrument called a *resectoscope* (rē-SĔK-tō-skōp) is inserted through the urethra to the prostate. Using the resectoscope, which functions as both a visual and surgical instrument, the physician removes the section of the prostate that is obstructing urine flow.

Vasectomy

A **vasectomy** is considered a permanent method of male contraception (Figure 8.15). During a vasectomy, the vas deferens from each testicle is clamped or cut, preventing the release of sperm. Vasectomy is one of the most commonly used surgical sterilization procedures for men. A vasectomy only prevents pregnancy; it offers no protection against STIs.

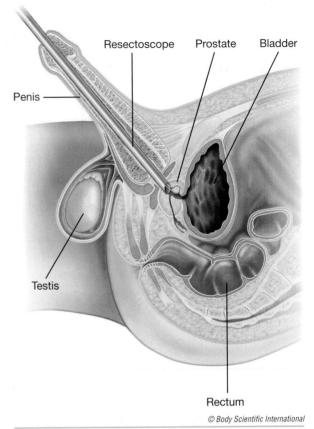

© Body Scientific International

Figure 8.14 Transurethral resection of the prostate (TURP) is performed to relieve moderate to severe urinary symptoms caused by an enlarged prostate.

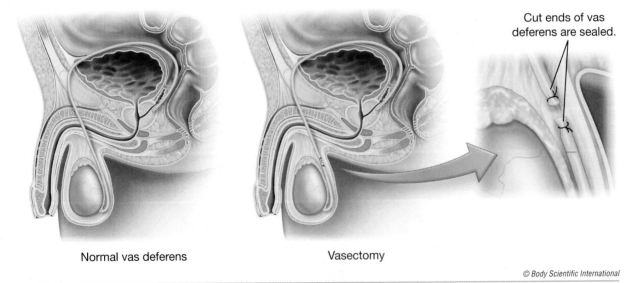

© Body Scientific International

Figure 8.15 Vasectomy is a permanent method of male contraception.

Tubal Ligation

Tubal ligation is a type of female contraception (birth control) that permanently prevents pregnancy (Figure 8.16). During tubal ligation, the uterine (fallopian) tubes are clamped, severed, or sealed. This procedure prevents ova from reaching the uterus for fertilization and blocks sperm from traveling up the uterine tubes to the egg. A tubal ligation does not affect the menstrual cycle, nor does it offer protection from sexually transmitted infections (STIs).

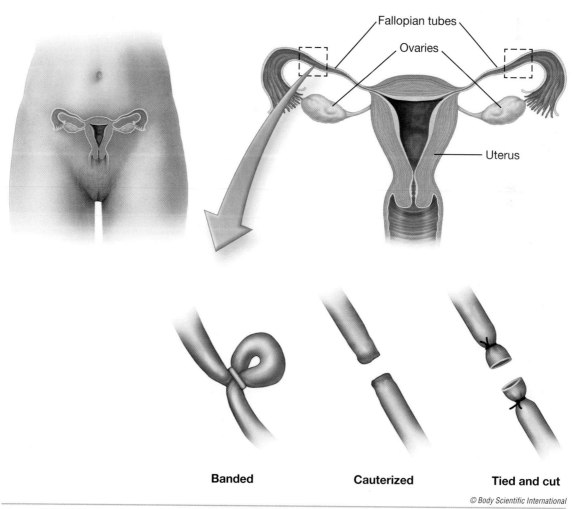

Banded **Cauterized** **Tied and cut**

© Body Scientific International

Figure 8.16 Tubal ligation is a permanent method of female birth control.

Multiple Choice: Diseases and Disorders

Directions: Choose the disease or disorder that matches each definition. You can also complete this activity online using *EduHub*.

_____ 1. Gonorrhea is
   a. found in women only.
   b. a benign tumor.
   c. passed to the fetus during pregnancy.
   d. a virus that lies dormant in the body and can reactivate several times a year.

_____ 2. a sexually transmitted infection that produces chancres
   a. urethritis   c. endometriosis
   b. cervicitis   d. syphilis

_____ 3. a common bacterial STI that can cause cervicitis in women and urethritis in men
   a. chlamydia
   b. genital herpes
   c. endometriosis
   d. benign prostatic hypertrophy

_____ 4. an infection of the female reproductive organs
   a. pelvic inflammatory disease
   b. syphilis
   c. endometriosis
   d. chlamydia

_____ 5. a highly contagious sexually transmitted infection caused by the herpes simplex virus (HSV)
   a. chlamydia   c. endometriosis
   b. genital herpes   d. gonorrhea

_____ 6. a disorder in which the tissue lining the inside of the uterus grows outside the uterus
   a. chlamydia
   b. endometriosis
   c. genital herpes
   d. pelvic inflammatory disease

_____ 7. a cancer that starts in the prostate gland
   a. genital herpes
   b. prostate cancer
   c. benign prostatic hypertrophy
   d. endometriosis

SCORECARD: How Did You Do?

Number correct (_____), divided by 7 (_____), multiplied by 100 equals _____ (your score)

Multiple Choice: Procedures and Treatments

Directions: Choose the procedure or treatment that matches each definition. You can also complete this activity online using *EduHub*.

_____ 1. surgical removal of the foreskin
   a. circumcision
   b. transurethral resection of the prostate gland
   c. vasectomy
   d. tubal ligation

_____ 2. surgery done to relieve moderate to severe urinary symptoms caused by an enlarged prostate
   a. prostectomy
   b. vasectomy
   c. transurethral resection of the prostate gland
   d. tubal ligation

_____ 3. permanent method of male birth control
   a. transurethral resection of the prostate gland
   b. circumcision
   c. tubal ligation
   d. vasectomy

_____ 4. microscopic examination of cells scraped from the cervix
   a. Pap test
   b. colposcopy
   c. dilation and curettage
   d. laparoscopic hysterectomy

_____ 5. dilation of the cervix and surgical removal of part of the lining of the uterus and uterine contents
    a. laparoscopic hysterectomy
    b. dilation and curettage
    c. Pap test
    d. colposcopy

_____ 6. diagnostic procedure for examining the cervix, vagina, and vulva
    a. Pap test
    b. dilation and curettage
    c. tubal ligation
    d. colposcopy

_____ 7. excision of the uterus
    a. circumcision
    b. laparoscopic hysterectomy
    c. vasectomy
    d. tubal ligation

_____ 8. permanent method of female birth control
    a. tubal ligation
    b. transurethral resection of the prostate gland
    c. vasectomy
    d. circumcision

SCORECARD: How Did You Do?

Number correct (_____), divided by 8 (_____), multiplied by 100 equals _____ (your score)

Assessment 8.11

Identifying Abbreviations

Directions: Supply the correct abbreviation for each medical term. You can also complete this activity online using *EduHub*.

Medical Term	Abbreviation
1. sexually transmitted infection	_____
2. herpes simplex virus	_____
3. pelvic inflammatory disease	_____
4. benign prostatic hypertrophy	_____
5. premenstrual syndrome	_____
6. transurethral resection of the prostate gland	_____
7. dilation and curettage	_____

SCORECARD: How Did You Do?

Number correct (_____), divided by 7 (_____), multiplied by 100 equals _____ (your score)

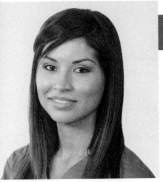

Analyzing the Intern Experience

In the Intern Experience described at the beginning of this chapter, we met Emily, an intern with the Village Square Institute. Emily was assigned to shadow Pam, a registered nurse (RN). Their first patient was Nancy Hopps, an older woman who recently discovered a lump in her right breast. Her primary care physician had referred Mrs. Hopps to the Village Square Institute for more in-depth clinical evaluation.

A doctor at the Institute examined Mrs. Hopps and obtained her personal and family health history. He then made a medical diagnosis and provided Mrs. Hopps with a treatment plan. Later, the doctor made a dictated recording of the patient's health information, which was subsequently transcribed into a chart note.

We will now learn more about Nancy Hopps's condition from a clinical perspective, interpreting the medical terms in the doctor's chart note as we analyze the scenario presented in the Intern Experience.

Audio Activity: Nancy Hopps's Chart Note

Directions: Access your *EduHub* subscription and listen to the recording of the physician reading Nancy Hopps's chart note. Read along with the physician and pay attention to the pronunciation of each medical term.

CHART NOTE

Patient Name: Hopps, Nancy
ID Number: HN 25780
Examination Date: January 12, 20xx

SUBJECTIVE
Mrs. Nancy Hopps is an 82-year-old female who is new to this practice. She was referred by her primary care physician after physical examination confirmed a lump in her right breast.

OBJECTIVE
Vital signs within normal limits, although **BP** is slightly elevated. Physical exam reveals a significant, easily **palpated** (lightly pressed with the palms and fingers) lump of the right breast that is somewhat hard with irregular borders.

ASSESSMENT
Possible breast **carcinoma**.

PLAN
Mammogram and a breast ultrasound will be performed in our office and sent to our radiology group for analysis.

Interpret Nancy Hopps's Chart Note

Directions: Access your *EduHub* subscription and listen to the recording of the physician reading Nancy Hopps's chart note. After listening to the recording, supply the medical term that matches each definition. You may encounter definitions and terms introduced in previous chapters.

Example: painful and difficult menstruation flow   *Answer:* dysmenorrhea

1. blood pressure

   _____

2. diagnostic procedure used to screen for
   breast cancer

   _____

3. examined by lightly pressing with the
   palms of the hands and the fingers

   _____

4. cancerous tumor

   _____

SCORECARD: How Did You Do?

Number correct (_____), divided by 4 (_____), multiplied by 100 equals _____ (your score)

Working with Medical Records

In this activity, you will interpret the medical records (chart notes) of patients with reproductive system disorders. These examples illustrate typical medical records prepared in a real-world healthcare environment. To interpret these chart notes, you will apply your knowledge of word elements (prefixes, combining forms, and suffixes), diseases and disorders, and procedures and treatments related to the male and female reproductive systems.

Audio Activity: Juan Forsum's Chart Note

Directions: Access your *EduHub* subscription and listen to the recording of the physician reading Juan Forsum's chart note. Read along with the physician and pay attention to the pronunciation of each medical term.

CHART NOTE

Patient Name: Forsum, Juan
ID Number: FJ 34896
Examination Date: April 4, 20xx

SUBJECTIVE
Juan returns to our office with continued problems of **nocturia**, urinary retention, and frequency. He returns due to increasing discomfort.

OBJECTIVE
The patient is a controlled diabetic with normal vital signs. **Digital rectal exam** revealed enlarged prostate.

ASSESSMENT
Benign prostatic hypertrophy

PLAN
Transurethral resection of the prostate (TURP)

Interpret Juan Forsum's Chart Note

Directions: Access your *EduHub* subscription and listen to the recording of the physician reading Juan Forsum's chart note. After listening to the recording, supply the medical term that matches each definition.

Example: inflammation of the prostate gland   *Answer:* prostatitis

1. noncancerous enlargement of the prostate gland
   _____

2. exam used to screen for BPH and prostate cancer
   _____

3. type of prostate surgery performed to relieve moderate to severe urinary symptoms caused by an enlarged prostate
   _____

4. frequent urination at night
   _____

SCORECARD: How Did You Do?

Number correct (_____), divided by 4 (_____), multiplied by 100 equals _____ (your score)

Audio Activity: Richard Thomas's Chart Note

Directions: Access your *EduHub* subscription and listen to the recording of the physician reading Richard Thomas's chart note. Read along with the physician and pay attention to the pronunciation of each medical term.

CHART NOTE

Patient Name: Thomas, Richard
ID Number: RT 69024
Examination Date: August 29, 20xx

SUBJECTIVE
Patient complains of **scrotal** and genital pain. There is also discomfort during urination often associated with a **purulent** discharge.

OBJECTIVE
Richard is a sexually active 17-year-old male who, by his own admission, does not routinely use a condom. Physical exam reveals small, palpable lump on **lateral** aspect of the left **testis**.

ASSESSMENT
Evaluate for **gonorrhea**.

PLAN
Culture test for gonorrhea.

Assessment 8.14

Interpret Richard Thomas's Chart Note

Directions: Access your *EduHub* subscription and listen to the recording of the physician reading Richard Thomas's chart note. After listening to the recording, supply the medical term that matches each definition. You may encounter definitions and terms introduced in previous chapters.

Example: excision of a vessel or duct   *Answer*: vasectomy

1. pertaining to the side   _____

2. curable sexually transmitted infection   _____

3. pertaining to pus   _____

4. male gonad   _____

5. pertaining to the sac in which the testes are suspended   _____

SCORECARD: How Did You Do?

Number correct (_____), divided by 5 (_____), multiplied by 100 equals _____ (your score)

Word Elements Summary

Prefixes

Prefix	Meaning
a-	not; without
dys-	painful; difficult
endo-	within
intra-	inside; within
trans-	across

Combining Forms

Root Word/Combining Vowel	Meaning
cervic/o	cervix; neck
colp/o	vagina
cyst/o	sac containing fluid; bladder
gynec/o	woman; female
hyster/o	uterus
lapar/o	abdomen
mamm/o	breast
mast/o	breast
men/o	menstruation
metr/o, metri/o	uterus
oophor/o	ovary
orchid/o	testes
prostat/o	prostate gland
salping/o	uterine tube; fallopian tube
scrot/o	scrotum
testicul/o	testes
ur/o	urine; urinary tract
vagin/o	vagina
vas/o	vessel; duct

Suffixes

Suffix	Meaning
-al	pertaining to
-algia	pain
-ectomy	surgical removal; excision
-gram	record; image
-graphy	process of recording an image
-ic	pertaining to
-itis	inflammation
-logist	specialist in the study and treatment of
-logy	study of
-osis	abnormal condition
-pexy	surgical fixation
-plasty	surgical repair
-rrhagia	bursting forth (of blood)
-rrhaphy	suture
-rrhea	discharge; flow
-rrhexis	rupture
-scope	instrument used to observe
-scopy	process of observing

More Practice: Activities and Games

The following activities will help you reinforce your skills and check your mastery of the medical terminology you learned in this chapter. Access your *EduHub* subscription to complete more activities and vocabulary games for mastering the word parts and terms you have learned.

Break It Down

Directions: Dissect each medical term into its word parts (prefix, root word, combining vowel, and suffix) using one or more slashes. Then define each term.

Example:
Medical Term: oophorectomy
Dissection: oophor/ectomy
Definition: excision of the ovary

Medical Term	Dissection
1. prostatocystitis	p r o s t a t o c y s t i t i s

Definition: _____

_____

2. metrosalpingography   m e t r o s a l p i n g o g r a p h y

Definition: _____

_____

3. mastalgia   m a s t a l g i a

Definition: _____

_____

4. intracervical   i n t r a c e r v i c a l

Definition: _____

_____

5. orchidopexy   o r c h i d o p e x y

Definition: _____

_____

6. mammoplasty   m a m m o p l a s t y

Definition: _____

_____

Medical Term	Dissection
7. laparoscope	l a p a r o s c o p e

Definition: _____

_____

| 8. hysterorrhaphy | h y s t e r o r r h a p h y |

Definition: _____

_____

| 9. colporrhexis | c o l p o r r h e x i s |

Definition: _____

_____

Audio Activity: Tyra McNamara's Chart Note

Directions: Access your *EduHub* subscription and listen to the recording of the physician reading Tyra McNamara's chart note. Read along with the physician and pay attention to the pronunciation of each medical term.

CHART NOTE

Patient Name: McNamara, Tyra
ID Number: MT 33412
Examination Date: July 28, 20xx

SUBJECTIVE
This newly married patient complains of painful intercourse, which is often associated with her **menstrual** period. She has random episodes of pain with urination and bowel movements.

OBJECTIVE
Patient had one child delivered vaginally. No history of **STIs** or cancer. **Dysmenorrhea** and **menorrhagia**.

ASSESSMENT
Probable **endometriosis**

PLAN
Patient prescribed hormonal contraceptives and ibuprofen to help reduce pelvic pain. Patient to return for follow-up.

Interpret Tyra McNamara's Chart Note

Directions: Access your *EduHub* subscription and listen to the recording of the physician reading Tyra McNamara's chart note. After listening to the recording, supply the medical term that matches each definition. You may encounter definitions and terms introduced in previous chapters.

Example: excision of the ovary   *Answer*: oophorectomy

1. pertaining to menstruation   _____

2. sexually transmitted infections   _____

3. painful menstruation   _____

4. excessively heavy periods (bursting forth of menstruation)   _____

5. disorder in which the tissue that lines the inside of the uterus grows outside of it   _____

Spelling

Directions: For each medical term, indicate the correct spelling.

1.	dysmenarrhea	dysmenorrea	dysmenorrhea	dysmenerrhea
2.	hysterorrhaphy	hysteroraphy	hysterorraphy	hysterrorphy
3.	endometreosis	endometriosis	endommetriosis	endomietriosis
4.	menorrhagea	mennoragea	menorrhagia	menoragia
5.	orophorectomy	ooforectomy	oophoroctomy	oophorectomy
6.	salpingitis	salpinjitis	selpingitis	salpingittis
7.	urrology	urology	eurology	eurollogy
8.	orchidopeksy	orchydopexy	orchidopeksia	orchidopexy
9.	prostotectomy	prostytectomy	prostatectomy	prostetectomy
10.	mastectomy	masstectomy	mastechtomy	mastyctomy
11.	cervicol	cervicall	cervical	cervichal
12.	gynecology	guynecology	gyneccology	gynnecology

Dictionary Skills

Directions: Using a medical dictionary, such as *Taber's Cyclopedic Medical Dictionary*, look up the term *mastitis*. For each medical term, indicate whether the term appears on the same page as *mastitis* (O), before the page (B), or after the page (A). Then define each term.

Medical Term	O, B, A
1. mammography	_____

Definition: _____

_____

2. mastoid	_____

Definition: _____

_____

3. mastopexy	_____

Definition: _____

_____

4. mastalgia	_____

Definition: _____

_____

5. mastopathy	_____

Definition: _____

_____

6. mastology	_____

Definition: _____

_____

Chapter 9
The Respiratory System

pulmon / o / logy = the study of the lungs

Chapter Organization

- Intern Experience
- Overview of Respiratory System Anatomy and Physiology
- Word Elements
- Breaking Down and Building Respiratory System Terms
- Diseases and Disorders
- Procedures and Treatments
- Working with Medical Records
- Chapter Review

Chapter Objectives

After completing this chapter, you will be able to

1. label an anatomical diagram of the respiratory system;
2. dissect and define common medical terminology related to the respiratory system;
3. build terms used to describe respiratory system diseases and disorders, diagnostic procedures, and therapeutic treatments;
4. pronounce and spell common medical terminology related to the respiratory system;
5. understand that the process of building and dissecting a medical term based on its prefix, root word, and suffix enables you to analyze an extremely large number of medical terms beyond those presented in this chapter;
6. interpret the meaning of abbreviations associated with the respiratory system; and
7. interpret medical records containing terminology and abbreviations related to the respiratory system.

Your *EduHub* subscription that accompanies this text provides access to online assessments, assignments, activities, and resources. Throughout this chapter, access *EduHub* to

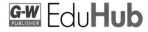

- use e-flash cards to review the medical terminology and word parts you learn;
- listen to the correct pronunciations of medical terms; and
- complete medical terminology activities and assignments.

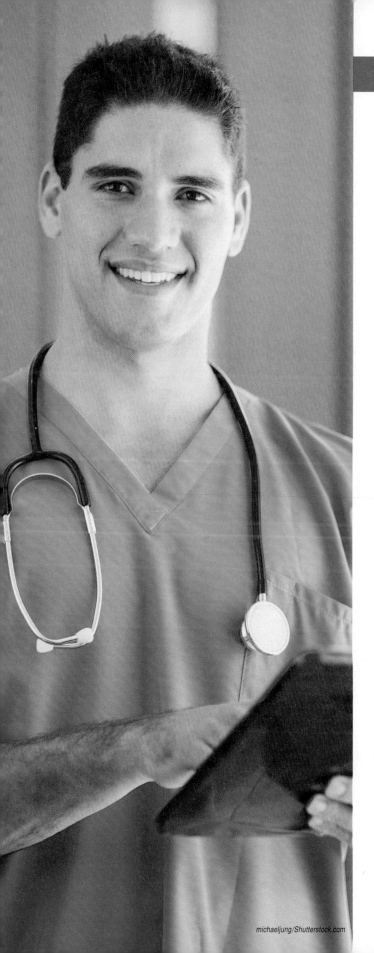

Intern Experience

Mark Lungus, an intern with the Oak Forest Urgent Care Center, has been assigned to shadow (observe and assist) Dr. Connor Wiley today. Mark and Dr. Wiley enter exam room 2, where they meet David, their first patient. David, a high school lacrosse player, was brought to the clinic after collapsing during a practice session.

David explains to Dr. Wiley that "it hurts to breathe" and he is "so tired." Lacrosse practice, rehearsals for the school play, and late nights spent studying and writing a research paper have been wearing him down. Running late for lacrosse practice this afternoon, David breathlessly dashed onto the field and lined up with his teammates. The coach ordered them to run a series of grueling sprints and offense drills. At one point, David's opponent pivoted and pushed off hard, slamming his lacrosse stick into David's chest. David could not catch his breath. The pain in his chest was so intense that he collapsed onto the grass, gasping for air. He could see the coach and the trainer rushing over to him.

David is suffering from an injury that has affected his respiratory system. To help you understand his health problem, this chapter will present word elements (combining forms, prefixes, and suffixes) that make up medical terms related to the respiratory system. As you learn these terms, you will recognize many common word elements from your study of body systems covered in previous chapters—particularly prefixes and suffixes, which are universal word elements.

We will begin our study of the respiratory system with a brief overview of its anatomy and physiology. Later in the chapter, you will learn about some common pathological conditions of the respiratory system, tests and procedures used to diagnose these conditions, and treatment methods.

Overview of Respiratory System Anatomy and Physiology

Breathing is essential to life. You can live a few weeks without food and a few days without water, but only a few minutes without oxygen. The respiratory system carries oxygen into the body and removes carbon dioxide. These processes occur in three steps:

- **ventilation**, which is normally accomplished by *inspiration* (drawing air into the lungs) and *expiration* (expelling air from the lungs);

- **exchange of gases**, which occurs in the lungs as (1) oxygen diffuses from the air sacs into the blood, and (2) carbon dioxide diffuses out of the blood as a waste product to be eliminated; and

- **transport** of oxygen from the lungs throughout the body and of carbon dioxide out of the body with the help of the cardiovascular (circulatory) system.

Major Organs and Structures of the Respiratory System

The major organs of the respiratory system include the nose, **pharynx** (throat), **trachea** (windpipe), and **lungs** (Figure 9.1). The lungs are the primary organs of *respiration*, or breathing. Air flows into the nose, through the pharynx,

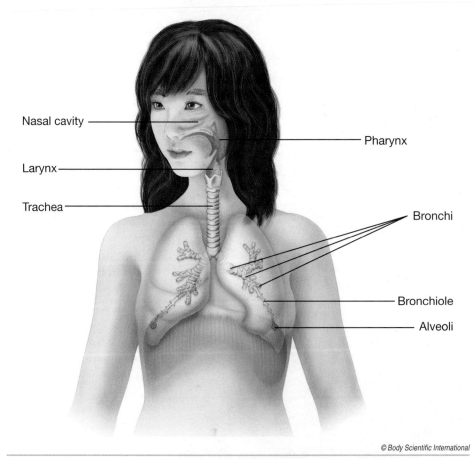

Nasal cavity

Larynx

Trachea

Pharynx

Bronchi

Bronchiole

Alveoli

Figure 9.1 Major organs and structures of the respiratory system

and into the trachea. The trachea branches off into the **bronchi** (BRŎNG-kē), tubes that carry air directly into the lungs. (The singular form of *bronchi* is *bronchus*.) Your lungs are enveloped by the **pleura**, a thin membrane of tissue that also lines the chest cavity. The diameters of the bronchi grow increasingly smaller until the bronchi divide into tiny **bronchioles** ("little bronchi"). The bronchioles terminate at the **alveoli** (ăl-VĒ-ō-lē), where the oxygen from the air is exchanged for carbon dioxide, a waste product.

Functions of the Respiratory System

The human respiratory system serves three primary functions:

1. **Gas exchange** — Every cell in your body needs oxygen and produces carbon dioxide. Oxygen from the air enters the blood, and carbon dioxide leaves the blood as a waste product that is expelled by the lungs.
2. **Regulation of acid-base (pH) levels** — The respiratory system maintains a normal acid-base balance by continually adjusting the carbon dioxide levels in the blood.
3. **Protection** — The respiratory system protects the body against "foreign invaders" by filtering out airborne pollutants and some microorganisms.

Pulmonology is the medical specialty concerned with the study, diagnosis, and treatment of diseases and disorders of the respiratory system. A **pulmonologist** is a physician who specializes in the study, diagnosis, and treatment of respiratory system diseases and disorders.

Anatomy and Physiology Vocabulary

Now that you have been introduced to the basic structure and functions of the respiratory system, we will explore in more detail the key terms presented in the introduction.

Key Term	Definition
alveoli	tiny, grape-like sacs in which the exchange of gases (oxygen and carbon dioxide) occurs
bronchi	tubes that carry air into the lungs
lungs	the primary organs of respiration (breathing)
pharynx	the throat
pleura	a thin, serous (watery) membrane that envelops each lung and also lines the chest cavity
pulmonologist	physician who specializes in the study and treatment of diseases and disorders of the respiratory system
pulmonology	the study of the respiratory system
trachea	windpipe

E-Flash Card Activity: Anatomy and Physiology Vocabulary

Directions: After you have reviewed the anatomy and physiology vocabulary related to the respiratory system, access your *EduHub* subscription and practice with the e-flash cards until you are comfortable with the spelling and definition of each term.

Identifying Major Organs and Structures of the Respiratory System

Directions: Label the diagram of the respiratory system. You can also complete this activity online using *EduHub*.

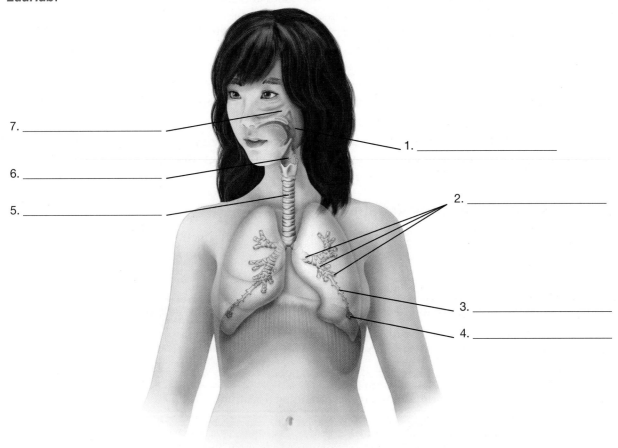

7. _____

6. _____

5. _____

1. _____

2. _____

3. _____

4. _____

© Body Scientific International

SCORECARD: How Did You Do?

Number correct (_____), divided by 7 (_____), multiplied by 100 equals _____ (your score)

Matching Anatomy and Physiology Vocabulary

Directions: Choose the correct vocabulary term for each meaning. You can also complete this activity online using *EduHub*.

_____ 1. tiny, grape-like sacs in which the exchange of gases (oxygen and carbon dioxide) occurs

_____ 2. tubes that carry air into the lungs

_____ 3. the primary organs of respiration (breathing)

_____ 4. a thin, serous (watery) membrane that envelops each lung and also lines the chest cavity

_____ 5. physician who specializes in the study and treatment of diseases and disorders of the respiratory system

_____ 6. the study of the respiratory system

_____ 7. windpipe

_____ 8. the throat

A. pharynx
B. trachea
C. pleura
D. bronchi
E. alveoli
F. pulmonologist
G. pulmonology
H. lungs

SCORECARD: How Did You Do?

Number correct (_____), divided by 8 (_____), multiplied by 100 equals _____ (your score)

Word Elements

In this section, you will learn word elements—prefixes, combining forms, and suffixes—that are common to the respiratory system. By learning these word elements and understanding how they are combined to build medical terms, you will be able to analyze David's health condition (described in the Intern Experience at the beginning of this chapter) and identify a large number of terms associated with the respiratory system.

E-Flash Card Activity: Word Elements

Directions: Review the word elements in the tables that follow. Then, access your *EduHub* subscription and practice with the e-flash cards until you are able to quickly recognize the different word parts (prefixes, combining forms, and suffixes) and their meanings. The e-flash cards are grouped together by prefixes, combining forms, and suffixes, followed by a cumulative review of all the word elements you are learning in this chapter.

Prefixes

Let's begin our study of word elements by looking at the prefixes listed in the table below. There is only one new prefix in this list; the others were introduced in previous chapters.

Prefix	Meaning
a-	not; without
an-	not; without
brady-	slow
dys-	painful; difficult
endo-	within
hyper-	above; above normal
hypo-	below; below normal
tachy-	fast

Combining Forms

Listed below are combining forms that appear in medical terms used to describe the respiratory system. Which of these combining forms have you already mastered?

Root Word/Combining Vowel	Meaning
bronch/o, bronchi/o	bronchial tube; bronchus
cyan/o	blue
embol/o	plug; embolus
hem/o	blood
lob/o	lobe (a defined portion of an organ or structure)
ox/o	oxygen
pharyng/o	pharynx; throat
pleur/o	pleura
pneum/o, pneumon/o	lung; air

(Continued)

Root Word/Combining Vowel	Meaning
pulmon/o	lung
rhin/o	nose
spir/o	breathe; breathing
sten/o	narrow; constricted
thorac/o	chest
trache/o	trachea; windpipe

Suffixes

Listed below are suffixes that appear in medical terms pertaining to the respiratory system. You are already familiar with most of these suffixes from your study of other body systems covered in previous chapters.

Suffix	Meaning
-al	pertaining to
-algia	pain
-centesis	surgical puncture to remove fluid
-ectasis	dilatation; dilation; expansion
-ectomy	surgical removal; excision
-gram	record; image
-ia	condition
-itis	inflammation
-logist	specialist in the study and treatment of
-logy	study of
-meter	measure
-osis	abnormal condition
-pnea	breathing
-scope	instrument used to observe
-thorax	chest; pleural cavity
-tomy	incision; cut into

Matching Prefixes, Combining Forms, and Suffixes

Directions: Choose the correct meaning for each word element. Some meanings may be used more than once. You can also complete this activity online using *EduHub*.

Prefixes

_____ 1. brady-

_____ 2. tachy-

_____ 3. a-

_____ 4. hypo-

_____ 5. endo-

_____ 6. an-

_____ 7. dys-

_____ 8. hyper-

A. above; above normal

B. not; without

C. slow

D. painful; difficult

E. fast

F. below; below normal

G. within

Combining Forms

_____ 1. thorac/o

_____ 2. pharyng/o

_____ 3. pneumon/o

_____ 4. lob/o

_____ 5. trache/o

_____ 6. bronchi/o

_____ 7. spir/o

_____ 8. embol/o

_____ 9. rhin/o

_____ 10. ox/o

_____ 11. pulmon/o

_____ 12. bronch/o

_____ 13. pneum/o

_____ 14. cyan/o

_____ 15. pleur/o

_____ 16. hem/o

_____ 17. sten/o

A. blue

B. oxygen

C. nose

D. chest

E. plug; embolus

F. pleura

G. blood

H. lung

I. lung; air

J. bronchial tube; bronchus

K. trachea; windpipe

L. breathe; breathing

M. pharynx; throat

N. lobe

O. narrow; constricted

Suffixes

_____ 1. -meter
_____ 2. -ectomy
_____ 3. -itis
_____ 4. -al
_____ 5. -tomy
_____ 6. -pnea
_____ 7. -centesis
_____ 8. -osis
_____ 9. -thorax
_____ 10. -logist
_____ 11. -ectasis
_____ 12. -ia
_____ 13. -algia
_____ 14. -logy
_____ 15. -scope
_____ 16. -gram

A. record; image
B. surgical puncture to remove fluid
C. pertaining to
D. condition
E. surgical removal; excision
F. dilatation; dilation; expansion
G. measure
H. breathing
I. inflammation
J. instrument used to observe
K. specialist in the study and treatment of
L. study of
M. incision; cut into
N. pain
O. chest; pleural cavity
P. abnormal condition

SCORECARD: How Did You Do?

Number correct (_____), divided by 41 (_____), multiplied by 100 equals _____ (your score)

Breaking Down and Building Respiratory System Terms

Now that you have mastered the prefixes, combining forms, and suffixes for medical terminology pertaining to the respiratory system, you have the ability to dissect and build a large number of terms related to this body system.

On the next page is a list of medical terms commonly used in pulmonology, the medical specialty concerning the study, diagnosis, and treatment of the respiratory system. For each term, a dissection has been provided, along with the meaning of each word element and the definition of the term as a whole.

Term	Dissection	Word Part/Meaning	Term Meaning
Note: *For simplification, combining vowels have been omitted from the Word Part/Meaning column.*			
1. **anoxia** (ăn-ŎK-sē-ă)	an/ox/ia	**an** = not; without **ox** = oxygen **ia** = condition	condition of without oxygen
2. **apnea** (ĂP-nē-ă)	a/pnea	**a** = not; without **pnea** = breathing	without breathing
3. **bradypnea** (brăd-ĭp-NĒ-ă)	brady/pnea	**brady** = slow **pnea** = breathing	slow breathing
4. **bronchiectasis** (BRŎNG-kē-ĕk-TĀ-sĭs)	bronchi/ectasis	**bronchi** = bronchial tube; bronchus **ectasis** = dilatation; dilation; expansion	dilatation of the bronchus
5. **bronchitis** (brŏng-KĪ-tĭs)	bronch/itis	**bronch** = bronchial tube; bronchus **itis** = inflammation	inflammation of the bronchus
6. **bronchogram** (BRŎNG-kō-grăm)	bronch/o/gram	**bronch** = bronchial tube; bronchus **gram** = record; image	record or image of the bronchus
7. **bronchopneumonia** (BRŎNG-kō-nū-MŌ-nē-ă)	bronch/o/pneumon/ia	**bronch** = bronchial tube; bronchus **pneumon** = lung; air **ia** = condition	condition of the bronchus and lung
8. **bronchoscope** (BRŎNG-kō-skōp)	bronch/o/scope	**bronch** = bronchial tube; bronchus **scope** = instrument used to observe	instrument used to observe the bronchus
9. **dyspnea** (DĬSP-nē-ă)	dys/pnea	**dys** = painful; difficult **pnea** = breathing	painful or difficult breathing
10. **hemothorax** (hē-mō-THOR-ăks)	hem/o/thorax	**hem** = blood **thorax** = chest; pleural cavity	blood in the pleural cavity
11. **hyperpnea** (hī-PĔRP-nē-ă)	hyper/pnea	**hyper** = above; above normal **pnea** = breathing	above-normal breathing
12. **hypopnea** (hī-PŎP-nē-ă)	hypo/pnea	**hypo** = below; below normal **pnea** = breathing	below-normal breathing
Prefixes = Green Root Words = Red Suffixes = Blue			

Term	Dissection	Word Part/Meaning	Term Meaning
13. **pharyngitis** (făr-ĭn-JĪ-tĭs)	pharyng/itis	**pharyng** = pharynx; throat **itis** = inflammation	inflammation of the throat
14. **pneumonia** (nū-MŌ-nē-ă)	pneumon/ia	**pneumon** = lung; air **ia** = condition	condition of the lung
15. **pneumonocentesis** (NŪ-mō-nō-sĕn-TĒ-sĭs)	pneumon/o/centesis	**pneumon** = lung; air **centesis** = surgical puncture to remove fluid	surgical puncture to remove fluid in the lung
16. **pneumothorax** (nū-mō-THOR-ăks)	pneum/o/thorax	**pneum** = lung; air **thorax** = chest; pleural cavity	air in the pleural cavity
17. **pulmonologist** (pŭl-mŏn-ŎL-ō-jĭst)	pulmon/o/logist	**pulmon** = lung **logist** = specialist in the study and treatment of	specialist in the study and treatment of the lungs
18. **pulmonology** (pŭl-mŏn-ŎL-ō-jē)	pulmon/o/logy	**pulmon** = lung **logy** = study of	study of the lungs
19. **rhinitis** (rī-NĪ-tĭs)	rhin/itis	**rhin** = nose **itis** = inflammation	inflammation of the nose
20. **spirometer** (spī-RŎM-ĕt-ĕr)	spir/o/meter	**spir** = breathe; breathing **meter** = measure	measure of breathing
21. **tachypnea** (tăk-ĭp-NĒ-ă)	tachy/pnea	**tachy** = fast **pnea** = breathing	fast breathing
22. **tracheal** (TRĀ-kē-ăl)	trache/al	**trache** = trachea **al** = pertaining to	pertaining to the trachea
23. **tracheitis** (trā-kē-Ī-tĭs)	trache/itis	**trache** = trachea **itis** = inflammation	inflammation of the trachea
24. **tracheostenosis** (TRĀ-kē-ō-stĕn-Ō-sĭs)	trache/o/sten/osis	**trache** = trachea **sten** = narrow; constricted **osis** = abnormal condition	abnormal condition of a narrow/constricted trachea
25. **tracheotomy** (trā-kē-ŎT-ō-mē)	trache/o/tomy	**trache** = trachea **tomy** = incision; cut into	incision to the trachea

Prefixes = Green   Root Words = Red   Suffixes = Blue

Using the pronunciation guide in the Breaking Down and Building chart, practice saying each medical term aloud. To hear the pronunciation of each term, complete the Pronounce It activity on the next page.

Audio Activity: Pronounce It

Directions: Access your *EduHub* subscription and listen to the correct pronunciations of the following medical terms. Practice pronouncing the terms until you are comfortable saying them aloud.

anoxia
(ăn-ŎK-sē-ă)

apnea
(ĂP-nē-ă)

bradypnea
(brăd-ĭp-NĒ-ă)

bronchiectasis
(BRŎNG-kē-ĕk-TĀ-sĭs)

bronchitis
(brŏng-KĪ-tĭs)

bronchogram
(BRŎNG-kō-grăm)

bronchopneumonia
(BRŎNG-kō-nū-MŌ-nē-ă)

bronchoscope
(BRŎNG-kō-skōp)

dyspnea
(DĬSP-nē-ă)

hemothorax
(hē-mō-THOR-ăks)

hyperpnea
(hī-PĔRP-nē-ă)

hypopnea
(hī-PŎP-nē-ă)

pharyngitis
(făr-ĭn-JĪ-tĭs)

pneumonia
(nū-MŌ-nē-ă)

pneumonocentesis
(NŪ-mō-nō-sĕn-TĒ-sĭs)

pneumothorax
(nū-mō-THOR-ăks)

pulmonologist
(pŭl-mŏn-ŎL-ō-jĭst)

pulmonology
(pŭl-mŏn-ŎL-ō-jē)

rhinitis
(rī-NĪ-tĭs)

spirometer
(spī-RŎM-ĕt-ĕr)

tachypnea
(tăk-ĭp-NĒ-ă)

tracheal
(TRĀ-kē-ăl)

tracheitis
(trā-kē-Ī-tĭs)

tracheostenosis
(TRĀ-kē-ō-stĕn-Ō-sĭs)

tracheotomy
(trā-kē-ŎT-ō-mē)

Assessment 9.4

Audio Activity: Spell It

Directions: Access your *EduHub* subscription and listen to the pronunciation for each number. As you hear each term, write its correct spelling.

1. _____
2. _____
3. _____
4. _____
5. _____
6. _____
7. _____
8. _____
9. _____
10. _____
11. _____
12. _____
13. _____
14. _____
15. _____
16. _____
17. _____
18. _____
19. _____
20. _____
21. _____
22. _____
23. _____
24. _____
25. _____

SCORECARD: How Did You Do?

Number correct (_____), divided by 25 (_____), multiplied by 100 equals _____ (your score)

Break It Down

Directions: Dissect each medical term into its word parts (prefix, root word, combining vowel, and suffix) using one or more slashes. Then define each term. You can also complete this activity online using *EduHub*.

Example:

Medical Term: pulmonologist

Dissection: pulmon/o/logist

Definition: specialist in the study and treatment of the lungs

Medical Term	Dissection
1. rhinitis	r h i n i t i s

Definition: _____

_____

| 2. pharyngitis | p h a r y n g i t i s |

Definition: _____

_____

| 3. hemothorax | h e m o t h o r a x |

Definition: _____

_____

| 4. pulmonology | p u l m o n o l o g y |

Definition: _____

_____

| 5. apnea | a p n e a |

Definition: _____

_____

Medical Term	Dissection
6. tachypnea	t a c h y p n e a

Definition: _____

_____

| 7. pneumonocentesis | p n e u m o n o c e n t e s i s |

Definition: _____

_____

| 8. bronchitis | b r o n c h i t i s |

Definition: _____

_____

| 9. tracheotomy | t r a c h e o t o m y |

Definition: _____

_____

| 10. anoxia | a n o x i a |

Definition: _____

_____

| 11. dyspnea | d y s p n e a |

Definition: _____

_____

| 12. pneumothorax | p n e u m o t h o r a x |

Definition: _____

_____

| 13. tracheostenosis | t r a c h e o s t e n o s i s |

Definition: _____

_____

Medical Term	Dissection
14. bronchiectasis	b r o n c h i e c t a s i s

Definition: _____

_____

15. spirometer   s p i r o m e t e r

Definition: _____

_____

16. tracheal   t r a c h e a l

Definition: _____

_____

17. bradypnea   b r a d y p n e a

Definition: _____

_____

18. bronchogram   b r o n c h o g r a m

Definition: _____

_____

19. tracheitis   t r a c h e i t i s

Definition: _____

_____

20. pneumonia   p n e u m o n i a

Definition: _____

_____

SCORECARD: How Did You Do?

Number correct (_____), divided by 20 (_____), multiplied by 100 equals _____ (your score)

Build It

Directions: Build the medical term that matches each definition by supplying the correct word parts. You can also complete this activity online using *EduHub*.

P (Prefixes) = Green
RW (Root Words) = Red
S (Suffixes) = Blue
CV (Combining Vowel) = Purple

1. air in the pleural cavity

    _____ _____ _____
    　　　　RW　　　　　　CV　　　S

2. above-normal breathing

    _____ _____
    　P　　　S

3. below-normal breathing

    _____ _____
    　P　　　S

4. blood in the pleural cavity

    _____ _____ _____
    　　　　RW　　　　　　CV　　　　　　　S

5. condition of the lung

    _____ _____
    　　　　RW　　　　　S

6. condition of the bronchus and lung

    _____ _____ _____ _____
    　　　　RW　　　　　　CV　　　　　RW　　　　　　S

7. slow breathing

    _____ _____
    　　　　RW　　　　　S

8. dilatation of the bronchus

    _____ _____
    　　　　RW　　　　　S

9. fast breathing

    _____ _____
    　P　　　S

10. incision to the trachea

‗‗‗‗‗‗‗‗‗‗‗‗‗‗‗‗ ‗‗‗‗‗‗ ‗‗‗‗‗‗
         RW   CV   S

11. inflammation of the bronchus

‗‗‗‗‗‗‗‗‗‗‗‗‗‗‗‗ ‗‗‗‗‗‗‗
         RW   S

12. inflammation of the nose

‗‗‗‗‗‗‗‗‗‗‗‗‗‗‗‗ ‗‗‗‗‗‗‗
         RW   S

13. inflammation of the throat

‗‗‗‗‗‗‗‗‗‗‗‗‗‗‗‗ ‗‗‗‗‗‗‗
         RW   S

14. inflammation of the trachea

‗‗‗‗‗‗‗‗‗‗‗‗‗‗‗‗ ‗‗‗‗‗‗‗
         RW   S

15. instrument used to observe the bronchus

‗‗‗‗‗‗‗‗‗‗‗‗‗‗‗‗ ‗‗‗‗‗‗ ‗‗‗‗‗‗
         RW   CV   S

16. measure of breathing

‗‗‗‗‗‗‗‗‗‗‗‗‗‗‗‗ ‗‗‗‗‗‗ ‗‗‗‗‗‗
         RW   CV   S

17. surgical puncture to remove fluid in the lung

‗‗‗‗‗‗‗‗‗‗‗‗‗‗‗‗ ‗‗‗‗‗‗ ‗‗‗‗‗‗
         RW   CV   S

18. record or image of the bronchus

‗‗‗‗‗‗‗‗‗‗‗‗‗‗‗‗ ‗‗‗‗‗‗ ‗‗‗‗‗‗
         RW   CV   S

19. specialist in the study and treatment of the lungs

‗‗‗‗‗‗‗‗‗‗‗‗‗‗‗‗ ‗‗‗‗‗‗ ‗‗‗‗‗‗
         RW   CV   S

20. without breathing

‗‗‗‗‗‗ ‗‗‗‗‗‗
  P   S

SCORECARD: How Did You Do?

Number correct (_____), divided by 20 (_____), multiplied by 100 equals _____ (your score)

Diseases and Disorders

Diseases and disorders of the respiratory system run the spectrum from the mild to the severe and have a number of different causes. In this section, we will briefly explore some common respiratory pathological conditions.

Asthma

As you learned in chapter 5, **asthma** is a disorder caused by inflammation of the bronchi (airways) in the lungs (Figure 9.2). When an asthma attack occurs, the muscles surrounding the bronchi constrict (narrow), and the lining (mucous membranes) of the bronchi swell. Both the constriction and swelling reduce the amount of air that can pass through the lungs. The result is wheezing, shortness of breath, coughing, and tightness in the chest. The etiology (cause) of asthma is unknown.

In people who are sensitive to environmental *allergens* (allergy-causing substances), inhalation can trigger asthma symptoms. Examples of common asthma-inducing allergens are dust, pet hair or dander, pollen, and mold. Even emotional stress can trigger an asthma attack. The duration of an asthma attack may be a few minutes or a few days.

Treatments for asthma include limiting exposure to irritants that can trigger an asthma attack and using prescription medications such as bronchodilators, anti-inflammatory drugs, and inhaled steroids. An asthma attack that severely restricts airflow is life-threatening and requires immediate medical intervention.

Pneumonia

Pneumonia is an inflammation in one or both lungs often caused by a bacterium or virus (Figure 9.3). *Exudate* (ĔKS-yū-dāt), fluid such as pus or cellular debris that leaks from blood vessels, clogs the air spaces of the lungs, preventing gas exchange. Symptoms of pneumonia include persistent cough, shortness of breath, chest pain, and fever with chills and sweating.

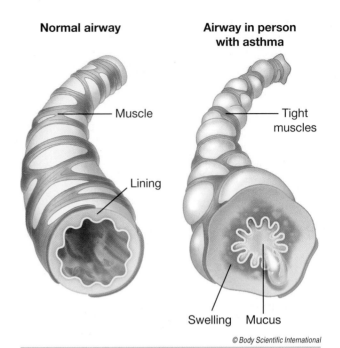

Normal airway — Muscle — Lining

Airway in person with asthma — Tight muscles — Swelling — Mucus

© Body Scientific International

Figure 9.2 During an asthma attack, the muscles surrounding the bronchi constrict, and the bronchial lining swells.

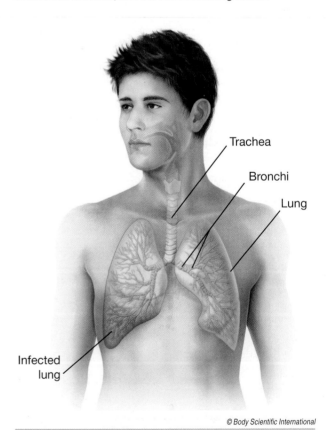

Trachea — Bronchi — Lung — Infected lung

© Body Scientific International

Figure 9.3 Pneumonia is an inflammation in one or both lungs caused by an infection.

Pneumothorax

A **pneumothorax** is a collapsed lung. It occurs when air escapes from the lung and collects in the pleural space, the small area between the lungs and thoracic cavity (Figure 9.4). This accumulation of air puts pressure on the lungs, preventing them from expanding. Symptoms of pneumothorax include shortness of breath and sharp pain in the chest upon deep breathing or coughing. The condition is caused by a penetrating chest injury, such as a gunshot or knife wound or a rib fracture that punctures the lung.

Bronchitis

Bronchitis is an inflammation of the lining of the bronchial tubes, which deliver air to and from the lungs (Figure 9.5). Bronchitis may be either *acute* (appearing suddenly and worsening quickly) or *chronic* (developing gradually and worsening over an extended period of time).

Acute bronchitis is a condition that can develop from a respiratory infection or the common cold. *Chronic bronchitis* is a more serious condition resulting from long-term irritation or inflammation of the bronchial tubes. Symptoms include fatigue, fever, chills, and a productive cough of *sputum*, mucus or fluid coughed up from the lungs. The sputum may be clear, white, or yellowish-green in color. Chronic bronchitis is one of the conditions included in the disease called chronic obstructive pulmonary disease (COPD), discussed on the next page.

Collapsed
left lung

© Body Scientific International

Figure 9.4 A pneumothorax is a collapsed lung.

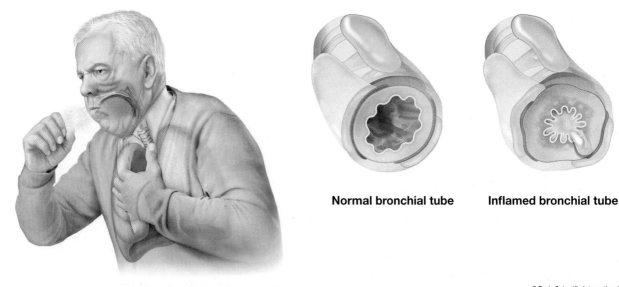

Normal bronchial tube   **Inflamed bronchial tube**

© Body Scientific International

Figure 9.5 Bronchitis is an inflammation of the lining of the bronchial tubes.

Chronic Obstructive Pulmonary Disease

Chronic obstructive pulmonary disease (COPD) is a progressive disease marked by difficulty breathing (Figure 9.6). It is caused by damage to the lungs over many years and is often, but not always, associated with smoking. Tobacco smoke irritates the bronchi and destroys the elastic fibers in the lungs, making it harder to breathe.

COPD is often a combination of two diseases: chronic bronchitis and emphysema. In **chronic bronchitis**, the bronchial tubes become inflamed and secrete excessive mucus. Bronchial inflammation and excessive mucous secretions can narrow or block the bronchial tubes, making breathing difficult.

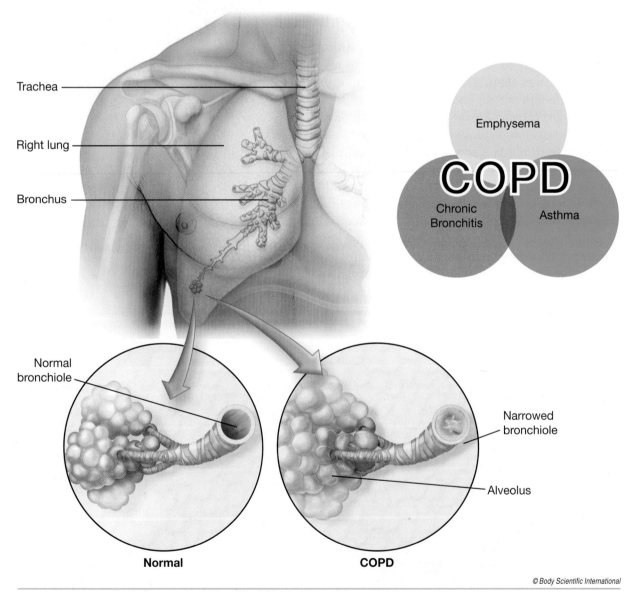

© Body Scientific International

Figure 9.6 COPD is often a combination of emphysema and chronic bronchitis. Although asthma is also marked by constricted bronchial airflow and inflammation, it is recognized as a distinct disease.

Chronic bronchitis is characterized by a long-term cough with mucus production. In **emphysema** (ĕm-fĭ-SĒ-mă), the walls of the alveoli (tiny air sacs in the lungs) have become damaged and lost their elasticity. Less air gets into and out of the lungs, causing **dyspnea** (DĬSP-nē-ă), or difficulty breathing, and lethargy. Because lung damage is irreversible, COPD worsens over time.

Croup

Croup (krūp) is difficulty breathing and a "barking" cough due to inflammation around the larynx (vocal cords) and trachea (Figure 9.7). It is common in infants and children. The cough reflex forces air through the swollen, constricted airway, causing the vocal cords to vibrate with a harsh sound similar to that of a barking seal. To diagnose croup, the physician listens through a stethoscope for a crackling or rattling sound during inspiration (breathing in) or expiration (breathing out). A rattle or crackle, medically described as *rales*, may be either a loud, low-pitched sound or a very short, high-pitched sound from the lungs.

Upper Respiratory Infection

An **upper respiratory infection (URI)** is any type of infection of the head and chest that is caused by a virus. It can affect the nose, throat, sinuses, and ears. It also can affect the eustachian tube (which connects the middle ear and throat), trachea, larynx, or bronchial tube.

A URI typically is referred to as the "common cold." It produces a collection of symptoms such as a cough, sore throat, headache, slight fever, ear congestion, and fatigue.

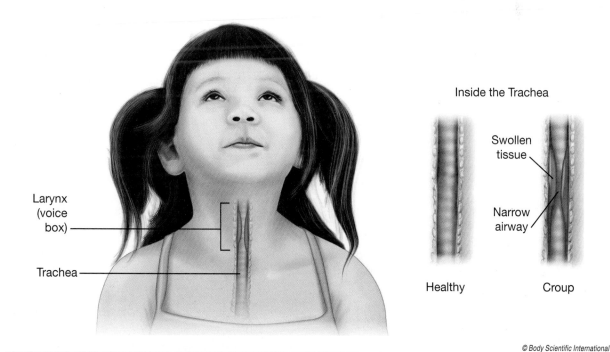

Inside the Trachea

Swollen tissue

Narrow airway

Larynx (voice box)

Trachea

Healthy

Croup

© Body Scientific International

Figure 9.7 Croup is marked by difficulty breathing and a "barking" cough due to inflammation around the larynx and trachea. The disease is common in infants and children.

Obstructive Sleep Apnea

Obstructive sleep apnea (commonly called "sleep apnea") is a condition in which airflow pauses or decreases during sleep due to narrowing or blockage of the airway. As a result, a person with obstructive sleep apnea often snores loudly. A pause in breathing is called an *apnea episode*. The reduced oxygen intake that occurs with sleep apnea causes the person to feel sleepy or drowsy throughout the day.

Pleural Effusion

A **pleural effusion** (ĕ-FYŪ-zhŭn) is an excessive accumulation of fluid between the pleurae, the layers of tissue that envelop the lungs and line the thoracic (chest) cavity (Figure 9.8).

During the act of respiration, the lungs expand, the ribs move out, and the diaphragm moves down. Your body naturally produces pleural fluid in small amounts to lubricate the tissue that surrounds the lungs and lines the thoracic cavity. This slippery fluid allows the two surfaces to slide easily against each other. An excessive amount of fluid impairs the ability of the lungs to expand and move, making breathing difficult and painful.

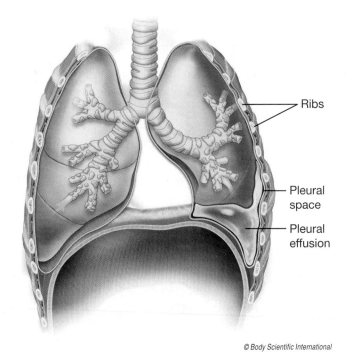

Ribs

Pleural space

Pleural effusion

© Body Scientific International

Figure 9.8 Pleural effusion is an excessive accumulation of fluid between the pleurae, the layers of tissue that surround the lungs and line the chest cavity.

Procedures and Treatments

We will now take a brief look at some diagnostic tests and procedures and therapeutic treatments common to the respiratory system.

Arterial Blood Gas

An **arterial blood gas (ABG) test** measures the levels of oxygen and carbon dioxide in the blood and determines the acidity (pH) of the blood (Figure 9.9). A blood sample typically is collected from the radial artery in the wrist. An ABG test evaluates how well the lungs move oxygen into the blood and remove carbon dioxide from the blood.

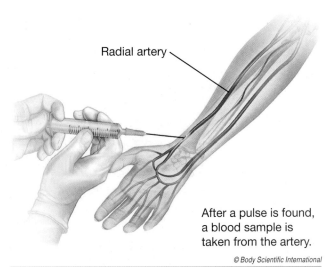

Radial artery

After a pulse is found, a blood sample is taken from the artery.

© Body Scientific International

Figure 9.9 An arterial blood gas (ABG) test is used to measure oxygen and carbon dioxide levels in the blood. It also helps determine the acidity (pH) of the blood.

Cardiopulmonary Resuscitation

Cardiopulmonary resuscitation (CPR) is a lifesaving technique used when cardiac arrest has occurred (breathing or heartbeat has stopped). When the heart stops, lack of oxygenated blood can cause brain damage in as few as four minutes. The American Heart Association recommends that CPR begin with chest compressions until emergency support arrives. CPR can keep oxygenated blood flowing to the brain and other vital organs until medical professionals can attempt to restore a normal heart rhythm.

Chest X-Ray

A **chest X-ray (CXR)** is a radiographic image of the structure of the thoracic cavity and its organs (Figure 9.10). A chest X-ray is typically taken in the posteroanterior (PA) and lateral positions to obtain detailed anatomical images. These images are analyzed to determine the presence of conditions such as pneumonia, lung disease, pleural effusion, or lung tumor.

Continuous Positive Airway Pressure

Continuous positive airway pressure (CPAP) is a treatment in which a machine is used to deliver a constant flow of mild air pressure through the airways (Figure 9.11). CPAP helps patients with breathing problems maintain adequate levels of arterial oxygen.

CPAP is used to treat conditions such as sleep apnea and respiratory distress syndrome in newborns. The continuous flow of mild air pressure helps keep the alveoli open at the end of exhalation, boosting oxygenation and decreasing the amount of effort needed to breathe. In patients with sleep apnea, CPAP is typically administered through a mask placed over the patient's nose or both the nose and the mouth.

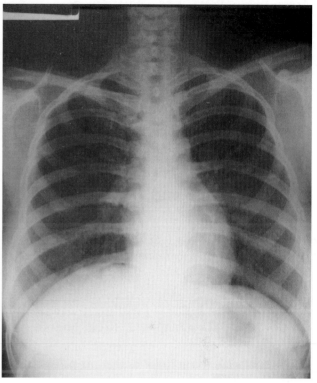

Santibhavank P/Shutterstock.com

Figure 9.10 A chest X-ray is a radiographic image of the structure of the thoracic cavity and its organs.

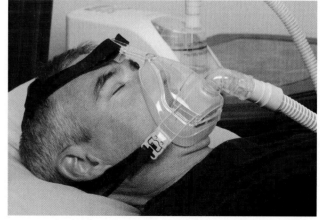

Brian Chase/Shutterstock.com

Figure 9.11 CPAP is a common treatment for sleep apnea.

Pulmonary Function Test

A **pulmonary function test (PFT)** is any of a group of tests that measures lung function (Figure 9.12). The patient breathes into an instrument called a *spirometer* (spī-RŎM-ĕt-ĕr), which determines lung capacity by measuring the volume of air taken in by the lungs during inhalation and released during exhalation. The spirometer records the rate at which air is taken in and expelled by the lungs. PFTs are used to evaluate a broad range of lung diseases, such as asthma, chronic bronchitis, and emphysema.

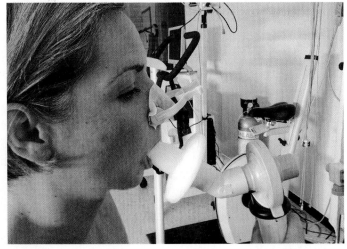

iStock.com/jgaunion

Figure 9.12 During a pulmonary function test, the patient breathes into a spirometer, which measures lung function.

Sputum Culture and Sensitivity

A **sputum culture and sensitivity (C&S)** involves two separate lab tests. In a *culture test*, microorganisms from a sample of a patient's sputum (mucus or fluid from the lungs) are placed in a culture medium and grown. Once a pathogen has been identified, a *sensitivity* test is done to determine what medicine (typically an antibiotic) will effectively treat a pulmonary infection.

In a manual sensitivity test, disks containing various antibiotics are placed on a culture plate along with a suspension of the isolated bacteria. If the infection is bacterial, the antibiotics that are most effective in treating the infection will inhibit bacterial growth near the disks.

Tuberculin Skin Test

The **tuberculin skin test**, or **TB skin test**, is used to determine whether or not a patient has been exposed to tuberculosis (TB), a highly contagious bacterial disease of the lungs (Figure 9.13). The TB skin test is also called the *PPD skin test* or the *Mantoux* (MÄN-tū) *test*. A sample of the TB bacillus (a purified protein derivative extracted from the disease-causing bacterium), abbreviated *PPD*, is injected intradermally (beneath the epidermis, or outer layer of skin). The skin test is interpreted 48 to 72 hours after the injection to detect exposure to TB.

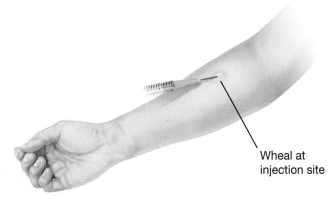

Wheal at injection site

© Body Scientific International

Figure 9.13 The tuberculin (TB) test helps determine whether or not a person has been exposed to the bacterium that causes tuberculosis.

Thoracentesis

Thoracentesis (THOR-ă-sĕn-TĒ-sĭs) is a procedure in which excess fluid is removed from the pleural space, or the area between the lungs and the chest wall (Figure 9.14). In certain respiratory disorders and diseases, abnormal fluid buildup in the pleural space puts pressure on the lungs, making breathing difficult.

As you learned earlier in this chapter, excessive buildup of pleural fluid is called *pleural effusion*. In thoracentesis, a thin needle or plastic tube is inserted into the pleural space to extract excess fluid, allowing the patient to breathe more easily. The fluid is often sent to a pathologist for analysis.

Ventilation/Perfusion Scan

A **ventilation/perfusion scan (VPS)** is also called a **lung scan** or **V/Q scan**. It is a diagnostic nuclear medicine test that measures airflow and blood flow in the lungs. It is used to help diagnose a variety of conditions such as pulmonary embolism, pleural effusion, and pulmonary edema.

During a ventilation/perfusion scan, the patient inhales radioactive gas, which is detected by a machine and converted into an image that reveals details about the patient's lung ventilation (airflow) and lung perfusion (blood flow).

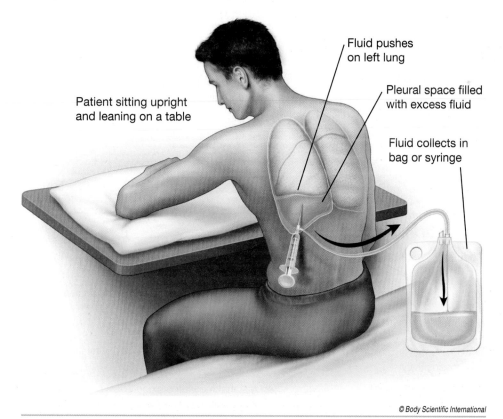

Patient sitting upright and leaning on a table

Fluid pushes on left lung

Pleural space filled with excess fluid

Fluid collects in bag or syringe

© Body Scientific International

Figure 9.14 Thoracentesis is a procedure for removing fluid buildup in the pleural space, the area between the lungs and chest wall.

Multiple Choice: Diseases and Disorders

Directions: Choose the disease or disorder that matches each definition. You can also complete this activity online using *EduHub*.

_____ 1. a combination of two diseases: chronic bronchitis and emphysema
   a. croup
   b. pleural effusion
   c. pneumothorax
   d. chronic obstructive pulmonary disease

_____ 2. inflammation of the lining of the bronchial tubes
   a. pneumonia   c. pleural effusion
   b. bronchitis   d. asthma

_____ 3. collapsed lung
   a. pleural effusion
   b. pneumonia
   c. pneumothorax
   d. chronic obstructive pulmonary disease

_____ 4. inflammation around the larynx and trachea
   a. croup   c. bronchitis
   b. pneumonia   d. pleural effusion

_____ 5. disorder caused by inflammation of the bronchi (airways of the lungs)
   a. pneumonia   c. pleural effusion
   b. pneumothorax   d. asthma

_____ 6. infection of the head and chest caused by a virus
   a. upper respiratory infection
   b. pleural effusion
   c. pneumothorax
   d. chronic obstructive pulmonary disease

_____ 7. excessive accumulation of fluid between the pleura, the layers of tissue that envelop the lungs and line the chest cavity
   a. pneumonia   c. pleural effusion
   b. bronchitis   d. asthma

_____ 8. condition in which airflow pauses or decreases during sleep due to narrowing or blockage of the airway
   a. pneumothorax
   b. pneumonia
   c. obstructive sleep apnea
   d. chronic obstructive pulmonary disease

_____ 9. inflammation of the lungs commonly caused by infection from a bacterium or virus
   a. upper respiratory infection
   b. pleural effusion
   c. pneumonia
   d. chronic obstructive pulmonary disease

SCORECARD: How Did You Do?

Number correct (_____), divided by 9 (_____), multiplied by 100 equals _____ (your score)

Multiple Choice: Procedures and Treatments

Directions: Choose the procedure or treatment that matches each definition. You can also complete this activity online using *EduHub*.

_____ 1. test used to determine if a patient has been exposed to tuberculosis
   a. pulmonary function test
   b. tuberculin skin test
   c. thoracentesis
   d. sputum culture and sensitivity

_____ 2. any of a group of tests that measures lung function
   a. pulmonary function test
   b. tuberculin skin test
   c. thoracentesis
   d. sputum culture and sensitivity

_____ 3. procedure in which excess fluid is removed from the pleural space
   a. thoracentesis
   b. chest X-ray
   c. sputum culture and sensitivity
   d. arterial blood gas test

_____ 4. test that measures blood levels of oxygen and carbon dioxide as well as the acidity of the blood
   a. pulmonary function test
   b. tuberculin skin test
   c. thoracentesis
   d. arterial blood gas test

5. treatment in which a machine is used to deliver a constant flow of mild air pressure through the airways
   a. thoracentesis
   b. constant positive airway pressure
   c. ventilation/perfusion scan
   d. cardiopulmonary resuscitation

6. test that identifies which bacterium, virus, or fungus is causing a pulmonary illness and helps determine the most effective antibiotic treatment
   a. pulmonary function test
   b. tuberculin skin test
   c. thoracentesis
   d. sputum culture and sensitivity

7. lifesaving technique involving the use of chest compressions following cardiac arrest
   a. thoracentesis
   b. constant positive airway pressure
   c. ventilation/perfusion scan
   d. cardiopulmonary resuscitation

SCORECARD: How Did You Do?

Number correct (_____), divided by 7 (_____), multiplied by 100 equals _____ (your score)

Identify Abbreviations

Directions: Supply the correct abbreviation for each medical term. You can also complete this activity online using *EduHub*.

Medical Term	Abbreviation
1. tuberculosis	_____
2. arterial blood gas	_____
3. culture and sensitivity	_____
4. upper respiratory infection	_____
5. pulmonary function test	_____
6. chest X-ray	_____
7. continuous positive airway pressure	_____
8. ventilation/perfusion scan	_____
9. cardiopulmonary resuscitation	_____
10. chronic obstructive pulmonary disease	_____

SCORECARD: How Did You Do?

Number correct (_____), divided by 10 (_____), multiplied by 100 equals _____ (your score)

Analyzing the Intern Experience

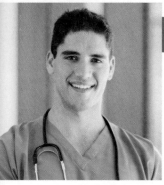

michaeljung/Shutterstock.com

In the Intern Experience described at the beginning of this chapter, we met Mark, a medical intern with the Oak Forest Urgent Care Center. Mark observed and assisted Dr. Connor Wiley as he examined and talked with David, a high school lacrosse player who came to the clinic because of chest pain and difficulty breathing.

After examining David and obtaining his personal and family health history, Dr. Wiley made a medical diagnosis and provided David with a treatment plan. Later, the physician made a dictated recording of the patient's health information, which was subsequently transcribed into a chart note.

We will now learn more about David's condition from a clinical perspective, interpreting the medical terms in his chart note as we analyze the scenario presented in the Intern Experience.

Audio Activity: David Marino's Chart Note

Directions: Access your *EduHub* subscription and listen to the recording of the physician reading David Marino's chart note. Read along with the physician and pay attention to the pronunciation of each medical term.

CHART NOTE

Patient Name: Marino, David
ID Number: DMM1782
Examination Date: September 7, 20xx

SUBJECTIVE
David is a 17-year-old high school student who complains of shortness of breath and sudden chest pain during lacrosse practice.

OBJECTIVE
Patient presents with pronounced **dyspnea** and elevated pulse and **BP**. Temperature is 101. The **pharynx** is clear. The right lung shows decreased breath sounds with air exchange. **Chest X-ray** reveals a collapsed lower lobe of the right lung.

ASSESSMENT
Pneumothorax due to blunt force rib fracture.

PLAN
Inserted chest tube to reinflate lung. Patient is stable and will be transferred by ambulance to General Hospital.

Interpret David Marino's Chart Note

Directions: Access your *EduHub* subscription and listen to the recording of the physician reading David Marino's chart note. After listening to the recording, supply the medical term that matches each definition. You may encounter definitions and terms introduced in previous chapters.

> *Example:* dilatation of the bronchus   *Answer:* bronchiectasis

1. collapsed lung   _____

2. the throat   _____

3. difficulty breathing   _____

4. radiographic image of the structure and
   organs of the thoracic cavity   _____

5. blood pressure   _____

SCORECARD: How Did You Do?

Number correct (_____), divided by 5 (_____), multiplied by 100 equals _____ (your score)

Working with Medical Records

In this activity, you will interpret the medical records (chart notes) of patients with respiratory system disorders. These examples illustrate typical medical records prepared in a real-world healthcare environment. To interpret these chart notes, you will apply your knowledge of word elements (prefixes, combining forms, and suffixes), diseases and disorders, and procedures and treatments related to the respiratory system.

Audio Activity: Emma LaCross's Chart Note

Directions: Access your *EduHub* subscription and listen to the recording of the physician reading Emma LaCross's chart note. Read along with the physician and pay attention to the pronunciation of each medical term.

CHART NOTE

Patient Name: LaCross, Emma
ID Number: YPU2975
Examination Date: June 10, 20xx

SUBJECTIVE
This 2-year-old female presents with a sore throat and cough that started last night and, according to the mother, "sounded quite croupy." The patient's temperature was not taken.

OBJECTIVE
Patient is alert, well hydrated, afebrile (without fever), and in no acute distress. Both **tympanic** (pertaining to the eardrum) membranes are clear. Throat is mildly injected (filled with fluid). No **exudate** or enlarged tonsils. Neck is supple without **adenopathy**. Lungs are clear with no wheezing or **rales**. Heart is without murmur (abnormal or extra sound heard during a heartbeat).

ASSESSMENT
Croup

PLAN
Mother will use a vaporizer, elevate the child's head when resting, and push fluids. Prescribed Robitussin® DM at bedtime only. Patient should return in 2–4 days if no improvement. Discussed with the mother the normal course of croup and suggested she return or visit an urgent care facility if the condition worsens.

Assessment 9.11

Interpret Emma LaCross's Chart Note

Directions: Access your *EduHub* subscription and listen to the recording of the physician reading Emma LaCross's chart note. After listening to the recording, supply the medical term that matches each definition. You may encounter definitions and terms introduced in previous chapters.

> *Example:* inflammation of the trachea   *Answer:* tracheitis

1. crackling or rattling sound heard in the lungs   _____

2. inflammation around the larynx and trachea   _____

3. disease of the glands   _____

4. pertaining to the eardrum   _____

5. fluid that leaks from blood vessels and clogs the air spaces of the lungs   _____

SCORECARD: How Did You Do?

Number correct (_____), divided by 5 (_____), multiplied by 100 equals _____ (your score)

Audio Activity: Azaria Taylor's Chart Note

Directions: Access your *EduHub* subscription and listen to the recording of the physician reading Azaria Taylor's chart note. Read along with the physician and pay attention to the pronunciation of each medical term.

CHART NOTE

Patient Name: Taylor, Azaria
ID Number: GLW0331
Examination Date: April 22, 20xx

SUBJECTIVE
This is a 9-year-old female who returns with about 10 days of nasal congestion, cough, and running a fever of 101–103°.

OBJECTIVE
Patient is cooperative, but subdued with mild, audible nasal congestion. Throat is clear and neck supple without adenopathy. Coarse **rales** heard in the left lung bases, both posteriorly and laterally. No wheezes or grunting. **CXR** results show consolidation (density) in the left middle lobe and infiltrate (fluid accumulation) in the left lower lobe.

ASSESSMENT
Left middle and lower lobe **pneumonia**.

PLAN
Augmentin® (antibiotic drug), 250 mg chewable, one t.i.d. (3 times a day) x 10 days. Patient should drink fluids for fever control. Recheck in 10 days. Repeat chest X-ray in 4 weeks to verify clearing.

Assessment 9.12

Interpret Azaria Taylor's Chart Note

Directions: Access your *EduHub* subscription and listen to the recording of the physician reading Azaria Taylor's chart note. After listening to the recording, supply the medical term that matches each definition.

Example: pain in the chest   *Answer:* thoracalgia

1. crackling or rattling sound heard in the lungs   _____

2. chest X-ray   _____

3. inflammation of the lungs usually caused by a bacterial or viral infection   _____

SCORECARD: How Did You Do?

Number correct (_____), divided by 3 (_____), multiplied by 100 equals _____ (your score)

Word Elements Summary

Prefixes

Prefix	Meaning
a-	not; without
an-	not; without
brady-	slow
dys-	painful; difficult
endo-	within
hyper-	above; above normal
hypo-	below; below normal
tachy-	fast

Combining Forms

Root Word/Combining Vowel	Meaning
bronch/o, bronchi/o	bronchial tube; bronchus
cyan/o	blue
embol/o	plug; embolus
hem/o	blood
lob/o	lobe (a defined portion of an organ or structure)
ox/o	oxygen
pharyng/o	pharynx; throat
pleur/o	pleura
pneum/o, pneumon/o	lung; air
pulmon/o	lung
rhin/o	nose
spir/o	breathe; breathing
sten/o	narrow; constricted
thorac/o	chest
trache/o	trachea; windpipe

Suffixes

Suffix	Meaning
-al	pertaining to
-algia	pain
-centesis	surgical puncture to remove fluid
-ectasis	dilatation; dilation; expansion
-ectomy	surgical removal; excision
-gram	record; image
-ia	condition
-itis	inflammation
-logist	specialist in the study and treatment of
-logy	study of
-meter	measure
-osis	abnormal condition
-pnea	breathing
-scope	instrument used to observe
-thorax	chest; pleural cavity
-tomy	incision; cut into

More Practice: Activities and Games

The following activities will help you reinforce your skills and check your mastery of the medical terminology you learned in this chapter. Access your *EduHub* subscription to complete more activities and vocabulary games for mastering the word parts and terms you have learned.

Audio Activity: Daniel Elliot's Chart Note

Directions: Access your *EduHub* subscription and listen to the recording of the physician reading Daniel Elliot's chart note. Read along with the physician and pay attention to the pronunciation of each medical term.

CHART NOTE

Patient Name: Elliot, Daniel
ID Number: FRU9764
Examination Date: January 30, 20xx

SUBJECTIVE

This is a 54-year-old male with **emphysema**, **dyspnea**, and increasing weakness. For the last 2 months, he has had recurring nocturnal (occurring at night) dyspnea up to 3 times a night, but denies problems of orthopnea (difficult breathing when lying flat). He states that he uses an albuterol inhaler for **asthma**, which seems to relieve the symptoms. He is barrel-chested with a productive cough of white **sputum**. Patient is a nonsmoker. **Afebrile** (without fever) with no chills or lower-extremity **edema**.

OBJECTIVE

Mr. Elliot is a thin, gaunt gentleman appearing older than his stated age. BP is 148/64. Pulse is 92. Respirations are 30. Heart is regular in rhythm. Lungs display good air movement with diffuse expiratory (pertaining to exhaling or breathing out) wheezing and prolongation of the expiratory phase. **CXR** reveals flattened diaphragm, increased AP (anteroposterior) diameter, and box-car lung shapes consistent with severe emphysema. **Pulmonary function test** before and after albuterol treatment shows severe obstructive changes with no improvement following treatment.

ASSESSMENT

Patient has shortness of breath secondary to **COPD** exacerbation (symptoms made worse by another disease).

PLAN

Refer patient to **pulmonary** medicine specialist.

Assessment

Interpret Daniel Elliot's Chart Note

Directions: Access your *EduHub* subscription and listen to the recording of the physician reading Daniel Elliot's chart note. After listening to the recording, supply the medical term that matches each definition. You may encounter definitions and terms introduced in previous chapters.

Example: condition of the bronchus and lung   *Answer:* bronchopneumonia

1. disorder caused by inflammation of the bronchi (airways) of the lungs   _____

2. pertaining to the lungs   _____

3. mucus or fluid coughed up from the lungs   _____

4. painful or difficult breathing   _____

5. chest X-ray   _____

(Continued on next page)

6. form of COPD in which the walls of the alveoli (tiny air sacs in the lungs) have become damaged and lost their elasticity

7. swelling

8. any of a group of tests that measures lung function

9. progressive lung disease marked by difficulty breathing; caused by damage to the lungs over a period of years

10. without fever

Break It Down

Directions: Dissect each medical term into its word parts (prefix, root word, combining vowel, and suffix) using one or more slashes. Then define each term.

Example:
Medical Term: hyperpnea
Dissection: hyper/pnea
Definition: above-normal breathing

Medical Term	Dissection
1. hyperoxia	h y p e r o x i a

Definition: _____

_____

2. bronchiectasis   b r o n c h i e c t a s i s

Definition: _____

_____

3. thoracalgia   t h o r a c a l g i a

Definition: _____

_____

Medical Term	Dissection
4. cyanosis	c y a n o s i s

Definition: _____

_____

5. endotracheal	e n d o t r a c h e a l

Definition: _____

_____

6. pleural	p l e u r a l

Definition: _____

_____

7. lobotomy	l o b o t o m y

Definition: _____

_____

8. thoracotomy	t h o r a c o t o m y

Definition: _____

_____

9. tachypnea	t a c h y p n e a

Definition: _____

_____

10. bronchostenosis	b r o n c h o s t e n o s i s

Definition: _____

_____

11. spirometer	s p i r o m e t e r

Definition: _____

_____

Identify the Medical Word Part

Directions: For each medical word part, identify the type of word part (prefix, root word, or suffix) and provide its meaning.

1. **hypo**   Prefix   Root Word   Suffix

   Meaning: _____

   _____

2. **centesis**   Prefix   Root Word   Suffix

   Meaning: _____

   _____

3. **pleur**   Prefix   Root Word   Suffix

   Meaning: _____

   _____

4. **pulmon**   Prefix   Root Word   Suffix

   Meaning: _____

   _____

5. **tachy**   Prefix   Root Word   Suffix

   Meaning: _____

   _____

6. **thorax**   Prefix   Root Word   Suffix

   Meaning: _____

   _____

7. **pnea**   Prefix   Root Word   Suffix

   Meaning: _____

   _____

8. **bronch**   Prefix   Root Word   Suffix

   Meaning: _____

   _____

Chapter 10

The Cardiovascular System

cardi / o / logy: the study of the heart

Chapter Organization

- Intern Experience
- Overview of Cardiovascular System Anatomy and Physiology
- Word Elements
- Breaking Down and Building Cardiovascular System Terms
- Diseases and Disorders
- Procedures and Treatments
- Analyzing the Intern Experience
- Working with Medical Records
- Chapter Review

Chapter Objectives

After completing this chapter, you will be able to

1. label an anatomical diagram of the cardiovascular system;

2. dissect and define common medical terminology related to the cardiovascular system;

3. build terms used to describe cardiovascular system diseases and disorders, diagnostic procedures, and therapeutic treatments;

4. pronounce and spell common medical terminology related to the cardiovascular system;

5. understand that the process of building and dissecting a medical term based on its prefix, root word, and suffix enables you to analyze an extremely large number of medical terms beyond those presented in this chapter;

6. interpret the meaning of abbreviations associated with the cardiovascular system; and

7. interpret medical records containing terminology and abbreviations related to the cardiovascular system.

Your *EduHub* subscription that accompanies this text provides access to online assessments, assignments, activities, and resources. Throughout this chapter, access *EduHub* to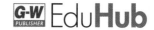

- use e-flash cards to review the medical terminology and word parts you learn;
- listen to the correct pronunciations of medical terms; and
- complete medical terminology activities and assignments.

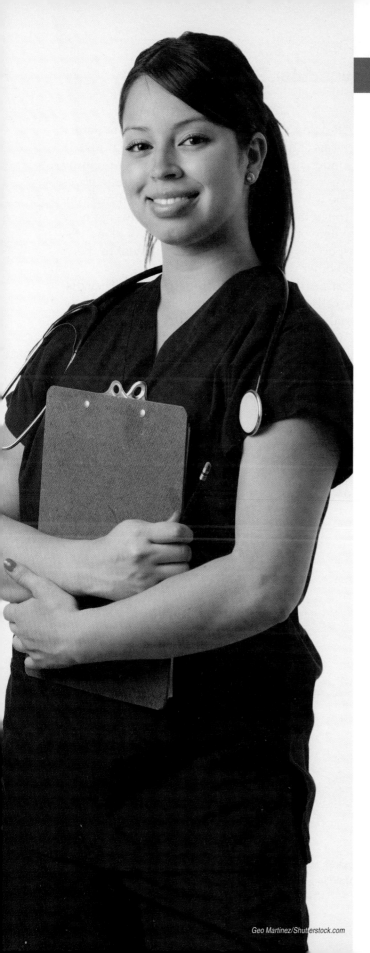
Geo Martinez/Shutterstock.com

Intern Experience

Layla Stern, an intern with Guardian Urgent Care Center, enters exam room 1, where a middle-aged man is lying on the examination table. He is pale and sweating profusely. A young woman who appears to be in her twenties is hovering near the man, and she is clearly distressed. When Layla begins the triage interview, she learns that Peggy, the young woman, had begged her father, Jim Flowers, to let her go to Citadel Stadium to see her favorite singer. Since Peggy's birthday was approaching, he agreed to take her and her best friend, Mira, to the concert. As they neared the stadium, Peggy was so excited that she didn't notice her father massaging his chest and left arm. When he missed the turn into the parking lot, Peggy yelled and then suddenly noticed that her father was "very pale and sweating a lot." Alarmed, she told him to pull the car over to the side of the road. She helped her father shift into the passenger seat and then drove him to the urgent care center only a few blocks from the stadium.

As you will learn later in this chapter, Jim Flowers has a health condition that has affected his heart, the organ that pumps blood throughout the body. You will have the opportunity to analyze and interpret Jim's patient chart note, the medical record dictated by his physician after the physical examination that Jim received.

In this chapter, you will learn common word elements (prefixes, combining forms, and suffixes) used to form medical terms pertaining to the cardiovascular system. Mastery of these terms and the word parts from which they are constructed will enable you to understand the health conditions, diagnostic procedures, and therapeutic treatments summarized in the patient chart notes presented throughout this chapter.

Let's begin our study of the cardiovascular system with a brief overview of its anatomy and physiology.

Overview of Cardiovascular System Anatomy and Physiology

The **cardiovascular** (KĂR-dē-ō-VĂS-kyū-lăr) system, or **circulatory** (SĔR-kyŭ-lă-TOR-ē) **system**, consists of the heart and blood vessels (Figure 10.1). This system is a huge transportation network. Think of it as a major highway system that transports substances necessary for our survival and also removes waste that is generated along the way. The cardiovascular system allows continuous movement of blood through the heart and blood vessels. This highway system is composed of a dense network of many different types of blood vessels that work together to transport oxygen and nutrients throughout the body and remove carbon dioxide and other waste products.

Arteries are blood vessels that carry blood away from the heart. They distribute oxygen and nutrients to cells, tissues, and organs throughout the body. Arterioles are very small arterial branches that connect arteries to capillaries. **Capillaries** (KĂP-ĭ-lăr-ēz) are tiny vessels in which the exchange of oxygen, nutrients, and waste products occurs. **Veins** are the blood vessels that carry blood toward the heart. They transport carbon dioxide and other waste products away from the cells, tissues, and organs. **Venules** (VĒN-yulz) are very small veins that connect capillaries to larger veins.

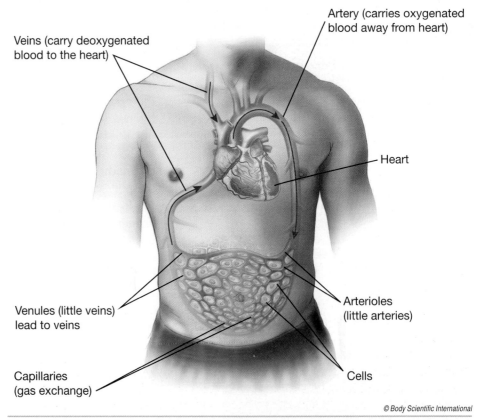

Veins (carry deoxygenated blood to the heart)

Artery (carries oxygenated blood away from heart)

Heart

Arterioles (little arteries)

Venules (little veins) lead to veins

Capillaries (gas exchange)

Cells

© Body Scientific International

Figure 10.1 The cardiovascular system is made up of the heart and a network of large and progressively smaller blood vessels.

While the arteries, veins, and capillaries make up the dense transportation network of the cardiovascular system, the **heart** functions as the muscular force behind this system. The heart pumps the blood that contains oxygen and nutrients, which our bodies need to survive. Blood also picks up waste products from the cells and delivers them to organs that can eliminate them from the body (for example, the lungs, kidneys, and intestines). Dysfunction within the cardiovascular system produces, at best, serious health issues; total failure results in death.

Cardiology (kär-dē-ŎL-ō-jē) is the medical specialty concerned with the study of the heart. A **cardiologist** (kär-dē-ŎL-ō-jĭst) is a physician who specializes in the study, diagnosis, and treatment of diseases and disorders of the heart—and, by extension, the cardiovascular system.

Anatomy and Physiology Vocabulary

Now that you have been introduced to the basic structure and functions of the cardiovascular system, we will explore in a bit more detail the key terms presented in the introduction.

Key Term	Definition
arteries	vessels that carry blood away from the heart and distribute oxygen and nutrients to cells, tissues, and organs
arterioles	very small arterial branches that connect arteries to capillaries
capillaries	tiny vessels in which the exchange of oxygen, nutrients, and waste products occurs
cardiovascular system	the body system that consists of the heart and blood vessels; *circulatory system*
circulatory system	another term for *cardiovascular system*
heart	muscular organ that pumps blood throughout the body
veins	vessels that carry blood toward the heart and remove carbon dioxide and other waste products from cells, tissues, and organs
venules	very small veins that connect capillaries to larger veins

E-Flash Card Activity: Anatomy and Physiology Vocabulary

Directions: After you have reviewed the anatomy and physiology vocabulary related to the cardiovascular system, access your *EduHub* subscription and practice with the e-flash cards until you are comfortable with the spelling and definition of each term.

Identifying Major Organs and Structures of the Cardiovascular System

Directions: Label the anatomical diagram of the cardiovascular system. You can also complete this activity online using *EduHub*.

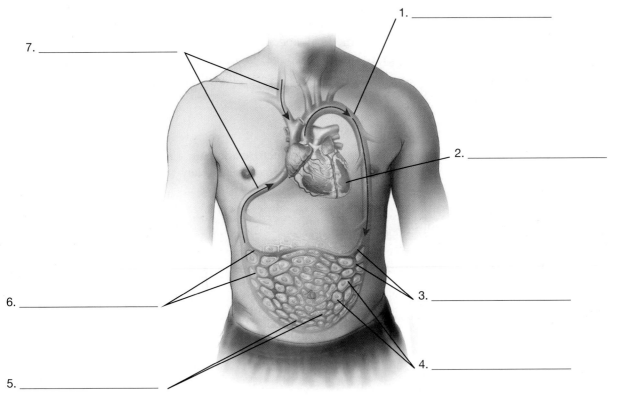

1. _____

7. _____

2. _____

6. _____

3. _____

4. _____

5. _____

© Body Scientific International

Matching Anatomy and Physiology Vocabulary

Directions: Choose the correct vocabulary term for each meaning. You can also complete this activity online using *EduHub*.

_____ 1. muscular organ that pumps blood throughout the body

_____ 2. very small veins that connect capillaries to larger veins

_____ 3. the body system that consists of the heart and blood vessels; *circulatory system*

_____ 4. another term for *cardiovascular system*

_____ 5. tiny vessels in which the exchange of oxygen, nutrients, and waste products occurs

_____ 6. vessels that carry blood toward the heart and transport carbon dioxide and other waste products away from the cells, tissues, and organs

_____ 7. very small arterial branches that connect arteries to capillaries

_____ 8. vessels that carry blood away from the heart and distribute oxygen and nutrients to cells, tissues, and organs

A. veins

B. arteries

C. cardiovascular system

D. capillaries

E. circulatory system

F. heart

G. venules

H. arterioles

SCORECARD: How Did You Do?

Number correct (_____), divided by 8 (_____), multiplied by 100 equals _____ (your score)

Word Elements

In this section, you will learn word elements—prefixes, combining forms, and suffixes—that are common to the cardiovascular system. By learning these word elements and understanding how they are combined to build medical terms, you will be able to analyze Jim's health condition (described in the Intern Experience at the beginning of this chapter) and identify a large number of terms associated with the cardiovascular system.

E-Flash Card Activity: Word Elements

Directions: Review the word elements in the tables that follow. Then, access your *EduHub* subscription and practice with the e-flash cards until you are able to quickly recognize the different word parts (prefixes, combining forms, and suffixes) and their meanings. The e-flash cards are grouped together by prefixes, combining forms, and suffixes, followed by a cumulative review of all the word elements you are learning in this chapter.

Prefixes

Let's begin our study of cardiovascular system word elements by looking at the prefixes listed in the table below. By now, you are familiar with all of these prefixes.

Prefix	Meaning
a-	not; without
brady-	slow
dys-	painful; difficult
hyper-	above; above normal
hypo-	below; below normal
intra-	inside; within
peri-	around
tachy-	fast

Combining Forms

Listed below are combining forms commonly used in medical terms related to the cardiovascular system.

Root Word/Combining Vowel	Meaning
angi/o	vessel
arteri/o	artery
ather/o	fatty substance
card/o, cardi/o	heart
coron/o	heart
cyan/o	blue
electr/o	electrical activity
hem/o, hemat/o	blood
isch/o	to keep back
my/o	muscle
phleb/o	vein
pulmon/o	lung
sten/o	narrow; constricted
tens/o	pressure; tension
thromb/o	clot
vas/o	vessel; duct
ven/o, ven/i	vein

Suffixes

Listed below are suffixes that appear in medical terms pertaining to the cardiovascular system. From your study of body systems covered in previous chapters, you are already familiar with most of these suffixes.

Suffix	Meaning
-ac	pertaining to
-al	pertaining to
-ary	pertaining to
-ation	process; condition; state of being or having
-emia	blood condition
-gram	record; image
-ia	condition
-ion	process
-itis	inflammation
-logist	specialist in the study and treatment of
-logy	study of
-megaly	large; enlargement
-oma	tumor; mass
-osis	abnormal condition
-ous	pertaining to
-pathy	disease
-penia	deficiency; abnormal reduction
-plasty	surgical repair
-pnea	breathing
-rrhage	bursting forth (of blood)
-rrhexis	rupture
-sclerosis	hardening
-stasis	stop; stand still
-tic	pertaining to
-tomy	incision; cut into
-trophy	development

Matching Prefixes, Combining Forms, and Suffixes

Directions: Choose the correct meaning for each word element. Some meanings may be used more than once. You can also complete this activity online using *EduHub*.

Prefixes

_____ 1. dys-

_____ 2. intra-

_____ 3. tachy-

_____ 4. brady-

_____ 5. a-

_____ 6. peri-

_____ 7. hyper-

_____ 8. hypo-

A. slow

B. above; above normal

C. not; without

D. painful; difficult

E. below; below normal

F. fast

G. inside; within

H. around

Combining Forms

_____ 1. isch/o

_____ 2. sten/o

_____ 3. pulmon/o

_____ 4. vas/o

_____ 5. thromb/o

_____ 6. phleb/o

_____ 7. hem/o

_____ 8. ven/o

_____ 9. angi/o

_____ 10. electr/o

_____ 11. arteri/o

_____ 12. my/o

_____ 13. coron/o

_____ 14. cardi/o

_____ 15. tens/o

_____ 16. cyan/o

_____ 17. ather/o

_____ 18. ven/i

_____ 19. hemat/o

A. artery

B. vein

C. blue

D. to keep back

E. muscle

F. electrical activity

G. vessel

H. heart

I. clot

J. narrow; constricted

K. blood

L. lung

M. pressure; tension

N. vessel; duct

O. fatty substance

Suffixes

_____ 1. -sclerosis

_____ 2. -ia

_____ 3. -itis

_____ 4. -logist

_____ 5. -logy

_____ 6. -megaly

_____ 7. -oma

_____ 8. -emia

_____ 9. -ous

_____ 10. -ac

_____ 11. -al

_____ 12. -gram

_____ 13. -plasty

_____ 14. -ary

_____ 15. -osis

_____ 16. -rrhexis

_____ 17. -pnea

_____ 18. -ation

_____ 19. -rrhage

_____ 20. -trophy

_____ 21. -pathy

_____ 22. -penia

_____ 23. -ion

_____ 24. -stasis

_____ 25. -tic

_____ 26. -tomy

A. pertaining to

B. specialist in the study and treatment of

C. development

D. condition

E. inflammation

F. tumor; mass

G. study of

H. abnormal condition

I. large; enlargement

J. disease

K. deficiency; abnormal reduction

L. surgical repair

M. bursting forth (of blood)

N. rupture

O. blood condition

P. hardening

Q. process; condition; state of being or having

R. record; image

S. breathing

T. stop; stand still

U. process

V. incision; cut into

SCORECARD: How Did You Do?

Number correct (_____), divided by 53 (_____), multiplied by 100 equals _____ (your score)

Breaking Down and Building Cardiovascular System Terms

Now that you have mastered the prefixes, combining forms, and suffixes for medical terminology pertaining to the cardiovascular system, you have the ability to dissect and build a large number of terms related to this body system.

Below is a list of medical terms commonly used in cardiology, the medical specialty concerning the study, diagnosis, and treatment of diseases and disorders of the cardiovascular system. For each term, a dissection has been provided, along with the meaning of each word element and the definition of the term as a whole.

Term	Dissection	Word Part/Meaning	Term Meaning
Note: *For simplification, combining vowels have been omitted from the Word Part/Meaning column.*			
1. **angioplasty** (ĂN-jē-ō-PLĂS-tē)	angi/o/plasty	**angi** = vessel **plasty** = surgical repair	surgical repair of a vessel
2. **arteriosclerosis** (är-TĒ-rē-ō-sklĕ-RŌ-sĭs)	arteri/o/sclerosis	**arteri** = artery **sclerosis** = hardening	hardening of the artery
3. **atherosclerosis** (ĂTH-ĕr-ō-sklĕ-RŌ-sĭs)	ather/o/sclerosis	**ather** = fatty substance **sclerosis** = hardening	hardening of a fatty substance
4. **bradycardia** (BRĀD-ē-KÄR-dē-ă)	brady/card/ia	**brady** = slow **card** = heart **ia** = condition	condition of a slow heart
5. **cardiac** (KÄR-dē-ăk)	cardi/ac	**cardi** = heart **ac** = pertaining to	pertaining to the heart
6. **cardiologist** (kär-dē-ŎL-ō-jĭst)	cardi/o/logist	**cardi** = heart **logist** = specialist in the study and treatment of	specialist in the study and treatment of the heart
7. **cardiology** (kär-dē-ŎL-ō-jē)	cardi/o/logy	**cardi** = heart **logy** = study of	study of the heart
8. **cardiomegaly** (KÄR-dē-ō-MĔG-ă-lē)	cardi/o/megaly	**cardi** = heart **megaly** = large; enlargement	enlargement of the heart
9. **cardiomyopathy** (KÄR-dē-ō-mī-ŎP-ă-thē)	cardi/o/my/o/pathy	**cardi** = heart **my** = muscle **pathy** = disease	disease of the heart muscle
10. **cardiopulmonary** (KÄR-dē-ō-PŬL-mō-nĕr-ē)	cardi/o/pulmon/ary	**cardi** = heart **pulmon** = lung **ary** = pertaining to	pertaining to the heart and lung
11. **coronary** (KOR-ō-nār-ē)	coron/ary	**coron** = heart **ary** = pertaining to	pertaining to the heart
12. **electrocardiogram** (ĕ-LĔK-trō-KÄR-dē-ō-gram)	electr/o/cardi/o/gram	**electr** = electrical activity **cardi** = heart **gram** = record; image	record of the electrical activity of the heart

Prefixes = **Green**   Root Words = **Red**   Suffixes = **Blue**

Term	Dissection	Word Part/Meaning	Term Meaning
13. **hemorrhage** (HĔM-ĕ-rĭj)	hem/o/rrhage	**hem** = blood **rrhage** = bursting forth (of blood)	bursting forth of blood
14. **hemostasis** (HĒ-mō-STĀ-sĭs)	hem/o/stasis	**hem** = blood **stasis** = stop; stand still	stop blood (flow)
15. **hypertension** (hī-pĕr-TĔN-shŭn)	hyper/tens/ion	**hyper** = above; above normal **tens** = pressure; tension **ion** = process	process of above-normal pressure/tension
16. **hypertrophy** (hī-PĔR-trŏ-fē)	hyper/trophy	**hyper** = above; above normal **trophy** = development	above-normal development
17. **hypotension** (hī-pō-TĔN-shun)	hypo/tens/ion	**hypo** = below; below normal **tens** = pressure; tension **ion** = process	process of below-normal pressure/tension
18. **myocardial** (mī-ō-KÄR-dē-ăl)	my/o/cardi/al	**my** = muscle **cardi** = heart **al** = pertaining to	pertaining to the heart muscle
19. **pericarditis** (PĔR-ĭ-kär-DĪ-tĭs)	peri/card/itis	**peri** = around **card** = heart **itis** = inflammation	inflammation around the heart
20. **phlebitis** (flĕ-BĪ-tĭs)	phleb/itis	**phleb** = vein **itis** = inflammation	inflammation of a vein
21. **stenotic** (stĕ-NŎT-ĭk)	sten/o/tic	**sten** = narrow; constricted **tic** = pertaining to	pertaining to (being) narrow/constricted
22. **tachycardia** (tăk-ē-KÄR-dē-ă)	tachy/card/ia	**tachy** = fast **card** = heart **ia** = condition	condition of a fast heart
23. **thrombophlebitis** (THRŎM-bō-flĕ-BĪ-tĭs)	thromb/o/phleb/itis	**thromb** = clot **phleb** = vein **itis** = inflammation	inflammation of a clot in a vein
24. **thrombosis** (thrŏm-BŌ-sĭs)	thromb/osis	**thromb** = clot **osis** = abnormal condition	abnormal condition of a clot
25. **venous** (VĒ-nŭs)	ven/ous	**ven** = vein **ous** = pertaining to	pertaining to the vein

Prefixes = Green   Root Words = **Red**   Suffixes = Blue

Using the pronunciation guide in the Breaking Down and Building chart, practice saying each medical term aloud. To hear the pronunciation of each term, complete the Pronounce It activity on the next page.

Audio Activity: Pronounce It

Directions: Access your *EduHub* subscription and listen to the correct pronunciations of the following medical terms. Practice pronouncing the terms until you are comfortable saying them aloud.

angioplasty
(ĂN-jē-ō-PLĂS-tē)

arteriosclerosis
(är-TĒ-rē-ō-sklĕ-RŌ-sĭs)

atherosclerosis
(ĂTH-ĕr-ō-sklĕ-RŌ-sĭs)

bradycardia
(BRĀD-ē-KĂR-dē-ă)

cardiac
(KĂR-dē-ăk)

cardiologist
(kär-dē-ŎL-ō-jĭst)

cardiology
(kär-dē-ŎL-ō-jē)

cardiomegaly
(KĂR-dē-ō-MĔG-ă-lē)

cardiomyopathy
(KĂR-dē-ō-mī-ŎP-ă-thē)

cardiopulmonary
(KĂR-dē-ō-PŬL-mō-nĕr-ē)

coronary
(KOR-ō-nār-ē)

electrocardiogram
(ĕ-LĔK-trō-KĂR-dē-ō-gram)

hemorrhage
(HĔM-ĕ-rĭj)

hemostasis
(HĒ-mō-STĀ-sĭs)

hypertension
(hī-pĕr-TĔN-shŭn)

hypertrophy
(hī-PĔR-trŏ-fē)

hypotension
(hī-pō-TĔN-shun)

myocardial
(mī-ō-KĂR-dē-ăl)

pericarditis
(PĔR-ĭ-kär-DĪ-tĭs)

phlebitis
(flĕ-BĪ-tĭs)

stenotic
(stĕ-NŎT-ĭk)

tachycardia
(tăk-ē-KĂR-dē-ă)

thrombophlebitis
(THRŎM-bō-flĕ-BĪ-tĭs)

thrombosis
(thrŏm-BŌ-sĭs)

venous
(VĒ-nŭs)

Audio Activity: Spell It

Directions: Access your *EduHub* subscription and listen to the pronunciation for each number. As you hear each term, write its correct spelling. You can also complete this activity online using *EduHub*.

1. _____
2. _____
3. _____
4. _____
5. _____
6. _____
7. _____
8. _____
9. _____
10. _____
11. _____
12. _____
13. _____

14. _____
15. _____
16. _____
17. _____
18. _____
19. _____
20. _____
21. _____
22. _____
23. _____
24. _____
25. _____

SCORECARD: How Did You Do?

Number correct (_____), divided by 25 (_____), multiplied by 100 equals _____ (your score)

Break It Down

Directions: Dissect each medical term into its word parts (prefix, root word, combining vowel, and suffix) using one or more slashes. Then define each term. You can also complete this activity online using *EduHub*.

Example:

Medical Term: cardiologist

Dissection: cardi/o/logist

Definition: specialist in the study and treatment of the heart

Medical Term   **Dissection**

1. venous   v e n o u s

Definition: _____

_____

2. cardiac   c a r d i a c

Definition: _____

_____

3. angioplasty   a n g i o p l a s t y

Definition: _____

_____

4. hypertension   h y p e r t e n s i o n

Definition: _____

_____

5. cardiopulmonary   c a r d i o p u l m o n a r y

Definition: _____

_____

6. pericarditis   p e r i c a r d i t i s

Definition: _____

_____

Medical Term	Dissection
7. stenotic	s t e n o t i c

Definition: _____

_____

| 8. arteriosclerosis | a r t e r i o s c l e r o s i s |

Definition: _____

_____

| 9. cardiology | c a r d i o l o g y |

Definition: _____

_____

| 10. hemostasis | h e m o s t a s i s |

Definition: _____

_____

| 11. hypotension | h y p o t e n s i o n |

Definition: _____

_____

| 12. thrombosis | t h r o m b o s i s |

Definition: _____

_____

| 13. myocardial | m y o c a r d i a l |

Definition: _____

_____

| 14. electrocardiogram | e l e c t r o c a r d i o g r a m |

Definition: _____

_____

Medical Term	Dissection
15. atherosclerosis	a t h e r o s c l e r o s i s

Definition: _____

_____

16. bradycardia   b r a d y c a r d i a

Definition: _____

_____

17. phlebitis   p h l e b i t i s

Definition: _____

_____

18. tachycardia   t a c h y c a r d i a

Definition: _____

_____

19. coronary   c o r o n a r y

Definition: _____

_____

20. thrombophlebitis   t h r o m b o p h l e b i t i s

Definition: _____

_____

SCORECARD: How Did You Do?

Number correct (_____), divided by 20 (_____), multiplied by 100 equals _____ (your score)

Build It

Directions: Build the medical term that matches each definition by supplying the correct word parts. You can also complete this activity online using *EduHub*.

P (Prefixes) = Green
RW (Root Words) = Red
S (Suffixes) = Blue
CV (Combining Vowel) = Purple

1. abnormal condition of a clot

   _____ _____
           RW   S

2. above-normal development

   _____ _____
      P   S

3. condition of a fast heart

   _____ _____ _____
      P   RW   S

4. condition of a slow heart

   _____ _____ _____
      P   RW   S

5. disease of the heart muscle

   _____ _____ _____ _____ _____
          RW   CV   RW   CV   S

6. bursting forth (of blood)

   _____ _____ _____
          RW   CV   S

7. hardening of a fatty substance

   _____ _____ _____
          RW   CV   S

8. hardening of the artery

   _____ _____ _____
          RW   CV   S

9. inflammation of a clot in a vein

   _____ _____ _____ _____
          RW   CV   RW   S

10. enlargement of the heart

_____ ____ ___
        RW   CV   S

11. process of above-normal pressure/tension

___ _____ _____
 P   RW   S

12. pertaining to (being) narrow/constricted

_____ ____ ___
        RW   CV   S

13. pertaining to the heart

_____ _____
        RW   S

14. pertaining to the heart and lung

_____ ____ _____ ____
        RW   CV   RW   S

15. pertaining to the vein

_____ _____
        RW   S

16. record of the electrical activity of the heart

_____ ____ _____ ____ ___
        RW   CV   RW   CV   S

17. stop blood (flow)

_____ ____ ___
        RW   CV   S

18. study of the heart

_____ ____ ___
        RW   CV   S

19. surgical repair of a blood vessel

_____ ____ ___
        RW   CV   S

SCORECARD: How Did You Do?

Number correct (_____), divided by 19 (_____), multiplied by 100 equals _____ (your score)

Diseases and Disorders

From the mild to the severe, diseases and disorders of the cardiovascular system have a variety of causes, some of which are rooted in genetics; others, in lifestyle habits. In this section, we will briefly explore some common pathological conditions of the cardiovascular system and their etiologies (causes).

Aneurysm

An **aneurysm** (ĂN-yū-rĭzm) is the *dilatation* (widening) and thinning of an artery due to a weakness in the arterial wall (Figures 10.2 and 10.3). Each time the heart beats, the thin, weakened wall of the artery balloons outward. Damage to the arterial wall may be congenital (present at birth) or the result of arteriosclerosis (discussed in the next entry). The continuous, repetitive force of each heartbeat can cause the thin blood vessel to rupture. If the aneurysm is located in a critical artery, such as in the brain or aorta (large, main artery of the body), sudden death can result.

Arteriosclerosis

Arteriosclerosis (är-TĒ-rē-ō-sklĕ-RŌ-sĭs) is commonly called "hardening of the arteries." As we age, our arteries naturally thicken, grow narrower, and lose their elasticity. Blood vessels affected by arteriosclerosis become less flexible and unable to accommodate increases in blood volume. This limited flexibility can lead to *hypertension* (high blood pressure) and clots that obstruct blood flow.

Atherosclerosis

Atherosclerosis (ĂTH-ĕr-ō-sklĕ-RŌ-sĭs), the most common form of arteriosclerosis, is a chronic (long-term) disease in which the arteries that supply blood to the heart muscle become *stenotic* (narrowed) from fatty deposits called *plaque* (Figure 10.4 on the next page). The fatty plaque builds up along the internal wall of the artery, slowing blood flow and depriving the heart of oxygenated blood, a condition called *ischemia* (ĭs-KĒ-mē-ă).

Ischemia causes cell death and damage to surrounding tissues. Myocardial ischemia, which affects the heart muscle, produces a condition called **angina pectoris** (ĂN-jĭ-nă PĔK-tō-rĭs), more commonly known as severe chest pain. The term *angina pectoris* is often shortened to *angina*.

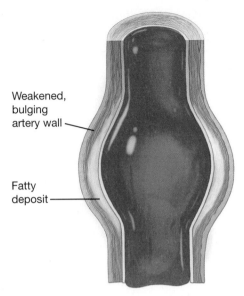

Weakened, bulging artery wall

Fatty deposit

© Body Scientific International

Figure 10.2 An aneurysm is the widening and thinning of an artery due to weakness in the arterial wall. It can be the result of accumulation of fatty deposits in the arterial wall.

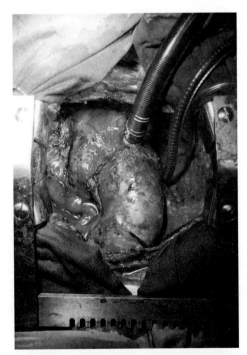

kalewa/Shutterstock.com

Figure 10.3 An aneurysm in one of the large arteries of the heart, shown during "open" surgical repair.

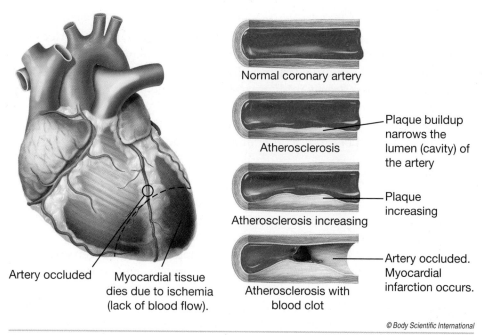

Normal coronary artery

Atherosclerosis

Plaque buildup narrows the lumen (cavity) of the artery

Atherosclerosis increasing

Plaque increasing

Atherosclerosis with blood clot

Artery occluded. Myocardial infarction occurs.

Artery occluded

Myocardial tissue dies due to ischemia (lack of blood flow).

© Body Scientific International

Figure 10.4 Atherosclerosis is marked by stenosis (narrowing) of the arteries that supply blood to the heart muscle. Stenosis is caused by buildup of fatty deposits in the arteries.

Congestive Heart Failure

Congestive heart failure (CHF) occurs when the heart muscle cannot pump enough oxygenated and nutrient-rich blood throughout the body (Figure 10.5). When the heart muscle becomes less effective, blood may back up within other areas of the body, causing fluid buildup in organs, tissues, and extremities. The patient may experience weakness, dyspnea (difficulty breathing), and edema (swelling).

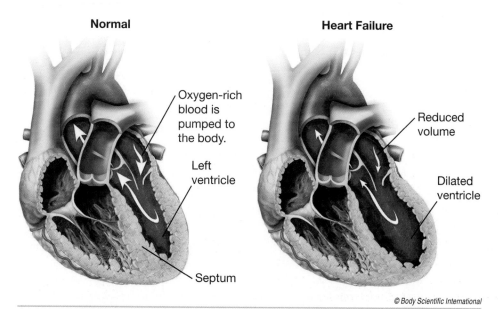

Normal

Heart Failure

Oxygen-rich blood is pumped to the body.

Left ventricle

Septum

Reduced volume

Dilated ventricle

© Body Scientific International

Figure 10.5 When the heart muscle fails to pump a sufficient amount of oxygenated blood throughout the body, the result is congestive heart failure.

The reduction of blood flow to the heart is called *coronary artery disease (CAD)*. As time progresses, conditions such as *stenosis* (narrowed arteries of the heart), coronary artery disease, or hypertension may weaken the heart, making it too stiff to pump efficiently. To compensate for this inefficiency, the heart undergoes *hypertrophy* (hī-PĔR-trŏ-fē), or enlargement. More specifically, the thickness of the heart muscle increases. Cardiac hypertrophy temporarily improves blood flow but leads to irregular heartbeat, fluid congestion in the lungs, and retention of fluid in other areas of the body.

Myocardial Infarction

An *infarct* (ĬN-färkt) is an area of tissue that has died due to a lack of oxygenated blood. A **myocardial infarction (MI)**, commonly called a *heart attack*, occurs when the heart muscle is deprived of oxygen (Figure 10.6).

Just like the rest of the body, the heart is supplied with oxygen and nutrients through the arteries. When a coronary artery is occluded (blocked) by a blood clot, for example, the heart is deprived of oxygen, resulting in death of a portion of the muscle (infarction). Heart tissue that dies during an MI does not regenerate, permanently affecting the heart's blood-pumping efficiency.

Signs of a Heart Attack

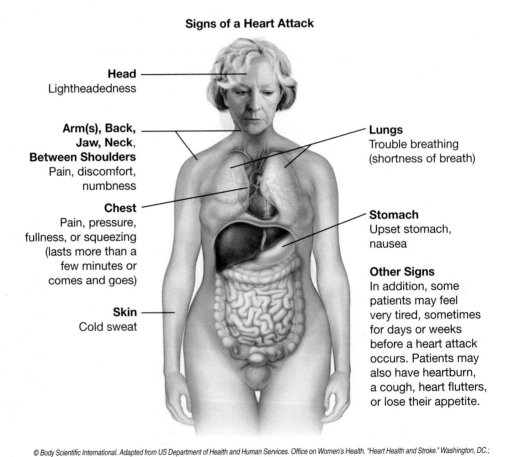

Head
Lightheadedness

Arm(s), Back, Jaw, Neck, Between Shoulders
Pain, discomfort, numbness

Chest
Pain, pressure, fullness, or squeezing (lasts more than a few minutes or comes and goes)

Skin
Cold sweat

Lungs
Trouble breathing (shortness of breath)

Stomach
Upset stomach, nausea

Other Signs
In addition, some patients may feel very tired, sometimes for days or weeks before a heart attack occurs. Patients may also have heartburn, a cough, heart flutters, or lose their appetite.

© Body Scientific International. Adapted from US Department of Health and Human Services. Office on Women's Health. "Heart Health and Stroke." Washington, DC.; available at http://womenshealth.gov/heart-health-stroke/signs-of-a-heart-attack/.

Figure 10.6 Common signs of myocardial infarction, or heart attack.

Varicose Veins

Varicose (VĂR-ĭ-kōs) **veins** are veins that have lost their elasticity (Figures 10.7 and 10.8). As a result, they appear *edematous* (ĕ-DĔM-ă-tŭs) (swollen) and tortuous (having many twists and turns). This appearance is due to the failure of valves within the veins to prevent the backflow of blood. Incompetent valves cause the blood to pool and the veins to swell. A varicose vein disorder can involve both deep veins and superficial (close to the surface) veins. Superficial varicose veins are called "spider veins" and often cause cosmetic embarrassment.

Procedures and Treatments

In this section, you will learn about tests and procedures used to help diagnose pathological conditions of the cardiovascular system, as well as therapeutic methods commonly used to treat certain conditions.

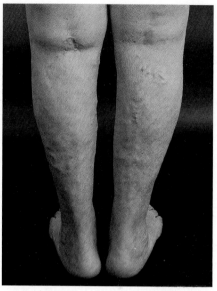

Josep Curto/Shutterstock.com

Figure 10.7 A patient with varicose veins in the legs, a common site of occurrence

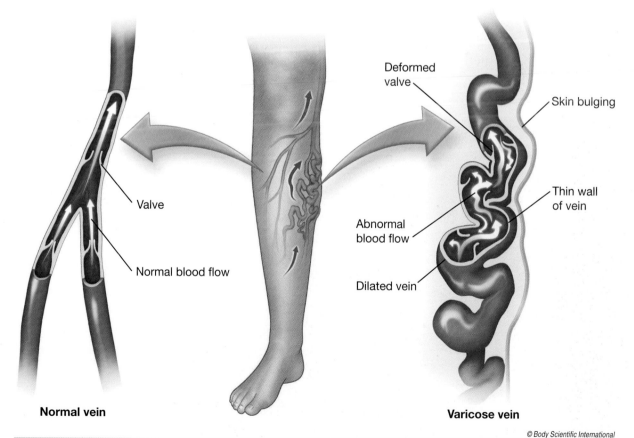

Normal vein

Valve

Normal blood flow

Deformed valve

Skin bulging

Abnormal blood flow

Thin wall of vein

Dilated vein

Varicose vein

© Body Scientific International

Figure 10.8 Varicose veins are marked by edema, loss of elasticity, and a tortuous appearance (having twists and turns).

Cardiac Catheterization

Cardiac catheterization (KĂTH-ĕ-tĕr-ĭ-ZĀ-shŭn) is a procedure in which a catheter (narrow, flexible tube) is inserted into a vein or artery leading to the heart (Figure 10.9). The catheter insertion usually originates in the groin. Frequently, the catheter is inserted in the femoral artery, yet may be introduced through the arm. A contrast agent is then injected through the catheter to "image" the heart, measure cardiac pressures, and withdraw blood samples for analysis (Figure 10.10).

Cardiopulmonary Resuscitation

Cardiopulmonary resuscitation, or **CPR**, is an emergency-response procedure used in an effort to resuscitate a patient who has had a myocardial infarction (heart attack). First responders apply chest compressions or, if available, use an *automated external defibrillator (AED)*. This machine delivers an electrical charge to the heart (*defibrillation*) that can restore normal heart rhythm.

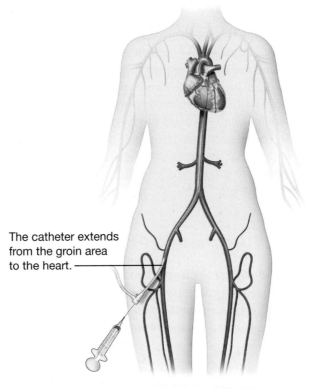

The catheter extends from the groin area to the heart.

© Body Scientific International

Figure 10.9 Cardiac catheterization is a procedure in which images are taken of the heart, cardiac pressures are measured, and blood is withdrawn for laboratory analysis.

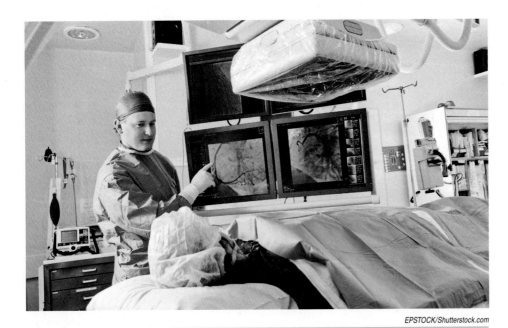

EPSTOCK/Shutterstock.com

Figure 10.10 A catheterization lab, or "cath" lab, in a modern hospital

Doppler Sonography

Doppler sonography is a technique used to measure blood flow and blood pressure by "bouncing" ultrasound (high-frequency sound waves) off red blood cells as they circulate through the body. Unlike standard sonography procedures, which cannot show blood flow, Doppler sonography shows images of body organs and tissues as well as blood flow.

During Doppler sonography, sound waves are directed toward the heart to detect and record cardiac anomalies (Figure 10.11). This imaging technique creates moving images of heart muscle contraction, heart valve movement, and blood flow. Doppler sonography is not only limited to the heart, but also is used extensively to evaluate venous and arterial blood flow in other areas of the body.

Electrocardiogram

An **electrocardiogram (ECG)** is a diagnostic procedure used to record the electrical activity of the heart (Figure 10.12). ECG aids in diagnosing dysfunction of, or damage to, cardiac tissue.

If a patient has intermittent yet persistent chest pain or *arrhythmia* (painful or irregular heart contractions), a cardiologist may instruct a patient to wear a device called a *Holter monitor*. Because heart irregularities are difficult to capture on a single ECG, the Holter monitor is worn by the patient for about 24 hours. The patient keeps track of all daily activities in a diary. Then the cardiologist compares this data to the electrical activity of the heart recorded by the Holter monitor. This comparison provides the cardiologist with further insight to help identify the etiology (cause) of the heart dysfunction or damage.

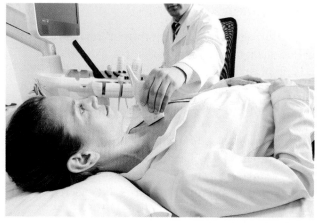

Lorena Fernandez/Shutterstock.com

Figure 10.11 In Doppler sonography, blood flow and blood pressure are measured by "bouncing" ultrasound (high-frequency sound waves) off red blood cells as they travel through the body.

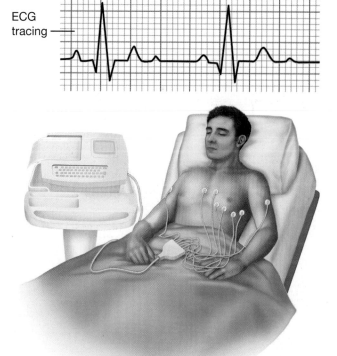

ECG tracing

© Body Scientific International

Figure 10.12 Electrocardiogram, or ECG, is a common procedure for identifying cardiac dysfunction or damage.

Pacemaker

An irregular rate or rhythm of the heart is called *arrhythmia*. *Bradycardia*, for example, is a type of arrhythmia in which the heart beats too slowly. *Tachycardia* is a form of arrhythmia in which the heart beats too fast.

Cardiac arrhythmia may be treated with the insertion of a **pacemaker** (Figures 10.13, 10.14, and 10.15). A pacemaker is a device that corrects arrhythmia by stimulating contraction of the heart muscle with mild electrical impulses.

In more severe cases of cardiac arrhythmia, or when a patient has suffered a heart attack or is at high risk of having one, an electronic device called an **implantable cardioverter defibrillator (ICD)** is surgically placed inside the chest cavity. The ICD has wires with electrodes that are attached to the heart. The high-energy electrical impulses delivered by the ICD will shock the heart if a life-threatening arrhythmia occurs or the heart stops beating.

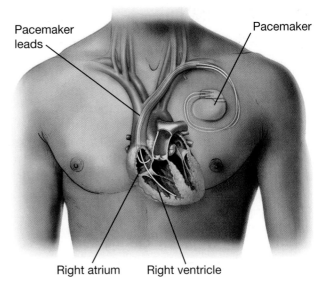

© Body Scientific International

Figure 10.13 A pacemaker, which helps maintain normal heart rhythm, typically has two leads: one that enters the right atrium (right upper chamber of the heart) and one that enters the right ventricle (lower right chamber of the heart). The pacemaker works by making contractions in these chambers occur "in sync" (together at the same rate).

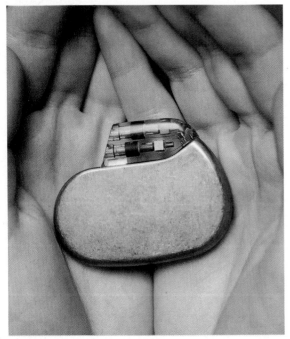

iStock.com/Fodor90

Figure 10.14 A pacemaker, shown here, is a device that helps correct arrhythmia.

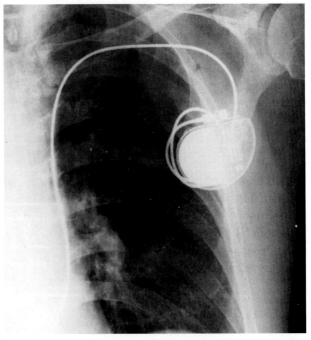

khuruzero/Shutterstock.com

Figure 10.15 An X-ray image of a pacemaker in a patient's chest cavity.

Multiple Choice: Diseases and Disorders

Directions: Choose the disease or disorder that matches each definition. You can also complete this activity online using *EduHub*.

_____ 1. disease in which the arteries thicken, narrow, and lose their elasticity
a. aneurysm
b. arteriosclerosis
c. congestive heart failure
d. varicose veins

_____ 2. event in which the heart muscle is deprived of oxygen
a. atherosclerosis
b. aneurysm
c. myocardial infarction
d. congestive heart failure

_____ 3. disease in which the heart muscle cannot pump enough oxygenated blood
a. congestive heart failure
b. atherosclerosis
c. aneurysm
d. myocardial infarction

_____ 4. dilatation and thinning of an artery due to weakness in the arterial wall
a. atherosclerosis
b. aneurysm
c. myocardial infarction
d. congestive heart failure

_____ 5. veins that have lost their elasticity and appear swollen and tortuous
a. atherosclerotic veins
b. arteriosclerotic veins
c. stenotic veins
d. varicose veins

_____ 6. chronic disease in which the arteries that supply blood to the heart muscle become narrowed from fatty deposits
a. aneurysm
b. myocardial infarction
c. atherosclerosis
d. varicose veins

SCORECARD: How Did You Do?

Number correct (_____), divided by 6 (_____), multiplied by 100 equals _____ (your score)

Multiple Choice: Procedures and Treatments

Directions: Choose the procedure or treatment that matches each definition. You can also complete this activity online using *EduHub*.

_____ 1. diagnostic procedure used to record the electrical activity of the heart
a. electrocardiogram
b. Doppler sonography
c. cardiopulmonary resuscitation
d. cardiac catheterization

_____ 2. procedure in which high-frequency sound waves are used to measure blood flow and blood pressure
a. cardiopulmonary resuscitation
b. Doppler sonography
c. cardiac catheterization
d. electrocardiogram

_____ 3. device that delivers mild electrical impulses to the heart to correct arrhythmia
a. pacemaker
b. Doppler sonography
c. electrocardiogram
d. cardiac catheterization

_____ 4 procedure in which a narrow, flexible tube is inserted into a vein or artery leading to the heart
a. Doppler sonography
b. cardiac catheterization
c. pacemaker
d. electrocardiogram

(Continued on next page)

_____ 5. emergency-response procedure used to try to revive a patient who has suffered a heart attack
   a. cardiac catheterization
   b. Doppler sonography
   c. cardiopulmonary resuscitation
   d. electrocardiogram

_____ 6. device surgically placed within the chest cavity to shock the heart when a dangerous arrhythmia occurs or the heart stops beating
   a. cardiac catheter
   b. implantable cardioverter defibrillator
   c. pacemaker
   d. cardiopulmonary resuscitator

SCORECARD: How Did You Do?

Number correct (_____), divided by 6 (_____), multiplied by 100 equals _____ (your score)

Assessment 10.9

Identifying Abbreviations

Directions: Supply the correct abbreviation for each medical term. You can also complete this activity online using *EduHub*.

Medical Term	Abbreviation
1. myocardial infarction	_____
2. congestive heart failure	_____
3. implantable cardioverter defibrillator	_____
4. electrocardiogram	_____
5. cardiopulmonary resuscitation	_____
6. coronary artery disease	_____
7. automated external defibrillator	_____

SCORECARD: How Did You Do?

Number correct (_____), divided by 7 (_____), multiplied by 100 equals _____ (your score)

Analyzing the Intern Experience

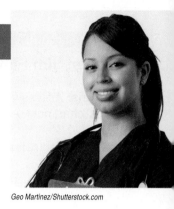

In the Intern Experience described at the beginning of this chapter, we met Layla, a medical intern with the Guardian Urgent Care Center. Layla shadowed (observed and assisted) the doctor as he examined and talked with Jim Flowers, a middle-aged man who came to the immediate-care center because of cardiac symptoms, including chest pain and profuse sweating.

After examining Mr. Flowers and obtaining his personal and family health history, the physician made a pending medical diagnosis of congestive heart failure and ordered a cardiac catheterization procedure. Later, the physician made a dictated recording of the patient's health information, which was subsequently transcribed into a chart note.

Geo Martinez/Shutterstock.com

We will now learn more about Jim Flowers' condition from a clinical perspective, interpreting the medical terms in his chart note as we analyze the scenario presented in the Intern Experience.

Audio Activity: Jim Flowers' Chart Note

Directions: Access your *EduHub* subscription and listen to the recording of the physician reading Jim Flowers' chart note. Read along with the physician and pay attention to the pronunciation of each medical term.

CHART NOTE

Patient Name: Flowers, Jim
ID Number: 95432
Examination Date: February 18, 20xx

SUBJECTIVE
Jim is a 55-year-old male who presents to the Guardian Urgent Care Clinic after an episode of intense chest pain and tingling and numbness of his left arm that occurred while driving his daughter to a concert. The pain was relieved by placing a nitroglycerin tablet under his tongue. Because of concerns from both his daughter and wife, he is here today for a follow-up.

OBJECTIVE
BP is 110/84, respirations 20, pulse is 90/min and regular. Temperature normal. His chest X-ray reveals a **pacemaker** on the left, **cardiomegaly**, and increased markings suggestive of **congestive heart failure**. The **ECG** reveals normal rate and rhythm.

ASSESSMENT
1. **Angina pectoris**.
2. Cardiomegaly.
3. Possible **CHF**.

PLAN
Admit patient to County Hospital for **cardiac catheterization**.

Interpret Jim Flowers' Chart Note

Directions: Access your *EduHub* subscription and listen to the recording of the physician reading Jim Flowers' chart note. After listening to the recording, supply the medical term that matches each definition.

Example: inflammation of a vein   *Answer:* phlebitis

1. disease in which the heart muscle cannot pump enough oxygenated and nutrient-rich blood throughout the body

   _____

2. procedure in which a narrow, flexible tube is inserted into a vein or artery leading to the heart

   _____

3. severe chest pain caused by myocardial ischemia (disruption of blood flow to the heart muscle caused by obstruction of a blood vessel)

   _____

4. diagnostic procedure used to record the electrical activity of the heart

   _____

5. enlargement of the heart

   _____

6. device that delivers mild electrical impulses to the heart to correct arrhythmia

   _____

7. abbreviation for *congestive heart failure*

   _____

SCORECARD: How Did You Do?

Number correct (_____), divided by 7 (_____), multiplied by 100 equals _____ (your score)

Working with Medical Records

In this activity, you will interpret the medical records (chart notes) of patients with cardiovascular system disorders. These examples illustrate typical medical records prepared in a real-world healthcare environment. To interpret these chart notes, you will apply your knowledge of word elements (prefixes, combining forms, and suffixes), diseases and disorders, and procedures and treatments related to the cardiovascular system.

Audio Activity: Carrie Geiger's Chart Note

Directions: Access your *EduHub* subscription and listen to the recording of the physician reading Carrie Geiger's chart note. Read along with the physician and pay attention to the pronunciation of each medical term.

CHART NOTE

Patient Name: Geiger, Carrie
ID Number: 67854
Examination Date: April 4, 20xx

SUBJECTIVE
Carrie is a 24-year-old female who presents with swelling, redness, and tenderness of the right **posterior** extremity, present for the past 72 hours and becoming more uncomfortable and swollen. She has some pain with walking. It is worse after being on her feet all day. She recalls no direct trauma to the area. She is on birth control pills. Nonsmoker.

OBJECTIVE
She has localized **erythema**, induration (areas of hardened tissue), tenderness, and **edema** along the right lower extremity. **Varicose veins** noted distally and proximally.

ASSESSMENT
Chronic **venous** insufficiency with superficial **thrombophlebitis**. No deep vein venous **thrombosis**.

PLAN
Ibuprofen 60 mg BID with food (take a 60-mg tablet of ibuprofen twice a day). Apply warm compresses to the affected area for 30–60 minutes TID (three times a day). Elevate leg as needed. Will recheck in 2–3 weeks or sooner if no improvement.

Assessment 10.11

Interpret Carrie Geiger's Chart Note

Directions: Access your *EduHub* subscription and listen to the recording of the physician reading Carrie Geiger's chart note. After listening to the recording, supply the medical term that matches each definition. You may encounter definitions and terms introduced in previous chapters.

Example: enlargement of the heart   *Answer:* cardiomegaly

1. pertaining to the veins   _____

2. abnormal condition of a clot   _____

3. veins that appear swollen and tortuous due to loss of elasticity   _____

4. inflammation of a clot in a vein   _____

5. redness of the skin   _____

6. swelling   _____

7. pertaining to the back (of the body)   _____

SCORECARD: How Did You Do?

Number correct (_____), divided by 7 (_____), multiplied by 100 equals _____ (your score)

Audio Activity: Richard Thomas's Chart Note

Directions: Access your *EduHub* subscription and listen to the recording of the physician reading Richard Thomas's chart note. Read along with the physician and pay attention to the pronunciation of each medical term.

CHART NOTE

Patient Name: Thomas, Richard
ID Number: 61842
Examination Date: July 19, 20xx

SUBJECTIVE
This 71-year-old male has a history of multiple episodes of **epistaxis** (nosebleeds). No history of nose trauma. **Hemorrhage** comes on spontaneously, usually at night or in the early morning. He may go a couple of months with one and then gets one every day for a few weeks. They start at rest and occasionally with exertion. He has been able to stop the bleeding by applying direct pressure to the nose. He has no other bleeding problems. He is currently taking antihypertensive (pertaining to preventing or controlling high blood pressure) medications.

OBJECTIVE
Blood pressure is 176/80; pulse 80. There is no active bleeding at this time. A small, dried blood clot is noted in the left nostril, which may be the bleeding site.

ASSESSMENT
1. **Hypertension**
2. Recurrent epistaxis

PLAN
Patient was given Procardia XL® sublingually (pertaining to under the tongue), with blood pressure dropping to 140/75. Vaseline® jelly was applied to the left nostril anteriorly. Patient was instructed in treatment of nosebleeds if they recur. Patient instructed to take Procardia XL once daily. Follow up for blood pressure check in 2 weeks.

Assessment 10.12

Interpret Richard Thomas's Chart Note

Directions: Access your *EduHub* subscription and listen to the recording of the physician reading Richard Thomas's chart note. After listening to the recording, supply the medical term that matches each definition.

Example: inflammation around the heart   *Answer:* pericarditis

1. bursting forth (excessive discharge) of blood   _____

2. process of above-normal pressure   _____

3. nosebleeds   _____

SCORECARD: How Did You Do?

Number correct (_____), divided by 3 (_____), multiplied by 100 equals _____ (your score)

Chapter Review

Word Elements Summary

Prefixes

Prefix	Meaning
a-	not; without
brady-	slow
dys-	painful; difficult
hyper-	above; above normal
hypo-	below; below normal
intra-	inside; within
peri-	around
tachy-	fast

Combining Forms

Root Word/Combining Vowel	Meaning
angi/o	vessel
arteri/o	artery
ather/o	fatty substance
card/o, cardi/o	heart
coron/o	heart
cyan/o	blue
electr/o	electrical activity
hem/o, hemat/o	blood
isch/o	to keep back
my/o	muscle
phleb/o	vein
pulmon/o	lung
sten/o	narrow; constricted
tens/o	pressure; tension
thromb/o	clot
vas/o	vessel; duct
ven/o, ven/i	vein

Suffixes

Suffix	Meaning
-ac	pertaining to
-al	pertaining to
-ary	pertaining to
-ation	process; condition; state of being or having
-emia	blood condition
-gram	record; image
-ia	condition
-ion	process
-itis	inflammation
-logist	specialist in the study and treatment of
-logy	study of
-megaly	large; enlargement
-oma	tumor; mass
-osis	abnormal condition
-ous	pertaining to
-pathy	disease
-penia	deficiency; abnormal reduction
-plasty	surgical repair
-pnea	breathing
-rrhage	bursting forth (of blood)
-rrhexis	rupture
-sclerosis	hardening
-stasis	stop; stand still
-tic	pertaining to
-tomy	incision; cut into
-trophy	development

More Practice: Activities and Games

The following activities will help you reinforce your skills and check your mastery of the medical terminology you learned in this chapter. Access your *EduHub* subscription to complete more activities and vocabulary games for mastering the word parts and terms you have learned.

Break It Down

Directions: Dissect each medical term into its word parts (prefix, root word, combining vowel, and suffix) using one or more slashes. Then define each term.

Example:

Medical Term: arteriosclerosis

Dissection: arteri/o/sclerosis

Definition: hardening of the arteries

Medical Term	Dissection
1. cardiorrhexis	c a r d i o r r h e x i s

Definition: _____

_____

| 2. hematoma | h e m a t o m a |

Definition: _____

_____

| 3. phlebography | p h l e b o g r a p h y |

Definition: _____

_____

| 4. ischemia | i s c h e m i a |

Definition: _____

_____

| 5. hemangioma | h e m a n g i o m a |

Definition: _____

_____

Medical Term	Dissection
6. phlebotomy	p h l e b o t o m y

Definition: _____

_____

7. arteriorrhexis   a r t e r i o r r h e x i s

Definition: _____

_____

8. thrombostasis   t h r o m b o s t a s i s

Definition: _____

_____

9. pericardial   p e r i c a r d i a l

Definition: _____

_____

10. stenocardia   s t e n o c a r d i a

Definition: _____

_____

11. thromboangiitis   t h r o m b o a n g i i t i s

Definition: _____

_____

12. angioma   a n g i o m a

Definition: _____

_____

Audio Activity: Samuel Gibson's Chart Note

Directions: Access your *EduHub* subscription and listen to the recording of the physician reading Samuel Gibson's chart note. Read along with the physician and pay attention to the pronunciation of each medical term.

CHART NOTE

Patient Name: Gibson, Samuel
ID Number: 25448
Date of Service: March 1, 20XX

SUBJECTIVE
Mr. Gibson is an obese 64-year-old male who is slightly **dyspneic** (pertaining to difficulty breathing) with a history of **hypertension** who yesterday experienced chest discomfort. The patient describes persistent pain across the upper chest with associated severe **dyspnea**. This occurred while walking his dog. Chest discomfort resolved after resting on a bench. The patient awoke today to chest pain and seeks advice.

OBJECTIVE
BP is 144/91 with a pulse of 80. Respiratory rate is 16/min. Heart is regular in rate and rhythm. **Cardiac** risk factors include hypertension, obesity, and a positive family history of **CAD**. **Electrocardiogram** is normal.

ASSESSMENT
1. Unstable **angina pectoris**
2. Hypertension

PLAN
Admit patient to County Hospital to exclude **myocardial infarction** and to initiate therapy with beta blockers (drugs used to reduce hypertension), aspirin, and heparin (blood thinner). The patient will also undergo **cardiac catheterization**.

Assessment

Interpret Samuel Gibson's Chart Note

Directions: Access your *EduHub* subscription and listen to the recording of the physician reading Samuel Gibson's chart note. After listening to the recording, supply the medical term that matches each definition. You may encounter definitions and terms introduced in previous chapters.

Example: disease of the heart muscle   *Answer:* cardiomyopathy

1. difficulty breathing   _____

2. above-normal blood pressure   _____

3. the reduction of blood flow to the heart; coronary artery disease   _____

(Continued)

4. record of the electrical activity of the heart   _____

5. procedure in which a narrow, flexible tube is inserted into a vein or artery leading to the heart   _____

6. severe chest pain   _____

7. pertaining to the heart   _____

8. event in which the heart muscle is deprived of oxygen   _____

9. pertaining to difficulty breathing   _____

10. blood pressure   _____

Spelling

Directions: For each medical term, indicate the correct spelling.

1.	cardiamegaly	chardiomegaly	cardiomegaly	cardioalmegaly
2.	hemostasis	hemastasis	haemastasis	hemmastasis
3.	periocarditis	peracarditis	pericharditis	pericarditis
4.	myacardial	myocardial	myocardeal	myochardial
5.	hypertrophy	hypertrophe	hyperotrophy	hypertroephy
6.	bradicardia	bradichardia	bradycardia	bradychardia
7.	cardiamyopathy	cardeomyopathy	cardialmyopathy	cardiomyopathy
8.	angioplasty	angialplasty	angeoplasty	anginoplasty
9.	phlobitis	phleabitis	phlebitis	phlebytis
10.	tachychardia	tachycardia	tachycardea	tachychardea
11.	thromboesis	thrombosis	thrombosys	thrombolsis
12.	venous	veinous	venious	veneous

Identify the Medical Word Part

Directions: For each medical word part, identify the type of word part (prefix, root word, or suffix) and provide its meaning.

1. **cardi**   Prefix   Root Word   Suffix

Meaning: _____

2. **ather**   Prefix   Root Word   Suffix

Meaning: _____

3. **emia**   Prefix   Root Word   Suffix

Meaning: _____

4. **tachy**   Prefix   Root Word   Suffix

Meaning: _____

5. **ation**   Prefix   Root Word   Suffix

Meaning: _____

6. **rrhage**   Prefix   Root Word   Suffix

Meaning: _____

7. **steno**   Prefix   Root Word   Suffix

Meaning: _____

8. **thromb**   Prefix   Root Word   Suffix

Meaning: _____

9. **tens**   Prefix   Root Word   Suffix

Meaning: _____

10. **pulmon**   Prefix   Root Word   Suffix

Meaning: _____

Cumulative Review

Chapters 8–10: Reproductive System, Respiratory System, and Cardiovascular System

Directions: Check your mastery of word elements used in medical terminology related to the male and female reproductive systems, respiratory system, and cardiovascular system by defining the following prefixes, combining forms, and suffixes.

Prefixes

a- _____

an- _____

brady- _____

dys- _____

endo- _____

hyper- _____

hypo- _____

intra- _____

peri- _____

tachy- _____

trans- _____

Combining Forms

angi/o _____

arteri/o _____

ather/o _____

bronch/o, bronchi/o _____

cardi/o _____

coron/o _____

cyan/o _____

cervic/o _____

colp/o   _____

cyst/o   _____

electr/o   _____

embol/o   _____

gynec/o   _____

hem/o, hemat/o _____

hyster/o   _____

isch/o   _____

lapar/o   _____

lob/o   _____

mamm/o   _____

mast/o   _____

men/o   _____

metr/o, metri/o _____

my/o   _____

oophor/o   _____

orchid/o   _____

ox/o   _____

pharyng/o   _____

phleb/o   _____

pleur/o   _____

pneum/o   _____

pneumon/o   _____

prostat/o   _____

pulmon/o   _____

rhin/o   _____

salping/o   _____

scrot/o   _____

spir/o _____

sten/o _____

tens/o _____

testicul/o _____

thorac/o _____

thromb/o _____

trache/o _____

ur/o _____

vagin/o _____

vas/o _____

ven/o, ven/i _____

Suffixes

-ac _____

-al _____

-algia _____

-ary _____

-ation _____

-centesis _____

-ectasis _____

-ectomy _____

-emia _____

-gram _____

-graphy _____

-ia _____

-ic _____

-ion _____

-itis _____

-logist _____

-logy _____

-megaly _____

-meter _____

-oma _____

-osis _____

-ous _____

-pathy _____

-penia _____

-pexy _____

-plasty _____

-pnea _____

-rrhage _____

-rrhagia _____

-rrhaphy _____

-rrhea _____

-rrhexis _____

-sclerosis _____

-scope _____

-scopy _____

-stasis _____

-thorax _____

-tic _____

-tomy _____

-trophy _____

Chapter 11

The Endocrine System

endo / crin / o / logy = the study of secretions within

Chapter Organization

- Intern Experience
- Overview of Endocrine System Anatomy and Physiology
- Word Elements
- Breaking Down and Building Endocrine System Terms
- Diseases and Disorders
- Tests and Procedures
- Analyzing the Intern Experience
- Working with Medical Records
- Chapter Review

Chapter Objectives

After completing this chapter, you will be able to

1. label an anatomical diagram of the endocrine system;
2. dissect and define common medical terminology related to the endocrine system;
3. build terms used to describe endocrine system diseases and disorders and diagnostic procedures;
4. pronounce and spell common medical terminology related to the endocrine system;
5. understand that the process of building and dissecting a medical term based on its prefix, root word, and suffix enables you to analyze an extremely large number of medical terms beyond those presented in this chapter;
6. interpret the meaning of abbreviations associated with the endocrine system; and
7. interpret medical records containing terminology and abbreviations related to the endocrine system.

Your *EduHub* subscription that accompanies this text provides access to online assessments, assignments, activities, and resources. Throughout this chapter, access *EduHub* to

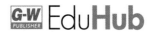

- use e-flash cards to review the medical terminology and word parts you learn;
- listen to the correct pronunciations of medical terms; and
- complete medical terminology activities and assignments.

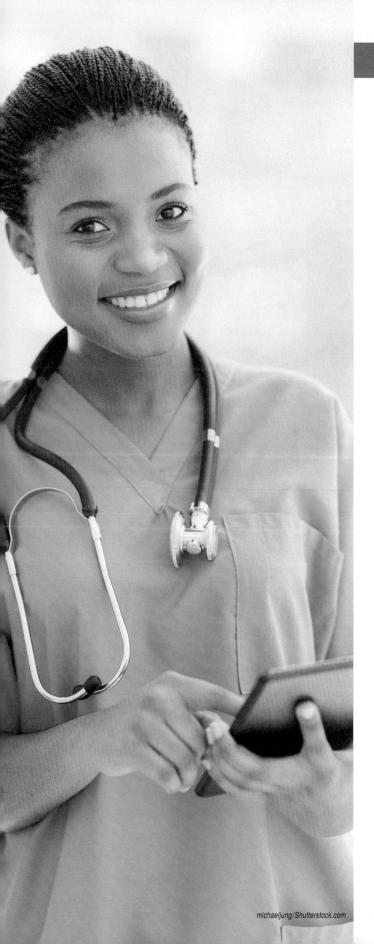

Intern Experience

Liza Stephens has just finished the "textbook learning" part of a medical assistant degree program, and she is eager to put her knowledge and skills to work. Liza has been assigned by the school to serve an internship with the Stringfield Medical Associates, an internal medicine practice. She is reporting to Jeff Blishmer, an LPN (licensed practical nurse) who assists Dr. Pitcher.

Today Liza meets Mrs. Kathryn Noah, a 78-year-old patient with poor ambulation (walking). Liza assists her into a wheelchair and pushes the chair into an exam room. Liza listens as Mrs. Noah tells the nurse that she has a fever and feelings of numbness and tingling in her left big toe. Jeff, the nurse, notes that the toe is bluish in color and accompanied by a foul-smelling discharge. After recording these details in Mrs. Noah's medical record, Jeff uses his laptop to electronically signal to the physician that the patient is ready to be seen.

As you will learn later in this chapter, Mrs. Noah is suffering from a condition that has affected her endocrine system. To help you understand her health problem, this chapter will present word elements (combining forms, prefixes, and suffixes) that make up medical terms related to the endocrine system. As you learn these terms, you will recognize many common word elements from your study of body systems covered in previous chapters—particularly prefixes and suffixes, which are universal word elements.

We will begin our study of the endocrine system with a brief overview of its anatomy and physiology. Later in the chapter, you will learn about some common endocrinological (ĔN-dō-krĭ-nō-LŎJ-ĭk-ăl) conditions and diagnostic tests.

Overview of Endocrine System Anatomy and Physiology

The **endocrine system** is composed of glands that are widely distributed throughout the body (Figure 11.1). The term *endocrine* means "to secrete within." Endocrine glands secrete chemicals called **hormones** directly within the bloodstream, which transports hormones to organs, glands, and tissues that need them to function properly. Endocrine glands play a vital role in maintaining *homeostasis*, a state of equilibrium within the body.

The endocrine system communicates with the nervous system to regulate bodily functions. While the nervous system responds rapidly to changes in both the internal environment (body) and the external environment (outside world), the endocrine system responds in a more measured fashion through hormonal secretions that effect longer-lasting physiological change.

Hormones are powerful chemical substances that travel through the bloodstream to targeted organs or glands. Excessive hormonal secretion (*hypersecretion*) or too little secretion (*hyposecretion*) disrupts the body's homeostatic state, causing the target gland or organ to malfunction. Endocrine disorders and diseases affect metabolism and other vital bodily functions, such as brain development, bone health, cardiovascular function, and digestion.

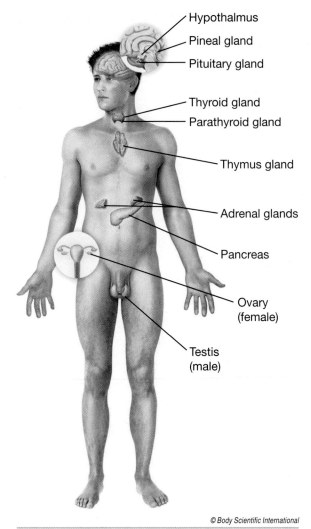

Hypothalmus
Pineal gland
Pituitary gland
Thyroid gland
Parathyroid gland
Thymus gland
Adrenal glands
Pancreas
Ovary (female)
Testis (male)

© Body Scientific International

Figure 11.1 The endocrine system is made up of glands that are distributed throughout the body.

Major Functions of the Endocrine System

The endocrine system regulates processes that occur slowly and effect long-lasting change within the body. These processes include

- growth and development of cells and tissues;
- metabolism (the process by which the body obtains energy from food);
- reproductive development and function; and
- mood.

Endocrinology (ĔN-dō-krĭ-NŎL-ō-jē) is the branch of medicine involving the study, diagnosis, and treatment of diseases and disorders of the endocrine glands. An **endocrinologist** (ĔN-dō-krĭ-NŎL-ō-jĭst) is a physician who specializes in treating diseases and disorders of the endocrine system.

Anatomy and Physiology Vocabulary

Now that you have been introduced to the basic structure and functions of the endocrine system, we will explore in more detail the key terms presented in the introduction.

Key Term	Definition
adrenal gland	triangle-shaped gland that sits atop each kidney; releases hormones that control metabolism, water and sodium levels, blood sugar levels, reproductive function, and response to stress
endocrine system	body system consisting of glands and hormones that maintain homeostasis (state of equilibrium)
endocrinologist	specialist in the study, diagnosis, and treatment of endocrine system diseases and disorders
endocrinology	the study of the endocrine system
homeostasis	a state of physiological equilibrium within the body
hormones	chemical substances that travel in the bloodstream to targeted glands or organs and are critical to homeostasis and normal body function
hypothalamus	the part of the anterior brain that regulates body temperature, hunger, thirst, sleep, and emotions
ovaries	female reproductive glands
pancreas	gland behind the stomach that regulates insulin and glucose production and secretes digestive enzymes
parathyroid glands	four glands situated behind the thyroid gland; help metabolize calcium and phosphorus
pineal gland	small, pinecone-shaped structure in the brain that secretes melatonin, a hormone that regulates sleep
pituitary gland	small, gray, rounded gland attached to the base of the brain; secretes hormones that regulate growth, reproduction, and various metabolic activities
testes	male reproductive glands
thymus gland	gland located above the heart; important in the development of immunity in newborns
thyroid gland	gland in the base of the neck, located in front of and on both sides of the upper part of the trachea (windpipe) and the lower part of the larynx (throat); plays a vital role in metabolism and other life-sustaining functions

E-Flash Card Activity: Anatomy and Physiology Vocabulary

Directions: After you have reviewed the anatomy and physiology vocabulary related to the endocrine system, access your *EduHub* subscription and practice with the e-flash cards until you are comfortable with the spelling and definition of each term.

Assessment 11.1

Identifying Major Glands of the Endocrine System

Directions: Label the anatomical diagram of the endocrine system. You can also complete this activity online using *EduHub*.

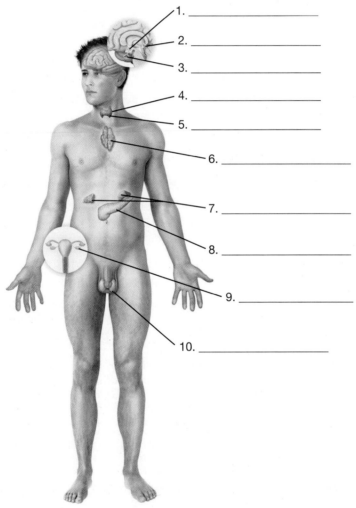

1. _____
2. _____
3. _____
4. _____
5. _____
6. _____
7. _____
8. _____
9. _____
10. _____

© Body Scientific International

SCORECARD: How Did You Do?

Number correct (_____), divided by 10 (_____), multiplied by 100 equals _____ (your score)

Matching Anatomy and Physiology Vocabulary

Directions: Choose the correct vocabulary term for each meaning. You can also complete this activity online using *EduHub*.

_____ 1. small, gray, rounded gland attached to the base of the brain; secretes hormones that regulate growth, reproduction, and various metabolic activities

_____ 2. male reproductive glands

_____ 3. gland in the base of the neck, located in front of and on both sides of the upper part of the trachea (windpipe) and the lower part of the larynx (throat); plays a vital role in metabolism and other life-sustaining functions

_____ 4. a state of physiological equilibrium within the body

_____ 5. triangle-shaped gland that sits atop each kidney; releases hormones that control metabolism, water and sodium levels, blood sugar levels, reproductive function, and response to stress

_____ 6. body system consisting of glands and hormones that maintain homeostasis in the body

_____ 7. small, pinecone-shaped structure in the brain that secretes melatonin, a hormone that regulates sleep

_____ 8. female reproductive glands

_____ 9. specialist in the study, diagnosis, and treatment of endocrine system diseases and disorders

_____ 10. gland located above the heart; important in the development of immunity in newborns

_____ 11. the part of the anterior brain that regulates body temperature, hunger, thirst, sleep, and emotions

_____ 12. the study of the endocrine system

_____ 13. large gland behind the stomach that regulates insulin and glucose production and secretes digestive enzymes

_____ 14. four glands situated behind the thyroid gland; involved in the metabolism of calcium and phosphorus

_____ 15. chemical substances that travel in the bloodstream to targeted glands or organs and are critical to homeostasis and normal body function

A. homeostasis
B. hypothalamus
C. adrenal gland
D. pineal gland
E. ovaries
F. endocrinologist
G. hormones
H. parathyroid glands
I. testes
J. thyroid gland
K. endocrinology
L. pancreas
M. pituitary gland
N. endocrine system
O. thymus gland

SCORECARD: How Did You Do?

Number correct (_____), divided by 15 (_____), multiplied by 100 equals _____ (your score)

Word Elements

In this section, you will learn word elements—prefixes, combining forms, and suffixes—that are common to the endocrine system. By learning these word elements and understanding how they are combined to build medical terms, you will be able to analyze Mrs. Noah's health condition (described in the Intern Experience at the beginning of this chapter) and identify a large number of terms associated with the endocrine system.

E-Flash Card Activity: Word Elements

Directions: Review the word elements in the tables that follow. Then, access your *EduHub* subscription and practice with the e-flash cards until you are able to quickly recognize the different word parts (prefixes, combining forms, and suffixes) and their meanings. The e-flash cards are grouped together by prefixes, combining forms, and suffixes, followed by a cumulative review of all the word elements you are learning in this chapter.

Prefixes

Let's begin our study of endocrine system word elements by looking at the prefixes listed in the table below. At this point in your studies, you have mastered all of these prefixes.

Prefix	Meaning
endo-	within
hyper-	above; above normal
hypo-	below; below normal
para-	beside; near
poly-	many; much

Combining Forms

The following combining forms appear in medical terms used to describe the endocrine system. Which of these have you already mastered?

Root Word/Combining Vowel	Meaning
acr/o	extremity
aden/o	gland
adren/o, adrenal/o	adrenal gland
carcin/o	cancer

(Continued)

Root Word/Combining Vowel	Meaning
crin/o	to secrete
dips/o	thirst
gluc/o	glucose; sugar
glyc/o	glucose; sugar
glycos/o	glucose; sugar
thym/o	thymus gland
thyr/o, thyroid/o	thyroid gland
ur/o	urine; urinary tract

Suffixes

Listed below are suffixes that appear in medical terms related to the endocrine system. From your study of body systems covered in previous chapters, you are already familiar with most of these suffixes.

Suffix	Meaning
-al	pertaining to
-e	noun suffix with no meaning
-ectomy	surgical removal; excision
-emia	blood condition
-ia	condition
-ic	pertaining to
-ism	condition; process
-itis	inflammation
-logist	specialist in the study and treatment of
-logy	study of
-megaly	large; enlargement
-oid	like; resembling
-oma	tumor; mass
-osis	abnormal condition
-pathy	disease
-phagia	eating; swallowing
-tomy	incision; cut into

Matching Prefixes, Combining Forms, and Suffixes

Directions: Choose the correct meaning for each word element. Some meanings may be used more than once. You can also complete this activity online using *EduHub*.

Prefixes

_____ 1. poly-

_____ 2. para-

_____ 3. hyper-

_____ 4. endo-

_____ 5. hypo-

A. above; above normal

B. within

C. below; below normal

D. many; much

E. beside; near

Combining Forms

_____ 1. glyc/o

_____ 2. acr/o

_____ 3. glycos/o

_____ 4. thym/o

_____ 5. aden/o

_____ 6. carcin/o

_____ 7. thyroid/o

_____ 8. crin/o

_____ 9. dips/o

_____ 10. ur/o

_____ 11. gluc/o

_____ 12. adren/o

_____ 13. thyr/o

A. extremity

B. gland

C. cancer

D. glucose; sugar

E. thirst

F. urine; urinary tract

G. adrenal gland

H. thymus gland

I. to secrete

J. thyroid gland

Suffixes

_____ 1. -megaly

_____ 2. -al

_____ 3. -oid

_____ 4. -ic

_____ 5. -phagia

_____ 6. -e

_____ 7. -logist

_____ 8. -emia

_____ 9. -logy

_____ 10. -ia

_____ 11. -itis

_____ 12. -ism

_____ 13. -ectomy

_____ 14. -pathy

_____ 15. -tomy

_____ 16. -osis

_____ 17. -oma

A. large; enlargement

B. specialist in the study and treatment of

C. study of

D. abnormal condition

E. like; resembling

F. disease

G. incision; cut into

H. condition; process

I. inflammation

J. surgical removal; excision

K. tumor; mass

L. pertaining to

M. eating; swallowing

N. noun suffix with no meaning

O. condition

P. blood condition

SCORECARD: How Did You Do?

Number correct (_____), divided by 35 (_____), multiplied by 100 equals _____ (your score)

Breaking Down and Building Endocrine System Terms

Now that you have mastered the prefixes, combining forms, and suffixes for medical terminology pertaining to the endocrine system, you have the ability to dissect and build a large number of terms related to this body system.

The chart that appears on the next two pages contains a list of medical terms commonly used in endocrinology, the medical specialty involving the study, diagnosis, and treatment of the endocrine system. For each term, a dissection has been provided, along with the meaning of each word element and the definition of the term as a whole.

Term	Dissection	Word Part/Meaning	Term Meaning
Note: *For simplification, combining vowels have been omitted from the Word Part/Meaning column.*			
1. **acromegaly** (ĂK-rō-MĔG-ă-lē)	acr/o/megaly	**acr** = extremity **megaly** = large; enlargement	large extremity; enlargement of an extremity
2. **adenocarcinoma** (ĂD-ĕ-nō-KĂR-sĭ-NŌ-mă)	aden/o/carcin/oma	**aden** = gland **carcin** = cancer **oma** = tumor; mass	cancerous tumor of a gland
3. **adenoid** (ĂD-ĕ-noyd)	aden/oid	**aden** = gland **oid** = like; resembling	resembling a gland
4. **adenoma** (ĂD-ĕ-NŌ-mă)	aden/oma	**aden** = gland **oma** = tumor; mass	tumor of a gland
5. **adenomegaly** (ĂD-ĕ-nō-MĔG-ă-lē)	aden/o/megaly	**aden** = gland **megaly** = large; enlargement	enlargement of a gland
6. **adrenal** (ă-DRĒ-năl)	adren/al	**adren** = adrenal gland **al** = pertaining to	pertaining to the adrenal gland
7. **adrenalectomy** (ă-DRĒ-năl-ĔK-tō-mē)	adrenal/ectomy	**adrenal** = adrenal gland **ectomy** = surgical removal; excision	excision of the adrenal gland
8. **adrenalopathy** (ă-DRĒ-nă-LŎP-ă-thē)	adrenal/o/pathy	**adrenal** = adrenal gland **pathy** = disease	disease of the adrenal gland
9. **endocrinologist** (ĔN-dō-krĭ-NŎL-ō-jĭst)	endo/crin/o/logist	**endo** = within **crin** = to secrete **logist** = specialist in the study and treatment of	specialist in the study and treatment of secretions within
10. **endocrinology** (ĔN-dō-krĭ-NŎL-ō-jē)	endo/crin/o/logy	**endo** = within **crin** = to secrete **logy** = study of	the study of secretions within
11. **endocrinopathy** (ĔN-dō-krĭ-NŎP-ă-thē)	endo/crin/o/pathy	**endo** = within **crin** = to secrete **pathy** = disease	disease of secretions within
12. **glycemia** (glī-SĒ-mē-ă)	glyc/emia	**glyc** = glucose; sugar **emia** = blood condition	blood condition of glucose (condition of glucose in the blood)
13. **hyperglycemia** (HĪ-pĕr-glī-SĒ-mē-ă)	hyper/glyc/emia	**hyper** = above; above normal **glyc** = glucose; sugar **emia** = blood condition	blood condition of above-normal glucose

Prefixes = Green   Root Words = **Red**   Suffixes = Blue

Term	Dissection	Word Part/Meaning	Term Meaning
14. **hyperthyroidism** (hī-per-THĪ-royd-ĭzm)	hyper/thyroid/ism	**hyper** = above; above normal **thyroid** = thyroid gland **ism** = condition; process	condition of above-normal thyroid gland
15. **hypoglycemia** (HĪ-pō-glī-SĒ-mē-ă)	hypo/glyc/emia	**hypo** = below; below normal **glyc** = glucose; sugar **emia** = blood condition	blood condition of below-normal glucose
16. **hypothyroidism** (HĪ-pō-THĪ-royd-ĭzm)	hypo/thyroid/ism	**hypo** = below; below normal **thyroid** = thyroid gland **ism** = condition; process	condition of below-normal thyroid gland
17. **polydipsia** (pŏl-ē-DĬP-sē-ă)	poly/dips/ia	**poly** = many; much **dips** = thirst **ia** = condition	condition of much (excessive) thirst
18. **polyphagia** (PŎL-ē-FĀ-jē-ă)	poly/phagia	**poly** = many; much **phagia** = eating; swallowing	much (excessive) eating
19. **polyuria** (pŏl-ē-YŪ-rē-ă)	poly/ur/ia	**poly** = many; much **ur** = urine; urinary tract **ia** = condition	condition of much (excessive) urine
20. **thymectomy** (thī-MĚK-tō-mē)	thym/ectomy	**thym** = thymus gland **ectomy** = surgical removal; excision	excision of the thymus gland
21. **thymic** (THĪ-mĭk)	thym/ic	**thym** = thymus gland **ic** = pertaining to	pertaining to the thymus gland
22. **thymoma** (thī-MŌ-mă)	thym/oma	**thym** = thymus gland **oma** = tumor; mass	tumor of the thymus gland
23. **thyroidectomy** (thī-roy-DĚK-tō-mē)	thyroid/ectomy	**thyroid** = thyroid gland **ectomy** = surgical removal; excision	excision of the thyroid gland
24. **thyroiditis** (THĪ-roy-DĪ-tĭs)	thyroid/itis	**thyroid** = thyroid gland **itis** = inflammation	inflammation of the thyroid gland
25. **thyromegaly** (THĪ-rō-MĚG-ă-lē)	thyr/o/megaly	**thyr** = thyroid gland **megaly** = large; enlargement	enlargement of the thyroid gland

Prefixes = Green   Root Words = **Red**   Suffixes = Blue

Using the pronunciation guide in the Breaking Down and Building chart, practice saying each medical term aloud. To hear the pronunciation of each term, complete the Pronounce It activity on the next page.

Audio Activity: Pronounce It

Directions: Access your *EduHub* subscription and listen to the correct pronunciations of the following medical terms. Practice pronouncing the terms until you are comfortable saying them aloud.

acromegaly
(ĂK-rō-MĔG-ă-lē)

adenocarcinoma
(ĂD-ĕ-nō-KĂR-sĭ-NŌ-mă)

adenoid
(ĂD-ĕ-noyd)

adenoma
(ĂD-ĕ-NŌ-mă)

adenomegaly
(ĂD-ĕ-nō-MĔG-ă-lē)

adrenal
(ă-DRĒ-năl)

adrenalectomy
(ă-DRĒ-năl-ĔK-tō-mē)

adrenalopathy
(ă-DRĒ-nă-LŎP-ă-thē)

endocrinologist
(ĔN-dō-krĭ-NŎL-ō-jĭst)

endocrinology
(ĔN-dō-krĭ-NŎL-ō-jē)

endocrinopathy
(ĔN-dō-krĭ-NŎP-ă-thē)

glycemia
(glī-SĒ-mē-ă)

hyperglycemia
(HĪ-pĕr-glī-SĒ-mē-ă)

hyperthyroidism
(hī-per-THĪ-royd-ĭzm)

hypoglycemia
(HĪ-pō-glī-SĒ-mē-ă)

hypothyroidism
(HĪ-pō-THĪ-royd-ĭzm)

polydipsia
(pŏl-ē-DĬP-sē-ă)

polyphagia
(PŎL-ē-FĀ-jē-ă)

polyuria
(pŏl-ē-YŪ-rē-ă)

thymectomy
(thī-MĔK-tō-mē)

thymic
(THĪ-mĭk)

thymoma
(thī-MŌ-mă)

thyroidectomy
(thī-roy-DĔK-tō-mē)

thyroiditis
(THĪ-roy-DĪ-tĭs)

thyromegaly
(THĪ-rō-MĔG-ă-lē)

Audio Activity: Spell It

Directions: Access your *EduHub* subscription and listen to the pronunciation for each number. As you hear each term, write its correct spelling.

1. _____

2. _____

3. _____

4. _____

5. _____

6. _____

7. _____

8. _____

9. _____

10. _____

11. _____

12. _____

13. _____

14. _____

15. _____

16. _____

17. _____

18. _____

19. _____

20. _____

21. _____

22. _____

23. _____

24. _____

25. _____

SCORECARD: How Did You Do?

Number correct (_____), divided by 25 (_____), multiplied by 100 equals _____ (your score)

Break It Down

Directions: Dissect each medical term into its word parts (prefix, root word, combining vowel, and suffix) using one or more slashes. Then define each term. You can also complete this activity online using *EduHub*.

Example:
Medical Term: adenomegaly
Dissection: aden/o/megaly
Definition: enlargement of a gland

Medical Term	Dissection
1. thyromegaly	t h y r o m e g a l y

Definition: _____

_____

| 2. glycemia | g l y c e m i a |

Definition: _____

_____

| 3. hyperglycemia | h y p e r g l y c e m i a |

Definition: _____

_____

| 4. thyroiditis | t h y r o i d i t i s |

Definition: _____

_____

| 5. adenoid | a d e n o i d |

Definition: _____

_____

Medical Term	Dissection
6. thyroidectomy	t h y r o i d e c t o m y

Definition: _____

_____

| 7. hyperthyroidism | h y p e r t h y r o i d i s m |

Definition: _____

_____

| 8. polyuria | p o l y u r i a |

Definition: _____

_____

| 9. adrenal | a d r e n a l |

Definition: _____

_____

| 10. endocrinologist | e n d o c r i n o l o g i s t |

Definition: _____

_____

| 11. acromegaly | a c r o m e g a l y |

Definition: _____

_____

| 12. polyphagia | p o l y p h a g i a |

Definition: _____

_____

SCORECARD: How Did You Do?

Number correct (_____), divided by 12 (_____), multiplied by 100 equals _____ (your score)

Build It

Directions: Build the medical term that matches each definition by supplying the correct word parts. You can also complete this activity online using *EduHub*.

P (Prefixes) = Green
RW (Root Words) = Red
S (Suffixes) = Blue
CV (Combining Vowel) = Purple

1. specialist in the study and treatment of secretions within

   _____ _____ _____ _____
   P   RW   CV   S

2. enlargement of the thyroid gland

   _____ _____ _____
        RW   CV   S

3. condition of much (excessive) urine

   _____ _____ _____
   P   RW   S

4. cancerous tumor of a gland

   _____ _____ _____ _____
        RW   CV   RW   S

5. blood condition of below-normal glucose

   _____ _____ _____
   P   RW   S

6. enlargement of a gland

   _____ _____ _____
        RW   CV   S

7. excision of the thyroid gland

   _____ _____
        RW   S

8. excision of the adrenal gland

   _____ _____
        RW   S

9. large extremity; enlargement of an extremity

_____ _____ _____
RW   CV   S

10. disease of the adrenal gland

_____ _____ _____
RW   CV   S

11. inflammation of the thyroid gland

_____ _____
RW   S

12. disease of secretions within

_____ _____ _____ _____
P   RW   CV   S

13. blood condition of glucose

_____ _____
RW   S

14. blood condition of above-normal glucose

_____ _____ _____
P   RW   S

15. resembling a gland

_____ _____
RW   S

16. condition of above-normal thyroid gland

_____ _____ _____
P   RW   S

17. condition of much (excessive) thirst

_____ _____ _____
P   RW   S

18. tumor of a gland

_____ _____
RW   S

Interpret the Pronunciation

Directions: For each pronunciation, supply the correct spelling of the medical term. You can also complete this activity online using *EduHub*.

1. ĂD-ĕ-noyd _____

2. glī-SĒ-mē-ă _____

3. HĪ-pō-THĪ-royd-ĭzm _____

4. ĔN-dō-krĭ-NŎL-ō-jĭst _____

5. pŏl-ē-DĬP-sē-ă _____

6. ĔN-dō-krĭ-NŎL-ō-jē _____

7. ă-DRĒ-nă-LŎP-ă-thē _____

8. THĪ-roy-DĪ-tĭs _____

9. ĂD-ĕ-nō-KĂR-sĭ-NŌ-mă _____

10. HĪ-pō-glī-SĒ-mē-ă _____

11. ĔN-dō-krĭ-NŎP-ă-thē _____

12. thī-MŌ-mă _____

13. ă-DRĒ-năl _____

14. PŎL-ē-FĀ-jē-ă _____

15. thī-MĔK-tō-mē _____

16. ĂD-ĕ-NŎP-ă-thē _____

17. THĪ-mĭk _____

18. hī-per-THĪ-royd-ĭzm _____

19. pŏl-ē-YŪ-rē-ă _____

20. THĪ-rō-MĔG-ă-lē _____

21. ă-DRĒ-năl-ĔK-tō-mē _____

Diseases and Disorders

Diseases and disorders of the endocrine system run the spectrum of the mild to the severe. Some diseases and disorders are congenital (present at birth); others are rooted in autoimmune dysfunction. In this section, we will briefly explore the major characteristics and causes of some common pathological conditions of the endocrine system.

Acromegaly

Acromegaly (ĂK-rō-MĔG-ă-lē) is a rare disorder that develops when the pituitary gland produces too much growth hormone (Figure 11.2). The result is increased bone growth and enlarged internal organs. A benign (noncancerous) tumor of the pituitary gland is the most common cause of acromegaly.

In adults, common signs of acromegaly include abnormally enlarged hands and feet; a broadened head; and a deepened, husky voice. In children, acromegaly is called *gigantism*. A common sign of acromegaly in children is excessive height caused by abnormally fast growth, unlike that which may occur during normal adolescent development.

Addison's Disease

When the adrenal glands produce an insufficient amount of the hormone cortisol, the result is **Addison's disease** (also called *Addison disease*). Cortisol affects almost every body system and is vital for a normal metabolism. Its most important job is to help the body respond to stress.

Symptoms of Addison's disease develop slowly and may include fatigue, low blood pressure, loss of appetite, weight loss, and hyperpigmentation (above-normal darkening of the skin) (Figure 11.3 on the next page). Patients with Addison's disease are treated with hormone replacement therapy.

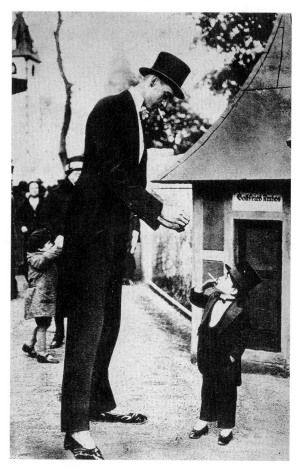

'Gigantism and ateleiosis, postcard. Tiny Town. 1927'. Credit: Wellcome Collection. CC BY

Figure 11.2 When the pituitary gland secretes an excessive amount of growth hormone, the result is acromegaly, a rare disorder.

Perhaps the most famous example of a person with Addison's disease was President John F. Kennedy, who also was diagnosed with hypothyroidism (discussed later in this section) after his 1960 election. Kennedy's well-known, year-round "tan" is probably attributable to Addison's hyperpigmentation.

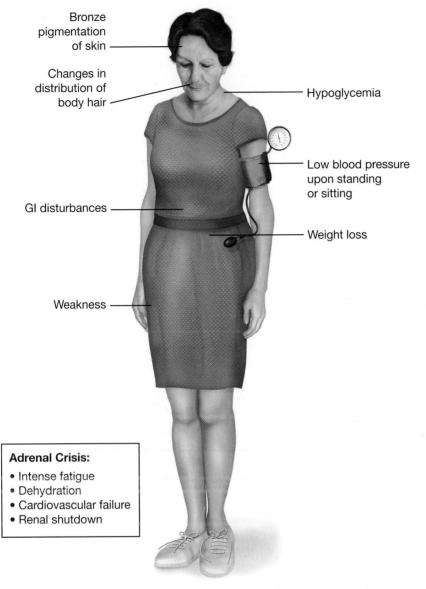

Bronze pigmentation of skin

Changes in distribution of body hair

Hypoglycemia

Low blood pressure upon standing or sitting

GI disturbances

Weight loss

Weakness

Adrenal Crisis:
- Intense fatigue
- Dehydration
- Cardiovascular failure
- Renal shutdown

© Body Scientific International

Figure 11.3 Common signs and symptoms of Addison's disease, the result of a deficiency in cortisol secretion by the adrenal glands

Cretinism

Cretinism (krĕ-tĭn-ĭzm), also known as *congenital hypothyroidism*, is a loss of thyroid function that is present from birth. The thyroid gland either is absent or fails to secrete thyroid hormones that are vital for brain development, physical growth, and metabolism. The result is a severe disruption in mental and physical growth in the infant.

Not all cases of cretinism are congenital in nature. This severe form of hypothyroidism may also be acquired later in life. Cretinism that develops during childhood or adulthood is called *myxedema* (MĬKS-ĕ-DĒ-mă).

Cushing's Syndrome

Cushing's syndrome (also called *Cushing syndrome*) is a disorder resulting from prolonged bodily exposure to high levels of the hormone cortisol. The hallmark signs of Cushing's syndrome include a fatty hump between the shoulders, obesity in the upper body, and a rounded face that is often described as a "moon face."

Weight gain in Cushing's syndrome stretches the already thin and weakened skin to hemorrhage, producing purple or red stretch marks called *striae* (STRĪ-ē), as shown in Figure 11.4. Cushing's syndrome may also develop from excessive use of steroids.

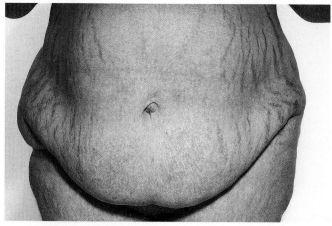

Mediscan/Alamy Stock Photos

Figure 11.4 In Cushing's syndrome, striae can form as a result of weight gain. As the skin stretches, hemorrhage leads to these purple or red marks.

Diabetes Mellitus

Diabetes mellitus (MĔL-ĭ-tŭs), or **DM**, is a disorder characterized by hyperglycemia due to a dysfunctional pancreas. The pancreas secretes both glucose and insulin. DM is a result of insulin deficiency or insulin ineffectiveness.

Physiological Overview

Insulin is the only hormone in the body that lowers blood sugar. Insulin helps transport glucose, the body's major source of energy, to the cells. Without glucose, the cells of the body cannot function or survive. Without insulin, they cannot absorb glucose. Insulin deficiency causes problems with metabolism of carbohydrates, proteins, and fats.

The physiological effects of insulin deficiency include polyuria (excessive urination), polydipsia (excessive thirst), and polyphagia (overeating) with unexplained weight loss (Figure 11.5 on the next page). Long-term complications of DM may include peripheral neuropathy (numbness and tingling in the feet and/or hands) and diabetic retinopathy (vision problems due to retinal disease). Uncontrolled diabetes may result in *gangrene*, death of tissues caused by a blood-supply decrease or absence. This metabolic disease is the leading cause of blindness, renal failure, and gangrene of the lower extremities.

Major Types of Diabetes Mellitus

There are two major types of diabetes mellitus. **Type 1 diabetes mellitus**, formerly known as *juvenile-onset diabetes* or *insulin-dependent diabetes mellitus (IDDM)*, typically develops before the age of 25 and is characterized by little to no insulin secretion. (The term *type 1 diabetes mellitus* is usually shortened to *type 1 diabetes*.)

Type 2 diabetes mellitus, formerly known as *adult-onset diabetes* or *non-insulin-dependent diabetes mellitus (NIDDM)*, occurs predominantly in adults.

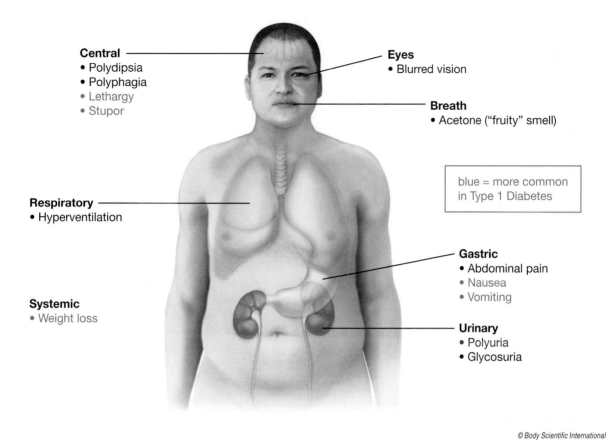

Central
- Polydipsia
- Polyphagia
- Lethargy
- Stupor

Eyes
- Blurred vision

Breath
- Acetone ("fruity" smell)

blue = more common
in Type 1 Diabetes

Respiratory
- Hyperventilation

Gastric
- Abdominal pain
- Nausea
- Vomiting

Systemic
- Weight loss

Urinary
- Polyuria
- Glycosuria

© Body Scientific International

Figure 11.5 Major signs and symptoms of diabetes mellitus

Insulin secretion is insufficient to meet bodily needs. Type 2 DM may be controlled by diet and oral medications. In some cases, however, insulin therapy may be required. The term *type 2 diabetes mellitus* is typically shortened to *type 2 diabetes*.

Diabetic patients who require insulin must monitor their blood glucose levels daily using a glucose meter (Figure 11.6). A small drop of blood is obtained by pricking the skin with a very small needle called a *lancet*. The blood drop is placed on a disposable test strip, which is read by the meter and used to calculate the patient's blood glucose level. Modern glucose meters are about the size of the palm of the hand and are battery-operated.

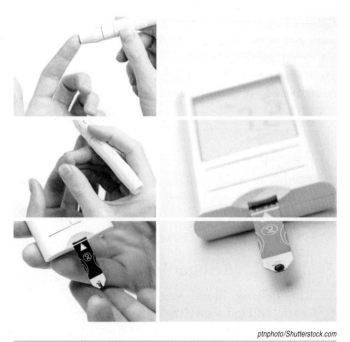

ptnphoto/Shutterstock.com

Figure 11.6 A patient performs a blood sugar test with a glucose meter.

Diabetes Insipidus

Diabetes insipidus (ĭn-SĬP-ĭ-dŭs), or **DI**, is not to be confused with diabetes mellitus. Diabetes insipidus is a rare disease in which the posterior pituitary gland produces an insufficient amount of antidiuretic hormone (ADH). DI is characterized by polyuria and polydipsia, which can lead to dehydration.

Graves' Disease

Graves' disease is an autoimmune disease in which the thyroid gland produces and releases excessive amounts of thyroid hormone into the blood, resulting in hyperthyroidism. Symptoms of Graves' disease include *exophthalmos* (ĔKS-ŏf-THĂL-mŏs), protruding or bulging of the eyes; a goiter (chronic enlargement of the thyroid gland); and edema in the lower extremities (Figure 11.7).

Hypothyroidism

Hypothyroidism, or *underactive thyroid*, is a disorder in which the thyroid gland does not produce a sufficient amount of thyroid hormone. Inadequate production of thyroid hormone decreases metabolism.

Symptoms of hypothyroidism, which develop gradually, may include weight gain, dry skin, bradycardia (slow heart rate), and lethargy (Figure 11.8 on the next page). Hormone replacement therapy, in the form of natural or synthetic thyroid hormone, is necessary.

Tests and Procedures

In this section, you will learn about tests and procedures used to help diagnose pathological conditions of the endocrine system.

Fasting Blood Sugar Test

The **fasting blood sugar (FBS) test** is a type of blood test that analyzes the amount of glucose in the blood after the patient has not eaten for at least eight

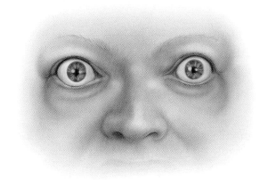

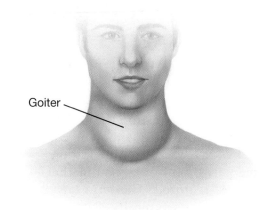

Goiter

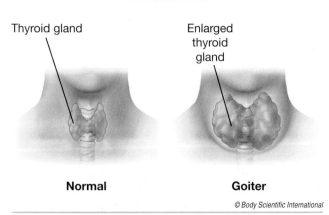

Thyroid gland

Enlarged thyroid gland

Normal

Goiter

© Body Scientific International

Figure 11.7 Bulging eyes and a goiter (enlarged thyroid gland) are typical of Graves' disease.

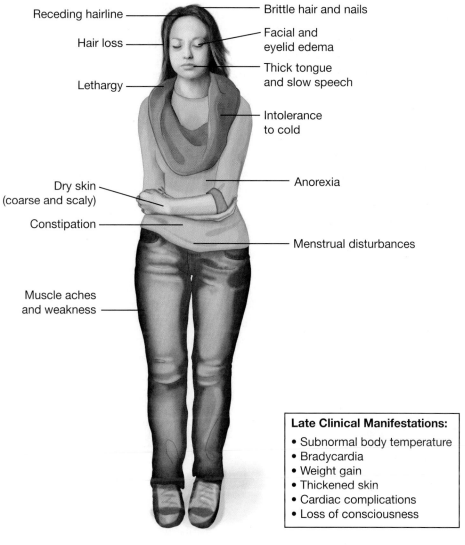

Receding hairline

Hair loss

Lethargy

Dry skin (coarse and scaly)

Constipation

Muscle aches and weakness

Brittle hair and nails

Facial and eyelid edema

Thick tongue and slow speech

Intolerance to cold

Anorexia

Menstrual disturbances

Late Clinical Manifestations:
- Subnormal body temperature
- Bradycardia
- Weight gain
- Thickened skin
- Cardiac complications
- Loss of consciousness

© Body Scientific International

Figure 11.8 Common signs and symptoms of hypothyroidism

hours (called *fasting*). A needle is inserted into a vein in the arm, and blood is withdrawn for analysis. The process of withdrawing blood from a vein for laboratory analysis is called *venipuncture*.

The fasting blood sugar test is a screening tool that aids in diagnosing diabetes. The FBS is also effective for the regular monitoring of diabetic patients' blood glucose levels.

Glucose Tolerance Test

The **glucose tolerance test (GTT)**, another type of fasting blood sugar test, determines how the body breaks down sugar. Like the fasting blood sugar test, the GTT requires a period of fasting, typically between eight and twelve hours.

Before the glucose tolerance test, a fasting blood sugar is drawn. Then the patient drinks a glucose (sugar) solution, and blood samples are drawn at timed intervals (Figure 11.9). An oral glucose tolerance test may take up to three hours to complete. This diagnostic test is often used to confirm a diagnosis of diabetes mellitus.

Thyroid Scan

A **thyroid scan** is a nuclear medicine imaging procedure that uses a radioactive iodine tracer to record the structure and function of the thyroid gland (Figure 11.10 on the next page). The scan shows the size and shape of the thyroid gland and is useful in detecting thyroid cysts or cancerous tumors.

Thyroid-Stimulating Hormone Test

The **thyroid-stimulating hormone test** is a laboratory test that measures the amount of thyroid-stimulating hormone (TSH) in the blood and the function of the thyroid gland. The TSH test is performed using venipuncture. It is given to patients with signs and symptoms of a thyroid disorder, such as hypothyroidism or hyperthyroidism.

Thyroid hormones control metabolism and regulate growth and development. TSH is manufactured by the pituitary gland, which "tells" the thyroid

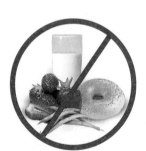

No food or drink 8 to 12 hours prior to test

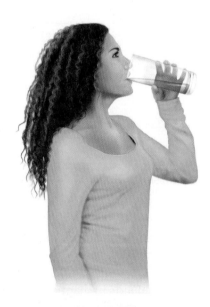

Drink glucose

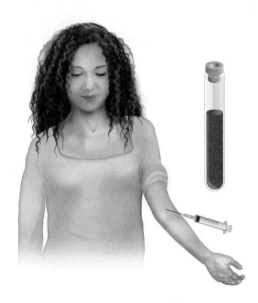

Blood tested at regular intervals

High glucose level = Potential diabetes

Figure 11.9 A glucose tolerance test is performed to confirm a diagnosis of diabetes. Before a glucose tolerance test, a fasting blood sugar is drawn. The patient drinks a sugar solution, and blood samples are taken at timed intervals.

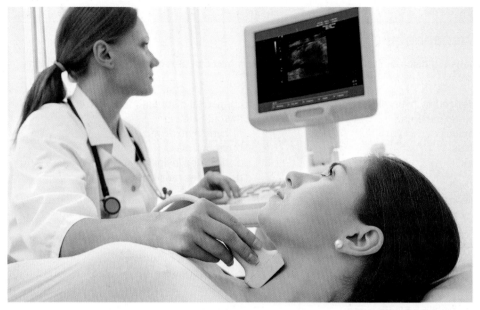

Figure 11.10 A technician performs a diagnostic thyroid scan on a patient.

gland to produce and release thyroid hormones (for example, thyroxine) into the blood (Figure 11.11). In other words, TSH controls production of the other thyroid hormones.

Thyroxine Test

Thyroxine (thī-RŎK-sēn or thī-RŎK-sĭn) is a hormone manufactured by the thyroid gland. It plays a vital role in brain development; bone health; metabolism; and cardiac, muscular, and digestive functions.

The **thyroxine test** analyzes thyroid function by measuring the amount of thyroxine in the blood. Like the thyroid-stimulating hormone (TSH) test, the thyroxine test is performed when a patient is suspected of having a disorder such as hyperthyroidism or hypothyroidism.

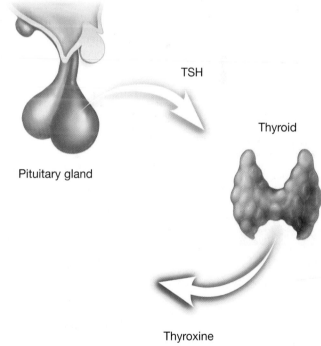

TSH

Thyroid

Pituitary gland

Thyroxine

Figure 11.11 Thyroid-stimulating hormone, or TSH, is made by the pituitary gland, which "tells" the thyroid gland to manufacture and secrete thyroid hormones into the bloodstream.

Multiple Choice: Diseases and Disorders

Directions: Choose the disease or disorder that matches each definition. You can also complete this activity online using *EduHub*.

_____ 1. disorder characterized by hyperglycemia from a dysfunctional pancreas
   a. diabetes insipidus
   b. diabetes mellitus
   c. hypothyroidism
   d. cretinism

_____ 2. rare hormonal disorder that develops when the pituitary gland produces excessive growth hormone
   a. Addison's disease
   b. acromegaly
   c. Cushing's syndrome
   d. Graves' disease

_____ 3. rare disorder in which the pituitary gland produces too little antidiuretic hormone, leading to polyuria and polydipsia
   a. hypothyroidism
   b. diabetes insipidus
   c. diabetes mellitus
   d. Addison's disease

_____ 4. disorder that arises when the adrenal glands produce an insufficient amount of cortisol
   a. Addison's disease
   b. acromegaly
   c. Graves' disease
   d. Cushing's syndrome

_____ 5. congenital disorder characterized by loss of thyroid function
   a. hypothyroidism
   b. cretinism
   c. diabetes insipidus
   d. diabetes mellitus

_____ 6. disorder characterized by a rounded face, upper-body obesity, and a fatty hump between the shoulders
   a. acromegaly
   b. Cushing's syndrome
   c. Addison's disease
   d. Graves' disease

_____ 7. disorder in which the thyroid gland fails to produce enough thyroid hormone
   a. cretinism
   b. Graves' disease
   c. hyperthyroidism
   d. diabetes mellitus

_____ 8. disease marked by excessive secretion of thyroid hormone into the blood
   a. Graves' disease
   b. hypothyroidism
   c. Cushing's syndrome
   d. Addison's disease

SCORECARD: How Did You Do?

Number correct (_____), divided by 8 (_____), multiplied by 100 equals _____ (your score)

Multiple Choice: Tests and Procedures

Directions: Choose the test or procedure that matches each definition. You can also complete this activity online using *EduHub*.

_____ 1. imaging procedure that uses a radioactive iodine tracer to detect cysts or cancerous tumors of the thyroid gland
   a. thyroid scan
   b. thyroxine test
   c. thyroid-stimulating hormone test
   d. glucose tolerance test

_____ 2. test that measures the amount of the thyroid hormone that plays an important role in brain development; bone health; metabolism; and heart, muscle, and digestive functions
   a. thyroxine test
   b. fasting blood sugar test
   c. thyroid scan
   d. glucose tolerance test

3. test that analyzes the amount of glucose in the blood
   a. glucose tolerance test
   b. fasting blood sugar test
   c. thyroxine test
   d. both a and b

4. laboratory test that measures the amount of a hormone produced and released into the bloodstream by the pituitary gland
   a. thyroid-stimulating hormone test
   b. thyroxine test
   c. thyroid scan
   d. glucose tolerance test

5. test that determines how the body breaks down sugar
   a. thyroxine test
   b. glucose tolerance test
   c. fasting blood sugar test
   d. thyroid-stimulating hormone test

SCORECARD: How Did You Do?

Number correct (_____), divided by 5 (_____), multiplied by 100 equals _____ (your score)

Assessment 11.10

Identifying Abbreviations

Directions: Supply the correct abbreviation for each medical term. You can also complete this activity online using *EduHub*.

Medical Term	Abbreviation
1. diabetes mellitus	_____
2. non-insulin-dependent diabetes mellitus	_____
3. diabetes insipidus	_____
4. insulin-dependent diabetes mellitus	_____
5. antidiuretic hormone	_____
6. fasting blood sugar	_____
7. glucose tolerance test	_____
8. thyroid-stimulating hormone	_____

SCORECARD: How Did You Do?

Number correct (_____), divided by 8 (_____), multiplied by 100 equals _____ (your score)

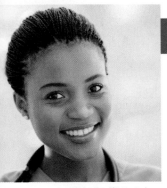

Analyzing the Intern Experience

In the Intern Experience described at the beginning of this chapter, we met Liza, who was assigned to an internship as a medical assistant with Stringfield Medical Associates. Liza listened and observed as the doctor talked with Mrs. Kathryn Noah, a 78-year-old patient with poor ambulation, fever, and sensations of numbness and tingling in her left big toe. The numbness and tingling were accompanied by a bluish discoloration and a foul-smelling discharge from the toe.

After examining Mrs. Noah, the physician made a diagnosis and a treatment plan. Later, he made a dictated recording of the patient's health information, which was subsequently transcribed into a chart note.

We will now learn more about Mrs. Noah's condition from a clinical perspective, interpreting the medical terms in her chart note as we analyze the scenario presented in the Intern Experience.

Audio Activity: Kathryn Noah's Chart Note

Directions: Access your *EduHub* subscription and listen to the recording of the physician reading Kathryn Noah's chart note. Read along with the physician and pay attention to the pronunciation of each medical term.

CHART NOTE

Patient Name: Noah, Kathryn
ID Number: 93654KN
Examination Date: February 12, 20xx

SUBJECTIVE
Kathryn is a 78-year-old patient who is here for a **diabetic** recheck. She rarely checks her blood sugars. She has not checked her sugar levels in the past 2 weeks and has lost 5–10 pounds since her last visit. Patient complains of numbness and tingling of the left great (big) toe with a foul-smelling discharge.

OBJECTIVE
She is inconsistent in taking her diabetic meds. **BP** is 140/98. Low-grade fever of 101. Eye exam is negative. Nose, mouth, neck, and **thyroid** exam are negative. Heart is without murmurs. Lungs are clear. Obese abdomen. Inflamed left great toe, bluish in color, with **purulent** discharge. The toe is cold to the touch with slight **sloughing** (falling off) of the skin.

ASSESSMENT
1. **Gangrene** of left great toe.
2. **Type 2 diabetes**, suboptimal control.
3. Obesity.

PLAN
Admit for amputation of left great toe due to gangrene.

Interpret Kathryn Noah's Chart Note

Directions: Access your *EduHub* subscription and listen to the recording of the physician reading Kathryn Noah's chart note. After listening to the recording, supply the medical term that matches each definition. You may encounter definitions and terms introduced in previous chapters.

Example: condition of below-normal thyroid gland   *Answer:* hypothyroidism

1. gland in the base of the neck; plays a vital role in metabolism and other life-sustaining functions

   _____

2. pertaining to pus

   _____

3. disorder characterized by hyperglycemia from a dysfunctional pancreas

   _____

4. falling off

   _____

5. death of tissue due to deficient blood supply

   _____

6. pertaining to diabetes

   _____

7. blood pressure

   _____

SCORECARD: How Did You Do?

Number correct (_____), divided by 7 (_____), multiplied by 100 equals _____ (your score)

Working with Medical Records

In this activity, you will interpret the medical records (chart notes) of patients with health conditions related to the endocrine system. These examples illustrate typical medical records prepared in a real-world healthcare environment. To interpret these chart notes, you will apply your knowledge of word elements (prefixes, combining forms, and suffixes), diseases and disorders, and tests and procedures related to the endocrine system.

Audio Activity: Dorothy Frederick's Chart Note

Directions: Access your *EduHub* subscription and listen to the recording of the physician reading Dorothy Frederick's chart note. Read along with the physician and pay attention to the pronunciation of each medical term.

CHART NOTE

Patient Name: Frederick, Dorothy
ID Number: 11472DR
Examination Date: November 23, 20xx

SUBJECTIVE
Dorothy is a 40-year-old music teacher here for follow-up of unusual irritability and fatigue over the past month. She also complains of anxiety and has noticed an intermittent rapid or irregular heartbeat. She said she always has a slight hand tremor, but it seems to be getting worse. She thinks the Paxil® (anti-anxiety medication) may be helping her sleep, but has not seen much of an improvement.

OBJECTIVE
Patient appears well. **HEENT** (head, eyes, ears, nose, and throat) are normal. A slightly enlarged **thyroid** is palpated. No **adenopathy**. There is a scar from a previous **lymphadenectomy**. Lungs are clear. **Tachycardia** noted. No **edema** of the lower extremities. Abdomen is soft and nontender. Lab report indicates a decreased **TSH** level. Other lab results were negative.

ASSESSMENT
Graves' disease

PLAN
Continue with Paxil for her anxiety and depression. She will be scheduled for a **thyroid scan** and **ECG**. I am referring her to an **endocrinologist** for further treatment.

Assessment 11.12

Interpret Dorothy Frederick's Chart Note

Directions: Access your *EduHub* subscription and listen to the recording of the physician reading Dorothy Frederick's chart note. After listening to the recording, supply the medical term that matches each definition.

Example: blood condition of above-normal glucose   *Answer:* hyperglycemia

1. excision of the lymph glands   _____

2. fast heartbeat   _____

3. thyroid-stimulating hormone   _____

4. autoimmune disease in which the thyroid gland secretes excessive amounts of thyroid hormone into the blood   _____

5. electrocardiogram   _____

6. disease of a gland   _____

7. head, eyes, ears, nose, and throat   _____

8. nuclear medicine imaging procedure that records the structure and function of the thyroid gland

_____

9. swelling

_____

10. specialist in the study and treatment of endocrine system diseases and disorders

_____

11. gland in the base of the neck; plays a vital role in metabolism and other life-sustaining functions

_____

SCORECARD: How Did You Do?

Number correct (_____), divided by 11 (_____), multiplied by 100 equals _____ (your score)

Audio Activity: Ralph Dixon's Chart Note

Directions: Access your *EduHub* subscription and listen to the recording of the physician reading Ralph Dixon's chart note. Read along with the physician and pay attention to the pronunciation of each medical term.

CHART NOTE

Patient Name: Dixon, Ralph
ID Number: 87457RD
Examination Date: August 4, 20xx

SUBJECTIVE
This is a **diabetic**, 20-year-old male patient who requests medical clearance to renew his driver's license.

OBJECTIVE
The patient states that he checks his glucose levels twice daily, which run in the 100–200 range. Further questioning reveals intermittent glucose levels in the 275–300 range. He states that he had **hyperglycemia**-like symptoms of **polydipsia** and **polyuria** twice last month. He had **hypoglycemic** symptoms consisting of weakness and inability to concentrate once in the last month. Vital signs are normal. Eye exam is negative. Examination of the feet shows some slight callous formation on the heels bilaterally (pertaining to both sides) with some cracked skin. No evidence of fungal infection or ulceration. Examination of feet normal and symmetric.

ASSESSMENT
Type 1 diabetes with suboptimal control.

PLAN
The importance of good **glycemic** control was discussed in detail with the patient. He is scheduled to see a diabetic nutritionist next week and was given information about local diabetic support groups. Return for a follow-up in one month or sooner if needed.

Interpret Ralph Dixon's Chart Note

Directions: Access your *EduHub* subscription and listen to the recording of the physician reading Ralph Dixon's chart note. After listening to the recording, supply the medical term that matches each definition.

Example: tumor of the thymus gland   *Answer:* thymoma

1. condition of much (excessive) thirst   _____

2. pertaining to glucose or sugar   _____

3. condition of above-normal glucose in the blood   _____

4. disorder characterized by hyperglycemia from a dysfunctional pancreas   _____

5. condition of much (excessive) urine   _____

6. pertaining to diabetes   _____

7. pertaining to below-normal glucose in the blood   _____

SCORECARD: How Did You Do?

Number correct (_____), divided by 7 (_____), multiplied by 100 equals _____ (your score)

Chapter Review

Word Elements Summary

Prefixes

Prefix	Meaning
endo-	within
hyper-	above; above normal
hypo-	below; below normal
para-	beside; near
poly-	many; much

Combining Forms

Root Word/Combining Vowel	Meaning
acr/o	extremity
aden/o	gland
adren/o, adrenal/o	adrenal gland
carcin/o	cancer
crin/o	to secrete
dips/o	thirst
gluc/o	glucose; sugar
glyc/o	glucose; sugar
glycos/o	glucose; sugar
thym/o	thymus gland
thyr/o, thyroid/o	thyroid gland
ur/o	urine; urinary tract

Suffixes

Suffix	Meaning
-al	pertaining to
-e	noun suffix with no meaning
-ectomy	surgical removal; excision
-emia	blood condition
-ia	condition
-ic	pertaining to

(Continued)

Suffix	Meaning
-ism	condition; process
-itis	inflammation
-logist	specialist in the study and treatment of
-logy	study of
-megaly	large; enlargement
-oid	like; resembling
-oma	tumor; mass
-osis	abnormal condition
-pathy	disease
-phagia	eating; swallowing
-tomy	incision; cut into

More Practice: Activities and Games

The following activities will help you reinforce your skills and check your mastery of the medical terminology you learned in this chapter. Access your *EduHub* subscription to complete more activities and vocabulary games for mastering the word parts and terms you have learned.

Break It Down

Directions: Dissect each medical term into its word parts (prefix, root word, combining vowel, and suffix) using one or more slashes. Then define each term.

Example:
Medical Term: polydipsia
Dissection: poly/dips/ia
Definition: condition of much (excessive) thirst

Medical Term

Dissection

1. parathyroidectomy   p a r a t h y r o i d e c t o m y

Definition: _____

_____

2. hypothymic   h y p o t h y m i c

Definition: _____

_____

Medical Term	Dissection
3. adenitis	a d e n i t i s

Definition: _____

_____

4. hypothyroidism	h y p o t h y r o i d i s m

Definition: _____

_____

5. adrenopathy	a d r e n o p a t h y

Definition: _____

_____

6. thyrotomy	t h y r o t o m y

Definition: _____

_____

7. hyperglycosuria	h y p e r g l y c o s u r i a

Definition: _____

_____

8. polyadenitis	p o l y a d e n i t i s

Definition: _____

_____

9. hyperadrenalism	h y p e r a d r e n a l i s m

Definition: _____

_____

10. endocrine	e n d o c r i n e

Definition: _____

_____

Medical Term	Dissection
11. hyperglycemia	h y p e r g l y c e m i a

Definition: _____

_____

| 12. thyromegaly | t h y r o m e g a l y |

Definition: _____

_____

Identifying Abbreviations

Directions: Supply the correct abbreviation for each medical term.

Medical Term	Abbreviation
1. fasting blood sugar	_____
2. thyroid-stimulating hormone	_____
3. diabetes mellitus	_____
4. glucose tolerance test	_____
5. diabetes insipidus	_____
6. antidiuretic hormone	_____
7. head, eyes, ears, nose, and throat	_____

Spelling

Directions: For each medical term that is misspelled, provide the correct spelling.

1. polidypsia   _____
2. thyramegaly   _____
3. endacrinologist   _____
4. adrenalapathy   _____
5. glycemea   _____
6. thiroyditis   _____
7. endochrinopathy   _____
8. polyphagea   _____
9. adinosis   _____
10. endalcrinology   _____
11. hypoglysemia   _____
12. polyurea   _____

Audio Activity: Pamela Rolf's Chart Note

Directions: Access your *EduHub* subscription and listen to the recording of the physician reading Pamela Rolf's chart note. Read along with the physician and pay attention to the pronunciation of each medical term.

CHART NOTE

Patient Name: Rolf, Pamela
ID Number: 54773EG
Examination Date: April 14, 20xx

SUBJECTIVE
Pamela has **edema** of the hands and legs. She complains of being constantly tired and cold. She still has problems with constipation and some weight gain. She has no hot flashes or depression. She has been on Synthroid® 110 mcg (micrograms) daily.

OBJECTIVE
BP is 124/76. Weight is 175 pounds, which is about 5 pounds heavier than a month ago. **HEENT** is normal. Chest, lungs, and heart rate are normal. **Thyroid** is clear to palpation. No goiter detected.

ASSESSMENT
Hypothyroidism

PLAN
Patient scheduled for **TSH test** next week. She will continue with Synthroid 110 mcg daily. She will return in 2 weeks to discuss her test results.

Assessment

Interpret Pamela Rolf's Chart Note

Directions: Access your *EduHub* subscription and listen to the recording of the physician reading Pamela Rolf's chart note. After listening to the recording, supply the medical term that matches each definition. You may encounter definitions and terms introduced in previous chapters.

> *Example:* inflammation of the thyroid gland   *Answer:* thyroiditis

1. disorder in which the thyroid gland does not produce a sufficient amount of thyroid hormone

   _____

2. lab test performed via venipuncture to measure the amount of thyroid-stimulating hormone in the blood

   _____

3. gland in the base of the neck; plays a vital role in metabolism and other life-sustaining functions

   _____

4. swelling

   _____

5. head, eyes, ears, nose, and throat

   _____

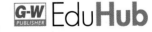

Chapter 12

The Urinary System

ur / o / logy: the study of urine and the urinary system

Chapter Organization

- Intern Experience
- Overview of Urinary System Anatomy and Physiology
- Word Elements
- Breaking Down and Building Urinary System Terms
- Diseases and Disorders
- Procedures and Treatments
- Analyzing the Intern Experience
- Working with Medical Records
- Chapter Review

Chapter Objectives

After completing this chapter, you will be able to

1. label an anatomical diagram of the urinary system;

2. dissect and define common medical terminology related to the urinary system;

3. build terms used to describe urinary system diseases and disorders and diagnostic procedures;

4. pronounce and spell common medical terminology related to the urinary system;

5. understand that the process of building and dissecting a medical term based on its prefix, root word, and suffix enables you to analyze an extremely large number of medical terms beyond those presented in this chapter;

6. interpret the meaning of abbreviations associated with the urinary system; and

7. interpret medical records containing terminology and abbreviations related to the urinary system.

Your *EduHub* subscription that accompanies this text provides access to online assessments, assignments, activities, and resources. Throughout this chapter, access *EduHub* to

- use e-flash cards to review the medical terminology and word parts you learn;
- listen to the correct pronunciations of medical terms; and
- complete medical terminology activities and assignments.

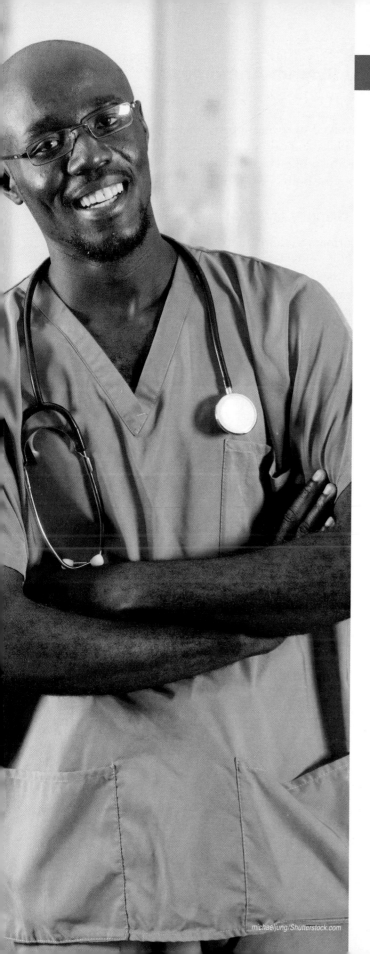

Intern Experience

Thomas O'Connor, an intern with Middletown Clinic, has been assigned this week to assist Dr. Nefron, a general practitioner. Their first patient is Shara, a college freshman with a complaint of bodily discomfort and fatigue. Thomas escorts Shara to exam room 4. "I've been feeling extremely tired," Shara says. Her roommate suggested that she visit the campus doctor; however, Shara did not go because she had to study for final exams. The symptoms did not go away, so after her exams, she came to the clinic.

Shara informs Thomas that, besides fatigue and a general feeling of unwellness, her urine has been red for three days. She has been urinating frequently, there is a burning sensation with urination, and she has lower back pain. She reveals that her family doctor has treated her for similar symptoms on several other occasions. Thomas notes these symptoms in Shara's chart and tells her that the doctor will want to do a urinalysis to help determine the cause of her symptoms.

As you will learn later in this chapter, Shara is suffering from a condition that has affected her urinary tract. To help you understand her health problem, this chapter will present word elements (combining forms, prefixes, and suffixes) that make up medical terms related to the urinary system. As you learn these terms, you will recognize many common word elements from your study of body systems covered in previous chapters—particularly prefixes and suffixes, which are universal word elements.

We will begin our study of the urinary system with a brief overview of its anatomy and physiology. Later in the chapter, you will learn about some common urinary conditions, diagnostic tests and procedures, and treatment methods.

Overview of Urinary System Anatomy and Physiology

The **urinary system** is involved in several processes necessary for maintaining *homeostasis*, a state of physiological equilibrium in the body. The urinary system removes waste products of metabolism from the blood in the form of urine, which is excreted from the body.

Main Functions of the Urinary System

The primary functions of the urinary system are to

1. remove nitrogenous (nī-TRŎJ-ĕ-nŭs) waste products such as urea, uric acid, ammonia, and creatinine (krē-ĂT-ĭ-nēn), which are chemical substances toxic to the human body;
2. help regulate the electrolyte content of the blood;
3. maintain normal pH levels—the acid/base balance of the blood; and
4. assist in the regulation of blood pressure and red blood cell production.

Major Organs and Structures of the Urinary System

The primary organs of the urinary system are

- the kidneys (2);
- the ureters (2);
- the urinary bladder (1); and
- the urethra (1).

The urinary system, or **urinary tract**, is composed of the kidneys, ureters (yū-RĒ-tĕrs), bladder, and urethra (yū-RĒ-thră) (Figure 12.1). The **kidneys** filter waste products from our blood, but also return substances that the body needs back into the circulatory (cardiovascular) system.

Nephrons (NĔF-rŏns) are the fundamental units within the kidneys that perform this filtration function. Each kidney contains nearly one million of these microscopic structures. After the nephrons have formed urine, the urine drains into the **renal pelvis**, a large, funnel-shaped cavity that narrows to form a pair of ureters.

The **ureters** are tube-like structures that carry urine from each kidney to the urinary bladder. Located at the floor of the pelvic cavity, the **urinary bladder** (more commonly called the **bladder**) is a hollow, muscular organ that temporarily stores urine. Just like the stomach, it has the ability to stretch. Its elastic walls expand to accommodate those four glasses of soda you can consume at a party, but shrivel when the bladder is empty.

The **urethra** is a muscular tube that drains urine from the bladder and transports it out of the body. It has both voluntary and involuntary, circular muscles called *sphincter muscles* that allow you to control your bladder function. At the end of the urethra is an opening called the **urinary meatus** (mē-Ā-tŭs) that expels urine to the outside of the body.

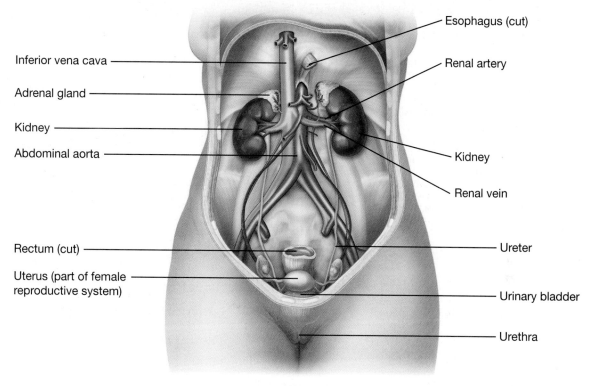

Inferior vena cava

Adrenal gland

Kidney

Abdominal aorta

Rectum (cut)

Uterus (part of female reproductive system)

Esophagus (cut)

Renal artery

Kidney

Renal vein

Ureter

Urinary bladder

Urethra

© Body Scientific International

Figure 12.1 Organs and structures of the urinary system

The act of excreting urine is called **urination**, **voiding**, or **micturition** (mĭk-tū-RĬ-shŭn). Sometimes a concentration of mineral salts forms a stone called a **calculus**, which blocks the passage of urine through the ureters. This condition is more commonly known as a "kidney stone." Kidney stones cause intense **flank** (lower back) pain accompanied by spasms, medically described as **renal colic**. Another common symptom of a kidney stone is urinary **frequency**—urinating often and usually in small amounts. (Urinary frequency may also be the result of other health conditions, such as a urinary tract infection.)

Urology (yū-RŎL-ō-jē) is the branch of medicine involving the study of urine and the urinary system and the diagnosis and treatment of **urological** (yū-rō-LŎJ-ĭ-kăl) conditions. A **urologist** (yū-RŎL-ō-jĭst) is a physician who specializes in the study, diagnosis, and treatment of urinary system diseases and disorders.

Anatomy and Physiology Vocabulary

Now that you have been introduced to the basic structure and functions of the urinary system, let's explore in more detail the key terms presented in the introduction.

Key Term	Definition
bladder	expandable pouch that stores urine; *urinary bladder*
calculus	stone
flank	lower back (area between the ribs and hips)
frequency	urinating often, usually in small amounts
kidney	organ of the urinary system that produces urine
micturition	act of expelling urine
nephron	microscopic, fundamental working unit of the kidney
renal colic	painful spasms in the lower back that are associated with calculus (kidney stone) formation
renal pelvis	funnel-shaped structure that collects urine and sends it to the ureter
ureter	tube that carries urine from the kidneys to the bladder
urethra	tube that transports urine to the outside of the body
urinary meatus	opening at the end of the urethra
urination	act of expelling urine
urine	water and waste products excreted by the kidneys
urologist	physician who specializes in the study, diagnosis, and treatment of urinary system diseases and disorders
urology	study of urine and the urinary system
voiding	act of expelling urine

E-Flash Card Activity: Anatomy and Physiology Vocabulary

Directions: After you have reviewed the anatomy and physiology vocabulary related to the urinary system, access your *EduHub* subscription and practice with the e-flash cards until you are comfortable with the spelling and definition of each term.

Identifying Major Organs and Structures of the Urinary System

Directions: Label the anatomical diagram of the urinary system. You can also complete this activity online using *EduHub*.

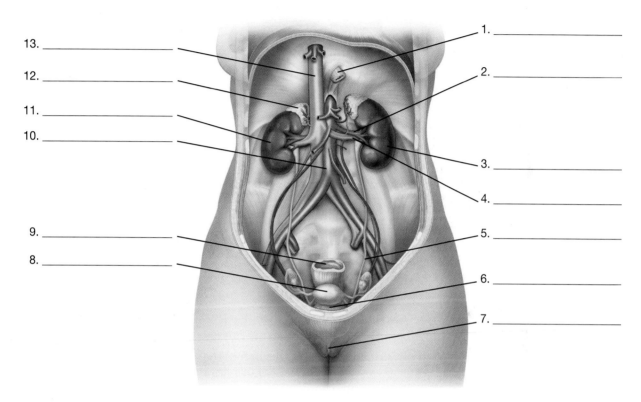

13. _____

12. _____

11. _____

10. _____

9. _____

8. _____

1. _____

2. _____

3. _____

4. _____

5. _____

6. _____

7. _____

© Body Scientific International

SCORECARD: How Did You Do?

Number correct (_____), divided by 13 (_____), multiplied by 100 equals _____ (your score)

Matching Anatomy and Physiology Vocabulary

Directions: Choose the correct vocabulary term for each meaning. You can also complete this activity online using *EduHub*.

_____ 1. urinating often

_____ 2. opening at the end of the urethra

_____ 3. microscopic, fundamental working unit of the kidney

_____ 4. funnel-shaped structure that collects urine and sends it to the ureter

_____ 5. tube that carries urine from the kidneys to the bladder

_____ 6. act of expelling urine

_____ 7. tube that transports urine to the outside of the body

_____ 8. expandable pouch that stores urine

_____ 9. water and waste products excreted by the kidneys

_____ 10. painful spasm

_____ 11. stone

_____ 12. organ of the urinary system that produces urine

_____ 13. lower back (area between the ribs and hips)

_____ 14. physician who specializes in the study, diagnosis, and treatment of urinary system diseases and disorders

_____ 15. study of urine and the urinary system

A. micturition
B. urine
C. urethra
D. kidney
E. bladder
F. nephron
G. ureter
H. renal pelvis
I. calculus
J. urinary meatus
K. renal colic
L. frequency
M. urology
N. flank
O. urologist

SCORECARD: How Did You Do?

Number correct (_____), divided by 15 (_____), multiplied by 100 equals _____ (your score)

Word Elements

In this section, you will learn word elements—prefixes, combining forms, and suffixes—that are common to the urinary system. By learning these word elements and understanding how they are combined to build medical terms, you will be able to analyze Shara's health condition (described in the Intern Experience at the beginning of this chapter) and identify a large number of terms associated with the urinary system.

E-Flash Card Activity: Word Elements

Directions: Review the word elements in the tables that follow. Then, access your *EduHub* subscription and practice with the e-flash cards until you are able to quickly recognize the different word parts (prefixes, combining forms, and suffixes) and their meanings. The e-flash cards are grouped together by prefixes, combining forms, and suffixes, followed by a cumulative review of all the word elements you are learning in this chapter.

Prefixes

Let's start our study of urinary system word elements by reviewing the prefixes listed in the table below.

Prefix	Meaning
a-	not; without
an-	not; without
dys-	painful; difficult
intra-	inside; within
peri-	around
poly-	many; much

Combining Forms

Listed below are combining forms that appear in medical terms used to describe the urinary system. Which of these are already familiar to you?

Root Word/Combining Vowel	Meaning
cyst/o	bladder; sac containing fluid
glyc/o	sugar; glucose
glycos/o	sugar; glucose
hem/o, hemat/o	blood
hydr/o	water
lith/o	stone
meat/o	opening
nephr/o	kidney
noct/o	night
olig/o	scanty; few
py/o	pus
pyel/o	renal pelvis
ren/o	kidney
son/o	sound
sten/o	narrow; constricted
ur/o	urine; urinary tract

(Continued)

Root Word/Combining Vowel	Meaning
ureter/o	ureter
urethr/o	urethra
urin/o	urine
vesic/o	bladder

Suffixes

Listed below are suffixes used in medical terms pertaining to the urinary system. You have also encountered these suffixes in your study of terms related to other body systems.

Suffix	Meaning
-al	pertaining to
-algia	pain
-cele	hernia; swelling; protrusion
-dipsia	thirst
-ectomy	surgical removal; excision
-emia	blood condition
-gram	record; image
-ia	condition
-iasis	abnormal condition
-itis	inflammation
-logist	specialist in the study and treatment of
-logy	study of
-lysis	destruction
-megaly	large; enlargement
-oma	tumor; mass
-osis	abnormal condition
-pexy	surgical fixation
-plasty	surgical repair
-ptosis	drooping; downward displacement
-rrhaphy	suture
-scope	instrument used to observe
-scopy	process of observing
-stomy	new opening
-tomy	incision; cut into
-tripsy	process of crushing

Matching Prefixes, Combining Forms, and Suffixes

Directions: Choose the correct meaning for each word element. Some meanings may be used more than once. You can also complete this activity online using *EduHub*.

Prefixes

_____ 1. a-
_____ 2. dys-
_____ 3. poly-
_____ 4. peri-
_____ 5. an-
_____ 6. intra-

A. inside; within
B. not; without
C. many; much
D. painful; difficult
E. around

Combining Forms

_____ 1. ureter/o
_____ 2. py/o
_____ 3. lith/o
_____ 4. hem/o
_____ 5. hydr/o
_____ 6. glyc/o
_____ 7. nephr/o
_____ 8. urin/o
_____ 9. sten/o
_____ 10. son/o
_____ 11. cyst/o
_____ 12. ren/o
_____ 13. glycos/o
_____ 14. urethr/o
_____ 15. ur/o
_____ 16. vesic/o
_____ 17. hemat/o
_____ 18. pyel/o
_____ 19. meat/o
_____ 20. olig/o
_____ 21. noct/o

A. narrow; constricted
B. water
C. night
D. pus
E. blood
F. scanty; few
G. sugar; glucose
H. sound
I. opening
J. renal pelvis
K. ureter
L. bladder
M. stone
N. urine; urinary tract
O. kidney
P. urethra

Suffixes

_____ 1. -ia	A. process of observing
_____ 2. -iasis	B. destruction
_____ 3. -pexy	C. pain
_____ 4. -ptosis	D. pertaining to
_____ 5. -osis	E. large; enlargement
_____ 6. -rrhaphy	F. instrument used to observe
_____ 7. -dipsia	G. tumor; mass
_____ 8. -tripsy	H. incision; cut into
_____ 9. -emia	I. new opening
_____ 10. -plasty	J. study of
_____ 11. -stomy	K. blood condition
_____ 12. -cele	L. specialist in the study and treatment of
_____ 13. -lysis	M. condition
_____ 14. -al	N. surgical repair
_____ 15. -algia	O. process of crushing
_____ 16. -itis	P. thirst
_____ 17. -logy	Q. drooping; downward placement
_____ 18. -megaly	R. suture
_____ 19. -tomy	S. surgical fixation
_____ 20. -oma	T. inflammation
_____ 21. -logist	U. record; image
_____ 22. -scope	V. surgical removal; excision
_____ 23. -gram	W. hernia; swelling; protrusion
_____ 24. -ectomy	X. abnormal condition
_____ 25. -scopy	

SCORECARD: How Did You Do?

Number correct (_____), divided by 52 (_____), multiplied by 100 equals _____ (your score)

Breaking Down and Building Urinary System Terms

Now that you have mastered the prefixes, combining forms, and suffixes for medical terminology pertaining to the urinary system, you have the ability to dissect and build a large number of terms related to this body system.

Below is a list of medical terms commonly used in *urology*, the medical specialty concerned with the study, diagnosis, and treatment of the urinary system. For each term, a dissection has been provided, along with the meaning of each word element and the definition of the term as a whole.

Term	Dissection	Word Part/Meaning	Term Meaning
Note: *For simplification, combining vowels have been omitted from the Word Part/Meaning column.*			
1. **anuria** (ăn-YŪ-rē-ă)	an/ur/ia	**an** = not; without **ur** = urine; urinary tract **ia** = condition	condition of without urine
2. **cystectomy** (sĭs-TĔK-tō-mē)	cyst/ectomy	**cyst** = bladder; sac containing fluid **ectomy** = surgical removal; excision	excision of the bladder
3. **cystitis** (sĭs-TĪ-tĭs)	cyst/itis	**cyst** = bladder; sac containing fluid **itis** = inflammation	inflammation of the bladder
4. **cystocele** (SĬS-tō-sēl)	cyst/o/cele	**cyst** = bladder; sac containing fluid **cele** = hernia; swelling; protrusion	hernia/swelling of the bladder
5. **cystolithiasis** (SĬS-tō-lĭ-THĪ-ă-sĭs)	cyst/o/lith/iasis	**cyst** = bladder; sac containing fluid **lith** = stone **iasis** = abnormal condition	abnormal condition of a stone in the bladder
6. **cystolithotomy** (SĬS-tō-lĭ-THŎT-ō-mē)	cyst/o/lith/o/tomy	**cyst** = bladder; sac containing fluid **lith** = stone **tomy** = incision; cut into	incision to the bladder for a stone
7. **cystoplasty** (SĬS-tō-PLĂS-tē)	cyst/o/plasty	**cyst** = bladder; sac containing fluid **plasty** = surgical repair	surgical repair of the bladder
Prefixes = Green Root Words = **Red** Suffixes = **Blue**			

Term	Dissection	Word Part/Meaning	Term Meaning
8. **cystoscope** (SĬS-tō-skōp)	cyst/o/scope	**cyst** = bladder; sac containing fluid **scope** = instrument used to observe	instrument used to observe the bladder
9. **cystoscopy** (sĭs-TŎS-kō-pē)	cyst/o/scopy	**cyst** = bladder; sac containing fluid **scopy** = process of observing	process of observing the bladder
10. **cystotomy** (sĭs-TŎT-ō-mē)	cyst/o/tomy	**cyst** = bladder; sac containing fluid **tomy** = incision; cut into	incision to the bladder
11. **dysuria** (dĭs-YŪ-rē-ă)	dys/ur/ia	**dys** = painful; difficult **ur** = urine; urinary tract **ia** = condition	condition of painful/difficult urination
12. **glycosuria** (GLĪ-kōs-YŪ-rē-ă)	glycos/ur/ia	**glycos** = glucose; sugar **ur** = urine; urinary tract **ia** = condition	condition of sugar in the urine
13. **hematuria** (HĒ-mă-TŪ-rē-ă)	hemat/ur/ia	**hemat** = blood **ur** = urine; urinary tract **ia** = condition	condition of blood in the urine
14. **hydronephrosis** (HĪ-drō-nĕ-FRŌ-sĭs)	hydr/o/nephr/osis	**hydr** = water **nephr** = kidney **osis** = abnormal condition	abnormal condition of water in the kidney
15. **lithotripsy** (LĬTH-ō-TRĬP-sē)	lith/o/tripsy	**lith** = stone **tripsy** = process of crushing	process of crushing a stone
16. **nephrectomy** (nĕ-FRĔK-tō-mē)	nephr/ectomy	**nephr** = kidney **ectomy** = surgical removal; excision	excision of the kidney
17. **nephritis** (nĕ-FRĪ-tĭs)	nephr/itis	**nephr** = kidney **itis** = inflammation	inflammation of the kidney
18. **nephrolithiasis** (NĔF-rō-lĭ-THĪ-ă-sĭs)	nephr/o/lith/iasis	**nephr** = kidney **lith** = stone **iasis** = abnormal condition	abnormal condition of a stone in the kidney
19. **nephroma** (nĕ-FRŌ-mă)	nephr/oma	**nephr** = kidney **oma** = tumor; mass	tumor of the kidney
20. **nephropexy** (NĔF-rō-PĔKS-ē)	nephr/o/pexy	**nephr** = kidney **pexy** = surgical fixation	surgical fixation of the kidney
21. **nephroplasty** (NĔF-rō-PLĂS-tē)	nephr/o/plasty	**nephr** = kidney **plasty** = surgical repair	surgical repair of the kidney

Prefixes = **Green**   Root Words = **Red**   Suffixes = **Blue**

Term	Dissection	Word Part/Meaning	Term Meaning
22. **nephroptosis** (NĔF-rŏp-TŌ-sĭs)	nephr/o/ptosis	**nephr** = kidney **ptosis** = drooping; downward displacement	drooping or downward displacement of the kidney
23. **nephrorrhaphy** (nĕf-ROR-ă-fē)	nephr/o/rrhaphy	**nephr** = kidney **rrhaphy** = suture	suture of the kidney
24. **nephrostomy** (nĕ-FRŎS-tō-mē)	nephr/o/stomy	**nephr** = kidney **stomy** = new opening	new opening in the kidney
25. **nephrotomy** (nĕ-FRŎT-ō-mē)	nephr/o/tomy	**nephr** = kidney **tomy** = incision; cut into	incision to the kidney
26. **nocturia** (nŏkt-YŪ-rē-ă)	noct/ur/ia	**noct** = night **ur** = urine; urinary tract **ia** = condition	condition of (producing) urine at night
27. **oliguria** (ŎL-ĭg-YŪ-rē-ă)	olig/ur/ia	**olig** = scanty; few **ur** = urine; urinary tract **ia** = condition	condition of scanty urine
28. **periurethral** (PĔR-ē-yū-RĒ-thrăl)	peri/urethr/al	**peri** = around **urethr** = urethra **al** = pertaining to	pertaining to around the urethra
29. **polydipsia** (PŎL-ē-DĬP-sē-ă)	poly/dipsia	**poly** = many; much **dipsia** = thirst	much thirst
30. **pyelogram** (PĪ-ĕ-lō-GRĂM)	pyel/o/gram	**pyel** = renal pelvis **gram** = record; image	record/image of the renal pelvis
31. **pyelonephritis** (PĪ-ĕ-lō-nĕ-FRĪ-tĭs)	pyel/o/nephr/itis	**pyel** = renal pelvis **nephr** = kidney **itis** = inflammation	inflammation of the kidney and renal pelvis
32. **pyelonephrosis** (PĪ-ĕ-lō-nĕ-FRŌ-sĭs)	pyel/o/nephr/osis	**pyel** = renal pelvis **nephr** = kidney **osis** = abnormal condition	abnormal condition of the kidney and renal pelvis
33. **pyonephritis** (PĪ-ō-nĕf-RĪ-tĭs)	py/o/nephr/itis	**py** = pus **nephr** = kidney **itis** = inflammation	inflammation and pus in the kidney
34. **pyuria** (pī-YŪ-rē-ă)	py/ur/ia	**py** = pus **ur** = urine; urinary tract **ia** = condition	condition of pus in the urine
35. **uremia** (yū-RĒ-mē-ă)	ur/emia	**ur** = urine; urinary tract **emia** = blood condition	blood condition of urine (waste products of urine in the blood)

Prefixes = Green   Root Words = Red   Suffixes = Blue

Term	Dissection	Word Part/Meaning	Term Meaning
36. **ureterolithiasis** (yū-RĒ-tĕr-ō-lĭth-Ī-ă-sĭs)	ureter/o/lith/iasis	**ureter** = ureter **lith** = stone **iasis** = abnormal condition	abnormal condition of a stone in the ureter
37. **ureteropyelonephritis** (yū-RĒ-tĕr-ō-PĪ-ĕl-ō-nĕf-RĪ-tĭs)	ureter/o/pyel/o/ nephr/itis	**ureter** = ureter **pyel** = renal pelvis **nephr** = kidney **itis** = inflammation	inflammation of the ureter, renal pelvis, and kidney
38. **ureterostenosis** (yū-RĒ-tĕr-ō-stĕn-Ō-sĭs)	ureter/o/sten/osis	**ureter** = ureter **sten** = narrow; constricted **osis** = abnormal condition	abnormal condition of a narrow or constricted ureter
39. **ureterovesicostomy** (yū-RĒ-tĕr-ō-vĕs-ĭ-KŎS-tō-mē)	ureter/o/vesic/o/ stomy	**ureter** = ureter **vesic** = bladder **stomy** = new opening	new opening in the ureter and bladder
40. **urethral** (yū-RĒ-thrăl)	urethr/al	**urethr** = urethra **al** = pertaining to	pertaining to the urethra
41. **urethralgia** (yū-rē-THRĂL-jē-ă)	urethr/algia	**urethr** = urethra **algia** = pain	pain in the urethra
42. **urethrocystitis** (yū-RĒ-thrō-sĭs-TĪ-tĭs)	urethr/o/cyst/itis	**urethr** = urethra **cyst** = bladder; sac containing fluid **itis** = inflammation	inflammation of the urethra and bladder
43. **urethroscope** (yū-RĒ-thrō-skōp)	urethr/o/scope	**urethr** = urethra **scope** = instrument used to observe	instrument used to observe the urethra
44. **urogram** (YŪ-rō-grăm)	ur/o/gram	**ur** = urine; urinary tract **gram** = record; image	record/image of the urinary tract
45. **urologist** (yū-RŎL-ō-jĭst)	ur/o/logist	**ur** = urine; urinary tract **logist** = specialist in the study and treatment of	specialist in the study and treatment of the urinary tract
46. **urology** (yū-RŎL-ō-jē)	ur/o/logy	**ur** = urine; urinary tract **logy** = study of	study of the urine and urinary tract

Prefixes = Green   Root Words = **Red**   Suffixes = Blue

Using the pronunciation guide in the Breaking Down and Building chart, practice saying each medical term aloud. To hear the pronunciation of each term, complete the Pronounce It activity on the next page.

Audio Activity: Pronounce It

Directions: Access your *EduHub* subscription and listen to the correct pronunciations of the following medical terms. Practice pronouncing the terms until you are comfortable saying them aloud.

anuria
(ăn-YŪ-rē-ă)

cystectomy
(sĭs-TĔK-tō-mē)

cystitis
(sĭs-TĪ-tĭs)

cystocele
(SĬS-tō-sēl)

cystolithiasis
(SĬS-tō-lĭ-THĪ-ă-sĭs)

cystolithotomy
(SĬS-tō-lĭ-THŎT-ō-mē)

cystoplasty
(SĬS-tō-PLĂS-tē)

cystoscope
(SĬS-tō-skōp)

cystoscopy
(sĭs-TŎS-kō-pē)

cystotomy
(sĭs-TŎT-ō-mē)

dysuria
(dĭs-YŪ-rē-ă)

glycosuria
(GLĪ-kōs-YŪ-rē-ă)

hematuria
(HĒ-mă-TŪ-rē-ă)

hydronephrosis
(HĪ-drō-nĕ-FRŌ-sĭs)

lithotripsy
(LĬTH-ō-TRĬP-sē)

nephrectomy
(nĕ-FRĔK-tō-mē)

nephritis
(nĕ-FRĪ-tĭs)

nephrolithiasis
(NĔF-rō-lĭ-THĪ-ă-sĭs)

nephroma
(nĕ-FRŌ-mă)

nephropexy
(NĔF-rō-PĔKS-ē)

nephroplasty
(NĔF-rō-PLĂS-tē)

nephroptosis
(NĔF-rŏp-TŌ-sĭs)

nephrorrhaphy
(nĕf-ROR-ă-fē)

nephrostomy
(nĕ-FRŎS-tō-mē)

nephrotomy
(nĕ-FRŎT-ō-mē)

nocturia
(nŏkt-YŪ-rē-ă)

oliguria
(ŎL-ĭg-YŪ-rē-ă)

periurethral
(PĔR-ē-yū-RĒ-thrăl)

polydipsia
(PŎL-ē-DĬP-sē-ă)

pyelogram
(PĪ-ĕ-lō-GRĂM)

pyelonephritis
(PĪ-ĕ-lō-nĕ-FRĪ-tĭs)

pyelonephrosis
(PĪ-ĕ-lō-nĕ-FRŌ-sĭs)

pyonephritis
(PĪ-ō-nĕf-RĪ-tĭs)

pyuria
(pī-YŪ-rē-ă)

uremia
(yū-RĒ-mē-ă)

ureterolithiasis
(yū-RĒ-tĕr-ō-lĭth-Ī-ă-sĭs)

ureteropyelonephritis
(yū-RĒ-tĕr-ō-PĪ-ĕl-ō-nĕf-RĪ-tĭs)

ureterostenosis
(yū-RĒ-tĕr-ō-stĕn-Ō-sĭs)

ureterovesicostomy
(yū-RĒ-tĕr-ō-vĕs-ĭ-KŌS-tō-mē)

urethral
(yū-RĒ-thrăl)

urethralgia
(yū-rē-THRĂL-jē-ă)

urethrocystitis
(yū-RĒ-thrō-sĭs-TĪ-tĭs)

urethroscope
(yū-RĒ-thrō-skōp)

urogram
(YŪ-rō-grăm)

urologist
(yū-RŎL-ō-jĭst)

urology
(yū-RŎL-ō-jē)

Assessment 12.4

Audio Activity: Spell It

Directions: Access your *EduHub* subscription and listen to the pronunciation for each number. As you hear each term, write its correct spelling.

1. _____
2. _____
3. _____
4. _____
5. _____
6. _____
7. _____
8. _____

9. _____
10. _____
11. _____
12. _____
13. _____
14. _____
15. _____
16. _____

17. _____	32. _____
18. _____	33. _____
19. _____	34. _____
20. _____	35. _____
21. _____	36. _____
22. _____	37. _____
23. _____	38. _____
24. _____	39. _____
25. _____	40. _____
26. _____	41. _____
27. _____	42. _____
28. _____	43. _____
29. _____	44. _____
30. _____	45. _____
31. _____	46. _____

SCORECARD: How Did You Do?

Number correct (_____), divided by 46 (_____), multiplied by 100 equals _____ (your score)

Assessment 12.5

Break It Down

Directions: Dissect each medical term into its word parts (prefix, root word, combining vowel, and suffix) using one or more slashes. Then define each term. You can also complete this activity online using *EduHub*.

Example:

Medical Term: nephropyelogram

Dissection: nephr/o/pyel/o/gram

Definition: record/image of the kidney and renal pelvis

Medical Term	Dissection
1. urogram	u r o g r a m

Definition: _____

_____

| 2. polydipsia | p o l y d i p s i a |

Definition: _____

_____

Medical Term	Dissection
3. nephrotomy	n e p h r o t o m y

Definition: _____

_____

4. nephroplasty	n e p h r o p l a s t y

Definition: _____

_____

5. cystoplasty	c y s t o p l a s t y

Definition: _____

_____

6. pyelonephritis	p y e l o n e p h r i t i s

Definition: _____

_____

7. nephrolithiasis	n e p h r o l i t h i a s i s

Definition: _____

_____

8. cystitis	c y s t i t i s

Definition: _____

_____

9. urethrocystitis	u r e t h r o c y s t i t i s

Definition: _____

_____

10. anuria	a n u r i a

Definition: _____

_____

Medical Term	Dissection
11. hydronephrosis	h y d r o n e p h r o s i s

Definition: _____

_____

| 12. cystoscopy | c y s t o s c o p y |

Definition: _____

_____

| 13. nephropexy | n e p h r o p e x y |

Definition: _____

_____

| 14. urology | u r o l o g y |

Definition: _____

_____

| 15. cystotomy | c y s t o t o m y |

Definition: _____

_____

| 16. cystectomy | c y s t e c t o m y |

Definition: _____

_____

| 17. nocturia | n o c t u r i a |

Definition: _____

_____

| 18. cystolithotomy | c y s t o l i t h o t o m y |

Definition: _____

_____

Medical Term	Dissection
19. glycosuria	g l y c o s u r i a

Definition: _____

_____

20. nephritis   n e p h r i t i s

Definition: _____

_____

21. cystoscope   c y s t o s c o p e

Definition: _____

_____

22. nephrorrhaphy   n e p h r o r r h a p h y

Definition: _____

_____

23. pyelonephrosis   p y e l o n e p h r o s i s

Definition: _____

_____

24. nephroma   n e p h r o m a

Definition: _____

_____

25. urethralgia   u r e t h r a l g i a

Definition: _____

_____

SCORECARD: How Did You Do?

Number correct (_____), divided by 25 (_____), multiplied by 100 equals _____ (your score)

Build It

Directions: Build the medical term that matches each definition by supplying the correct word parts. You can also complete this activity online using *EduHub*.

P (Prefixes) = Green
RW (Root Words) = Red
S (Suffixes) = Blue
CV (Combining Vowel) = Purple

1. abnormal condition of a narrow or constricted ureter

   _____ _____ _____ _____
   RW   CV   RW   S

2. condition of without urine

   _____ _____ _____
   P   RW   S

3. new opening in the ureter and bladder

   _____ _____ _____ _____ _____
   RW   CV   RW   CV   S

4. process of crushing a stone

   _____ _____ _____
   RW   CV   S

5. abnormal condition of a stone in the kidney

   _____ _____ _____ _____
   RW   CV   RW   S

6. incision to the bladder for a stone

   _____ _____ _____ _____ _____
   RW   CV   RW   CV   S

7. new opening in the kidney

   _____ _____ _____
   RW   CV   S

8. abnormal condition of a stone in the ureter

   _____ _____ _____ _____
   RW   CV   RW   S

9. incision to the kidney

_____ _____ ____
       RW   CV   S

10. blood condition of urine (waste products of urine in the blood)

_____   _____
       RW   S

11. hernia/swelling of the bladder

_____ _____ ____
       RW   CV   S

12. incision to the bladder

_____ _____ ____
       RW   CV   S

13. inflammation and pus in the kidney

_____ _____ _____ _____
       RW   CV   RW   S

14. abnormal condition of a stone in the bladder

_____ _____ _____ _____
       RW   CV   RW   S

15. inflammation of the urethra and bladder

_____ _____ _____ _____
       RW   CV   RW   S

16. excision of the kidney

_____   _____
       RW   S

17. inflammation of the ureter, renal pelvis, and kidney

_____ _____ _____ _____ _____ _____
       RW   CV   RW   CV   RW   S

SCORECARD: How Did You Do?

Number correct (_____), divided by 17 (_____), multiplied by 100 equals _____ (your score)

Diseases and Disorders

Diseases and disorders of the urinary system run the spectrum of the mild to the severe. In this section, we will briefly explore the major characteristics and causes of some common pathological conditions of this body system.

Urinary Tract Infection

When bacteria invade the urinary tract, they can cause a **urinary tract infection (UTI)**. Bacteria typically enter the bladder via the urethra. Cystitis and urethritis are two common types of lower urinary tract infections. Inflammation of the urethra is called **urethritis** (yū-rē-THRĪ-tĭs). Inflammation of the bladder is called **cystitis** (sĭs-TĪ-tĭs). Bladder inflammation caused by a bacterial infection is known as *bacterial cystitis*.

Symptoms of a UTI include fever, lower back pain, urinary frequency, and a sensation of burning during urination. The urine may appear dark yellow or even pink if blood is present. A urinalysis is often performed to determine the presence of bacteria and white blood cells in the urine.

If a bladder infection (cystitis) is left untreated, the infection can spread upward through the ureters and into the pelvis of the kidney, causing **pyelitis** (PĪ-ĕ-LĪ-tĭs). Thus, an infection of the kidneys that also involves the renal pelvis is called *pyelonephritis* (PĪ-ĕ-lō-nĕ-FRĪ-tĭs).

Cystitis

Cystitis (sĭs-TĪ-tĭs) is an inflammation of the urinary bladder, usually due to an ascending urinary tract infection. An ascending UTI is one in which bacteria travel from the bladder up through the ureter and into the kidney. Most cases of cystitis are caused by *Escherichia coli* (ĕsh-ĕr-ĪK-ē-ă KŌ-lī), a bacillus (type of bacteria) found in the lower gastrointestinal tract (stomach and intestines).

Cystitis is a common problem, especially in females. Because the urethra in the female is shorter than that in the male, bacteria do not have to travel very far to enter the bladder of a female. Urinary frequency, painful urination, chills, and fever are common symptoms of cystitis. A burning sensation during urination, which may or may not be accompanied by pyuria (pī-YŪ-rē-ă) (pus in the urine), may also be experienced.

Urinary Incontinence

Urinary incontinence is a disorder involving loss of bladder control. It can result in **enuresis** (ĕn-yū-RĒ-sĭs), commonly known as *bedwetting*.

Urinary incontinence (often shortened to the term *incontinence*) may be a symptom of an underlying medical condition or the result of everyday habits. Certain medications, foods, and beverages (such as caffeinated coffee, tea, and soda) can cause excessive urination and temporary urinary incontinence. Urinary tract infections often produce a strong urge to urinate, which can result in incontinence. Aging, pregnancy, and certain cancers can irritate the bladder, leading to urinary incontinence.

Urinary Retention

Urinary retention is the abnormal, involuntary holding of urine in the bladder, which leads to incomplete emptying of the bladder. Neurological dysfunction or an obstruction in the urinary tract can contribute to urinary retention. When a problem interferes with the nerve impulses reaching the bladder, a person is not aware that his or her bladder is full. Weak bladder muscles can also result in urinary retention. Other factors that can cause urinary retention include surgery, certain medications, and enlargement of the prostate gland.

Hydronephrosis

Hydronephrosis (HĪ-drō-nĕ-FRŌ-sĭs) is a condition that causes *distension* (inflation) and *dilation* (expansion) of the renal pelvis, resulting in enlargement of the kidney (Figure 12.2). It is usually caused by an obstructing stone or stricture (narrowing) in the ureter. It often leads to progressive atrophy (wasting away) of the kidney.

Kidney Stones

Kidney stones, also known as *renal calculi*, are small "pebbles" of salt and minerals that form inside the kidney. They can affect any part of the urinary tract from the kidneys to the bladder. Kidney stones are classified by their location in the kidney (*nephrolithiasis*), ureter (*ureterolithiasis*), or bladder (*cystolithiasis*).

Stones that obstruct the ureter or renal pelvis produce excruciating, intermittent pain that radiates from the flank to the groin. As described in the Overview of Urinary System Anatomy and Physiology earlier in this chapter, this phenomenon is clinically characterized as *renal colic*. Renal colic is commonly accompanied by urinary urgency, hematuria (blood in the urine), painful urination, fever, nausea, and vomiting.

A diagnosis of nephrolithiasis is made based on information obtained from a physical examination, personal and family health history, urinalysis, and radiographic studies. In addition, blood tests and ultrasound studies may aid in the diagnosis. Kidney stones occur more often in men than in women.

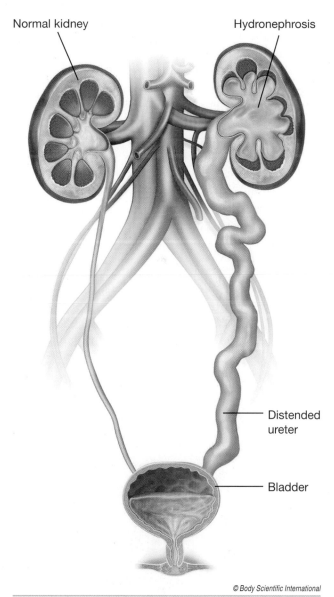

Normal kidney

Hydronephrosis

Distended ureter

Bladder

© Body Scientific International

Figure 12.2 Hydronephrosis, typically caused by an obstruction or a stricture in the ureter, causes the kidney to become enlarged.

Pyelonephritis

Pyelonephritis (PĪ-ě-lō-ně-FRĪ-tĭs) is an inflammation of the renal pelvis and kidney (Figure 12.3). It is often caused by a bacterial infection. Pyelonephritis can be described as an *ascending urinary tract infection* because the bacteria in the bladder ascend (travel up) the ureters to the kidneys.

Uremia

Uremia (yū-RĒ-mē-ă) is a condition associated with renal (kidney) failure. In uremia, the kidneys do not remove *urea* (yū-RĒ-ă), a waste product, from the blood. Thus, the blood is not completely cleansed of toxins and other substances that should have been excreted in the urine.

Uremia is a life-threatening condition that produces symptoms of low urine production (oliguria), tachycardia (rapid heart rate), edema (swelling), polydipsia (excessive thirst), dry mouth, fatigue, weakness, pallor (pale skin), confusion, and possible loss of consciousness.

Normal   **Chronic pyelonephritis**

© Body Scientific International

Figure 12.3 Pyelonephritis, an inflammation of the renal pelvis and the kidney, is frequently caused by a bacterial infection.

Cystocele

Cystocele (SĬS-tō-sēl) occurs when the urinary bladder *herniates* (protrudes) through the wall of the vagina (Figure 12.4). Doctors may refer to a cystocele as a *prolapsed bladder* because the vaginal wall has collapsed, causing the bladder to bulge downward into the vagina.

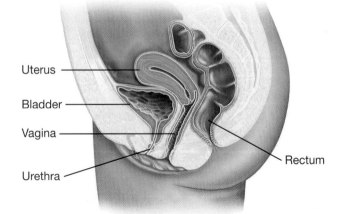

Normal female pelvic anatomy

Uterus
Bladder
Vagina
Urethra
Rectum

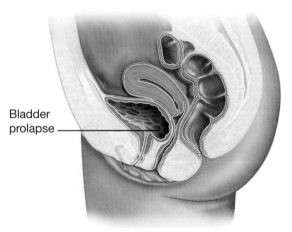

Cystocele

Bladder prolapse

© Body Scientific International

Figure 12.4 When the bladder protrudes through the vaginal wall, the result is a cystocele, or prolapsed bladder.

A cystocele is also known as a **vesicocele** (VĔS-ĭ-kō-SĒL). Patients with this condition may experience difficulty emptying their bladder, urinary incontinence, and repeated bladder infections.

Procedures and Treatments

In this section, we will briefly describe some diagnostic tests and procedures used to help identify disorders and diseases of the urinary system, as well as some common therapeutic procedures used to treat certain conditions.

Urinalysis

Urinalysis (YŪR-ĭ-NĂL-ĭ-sĭs), or **UA**, is a laboratory analysis of the urine, often performed in a doctor's office using a dipstick and/or microscopy. A *dipstick* is a plastic stick containing squares of many different colors (Figure 12.5). Each square contains a reagent, a chemical substance used to detect and measure other substances.

A dipstick is placed in a patient's urine specimen. When the urine interacts with the reagent, it changes color. All the reagent squares on the dipstick are compared to those on a color chart located on the container. The resulting color indicates various types of urinary problems. A dipstick urinalysis can help diagnose a urinary condition based on pH (acidity or alkalinity), specific gravity, or the content of substances such as blood, protein, glucose, ketones (a by-product of the breakdown of fat instead of glucose), or bilirubin (a substance produced when the liver breaks down old red blood cells).

Microscopic urinalysis provides more detailed information about a urine specimen when dipstick results are abnormal. The specimen is viewed under a high-magnification microscope (one with a high-powered field of view). More than four erythrocytes (red blood cells) seen in a high-powered field is an abnormal finding.

Culture and Sensitivity Test

A **culture and sensitivity (C&S)** involves a *culture test*, in which microorganisms from a sample of a patient's urine are placed in a culture medium in a petri dish. A *sensitivity test* determines what medicine (typically an antibiotic) will effectively treat a urinary tract infection (Figure 12.6).

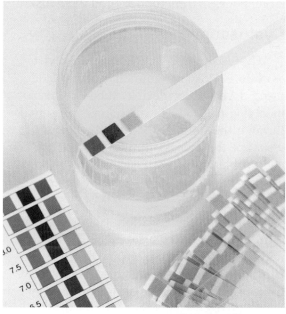

Christina Richards/Shutterstock.com

Figure 12.5 A urinalysis is often done in a doctor's office using a dipstick that contains chemical reagents, which help detect and measure the presence of other chemical substances.

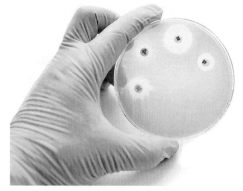

Jarun Ontakrai/Shutterstock.com

Figure 12.6 In this culture and sensitivity test, the clear rings around the antibiotic disks indicate that the antibiotic will be effective in treating an infection caused by the bacteria cultivated in the petri dish.

In a manual sensitivity test, disks with various antibiotics are placed on a culture plate along with a suspension of the isolated bacteria. If the infection is bacterial, the antibiotics most effective in treating the UTI will inhibit bacterial growth near the disks, and there will be larger zones of inhibition around these disks.

Cystoscopy

Cystoscopy (sĭs-TŎS-kō-pē), abbreviated as **cysto**, is a visual examination of the bladder using a very thin, flexible, tube-like instrument (Figure 12.7). The optic scope is inserted through the urethra and into the bladder to visualize the mucosa (lining) of the bladder and to obtain a biopsy if necessary.

Urinary Catheterization

Urinary catheterization (abbreviated as **cath**) involves placing a tube through the urinary meatus into the urethra and then manipulating the tube into the bladder (Figure 12.8). Urinary catheterization is commonly used for continuous drainage of the bladder. It may also be used to obtain a sterile urine sample or to *instill* (introduce) medications into the bladder.

An *indwelling catheter* drains urine from the bladder to a bag outside the body. It is held in place by a balloon tip filled with water and can be left inside the body for a longer period of time than a standard urinary catheter.

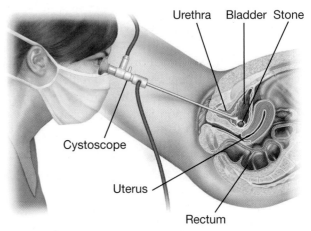

© Body Scientific International

Figure 12.7 Cystoscopy is the visual examination of the bladder using a cystoscope.

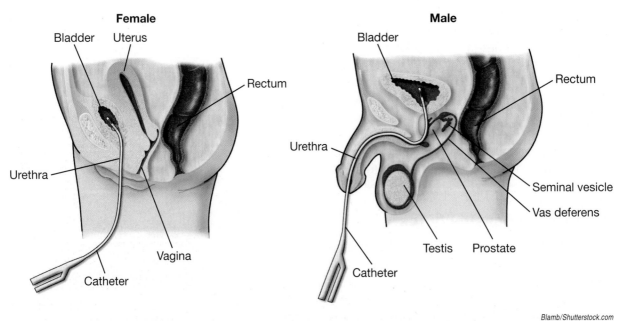

Blamb/Shutterstock.com

Figure 12.8 Urinary catheterization in the female and in the male

Intravenous Pyelogram

Intravenous pyelogram (PĪ-ĕ-lō-grăm), or **IVP**, is a radiographic procedure in which a contrast agent is injected into the body to visualize the urinary tract (Figure 12.9). A contrast agent, sometimes referred to as a *dye*, is often used in radiographic procedures. It allows visualization of bodily structures that are not dense enough to show up on routine X-rays.

Once the contrast agent has been injected into a vein, a rapid series of radiographs captures the visual progress of the agent through the kidneys, ureters, and bladder, providing information about their structure and function. Intravenous pyelogram is also called a *urogram*.

Renal Scan

A **renal scan** is a nuclear medicine imaging procedure that reveals the size, shape, position, and function of the kidneys. In this procedure, a radioactive isotope is injected intravenously into the patient. The isotope is absorbed by the kidneys and emits radioactive particles that are captured by a scanner. The scanner transforms the data collected into an image.

A renal scan is particularly useful when a person is allergic to the contrast material (dye) used in an intravenous pyelogram (IVP). Abnormal results of a renal scan are a sign of impaired kidney function.

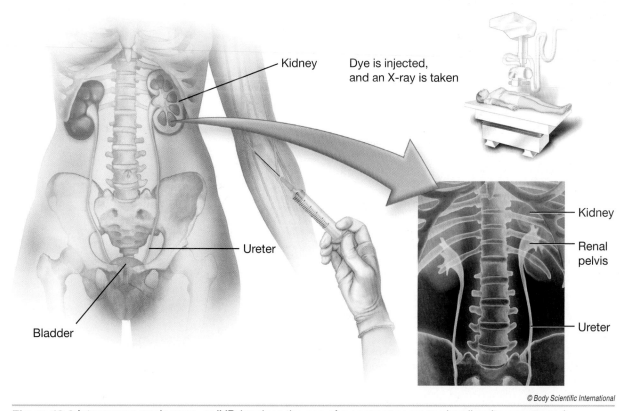

Figure 12.9 Intravenous pyelogram, or IVP, involves the use of a contrast agent to visualize the organs and structures of the urinary tract.

Renal Ultrasound

A **renal ultrasound** is an imaging technique that uses high-frequency sound waves and a computer to generate images of the kidneys. It is used to detect abnormal masses or blockages.

The renal ultrasound is a painless, noninvasive (does not pierce the skin) procedure that requires little preparation on the part of the patient. Because it does not involve exposure to radiation, it is an ideal diagnostic imaging method for the pregnant patient. A renal ultrasound is also called a *renal sonogram.*

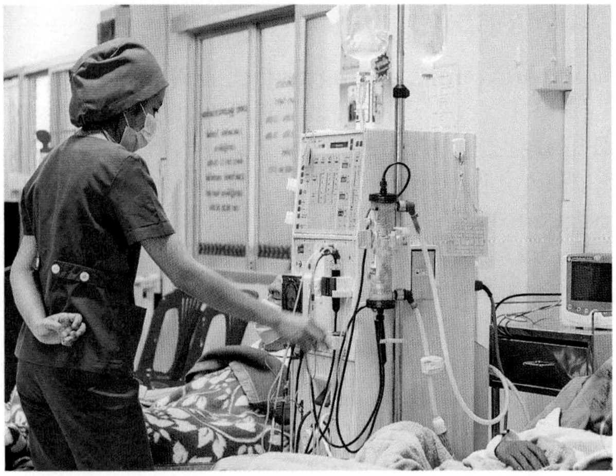

Renal Dialysis

Renal dialysis is an artificial method of filtration used to remove waste products and excess water from the body when the kidneys fail to perform this function (Figure 12.10). There are two main types of dialysis: *hemodialysis* and *peritoneal dialysis.* Both methods rid the body of harmful wastes by filtering the blood.

Hemodialysis, the more common dialysis method for renal failure, accomplishes the task of filtration using a machine called a *dialyzer* (Figure 12.11). In peritoneal dialysis, the lining of the patient's own abdomen (the *peritoneal membrane*) is used to filter the blood.

nittaya12122508/Shutterstock.com

Figure 12.10 Renal dialysis removes waste products and excess water from the body.

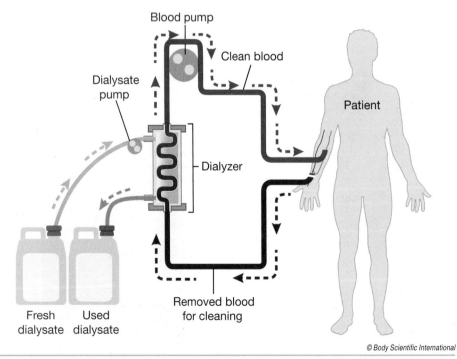

© Body Scientific International

Figure 12.11 In hemodialysis, the more common treatment method for kidney failure, a dialyzer cleanses the patient's blood and returns clean blood back into the body.

Multiple Choice: Diseases and Disorders

Directions: Choose the disease or disorder that matches each definition. You can also complete this activity online using *EduHub*.

_____ 1. the abnormal, involuntary holding of urine in the bladder
   a. urinary incontinence
   b. urinary retention
   c. polyuria
   d. oliguria

_____ 2. inflammation of the kidney and renal pelvis
   a. hydronephrosis
   b. pyonephrosis
   c. pyelonephritis
   d. nephrolithiasis

_____ 3. disorder characterized by loss of bladder control
   a. urinary incontinence
   b. urinary frequency
   c. nocturia
   d. polyuria

_____ 4. inflammation of the bladder due to an ascending urinary tract infection
   a. hydronephrosis
   b. hydronephritis
   c. cystitis
   d. uremia

_____ 5. condition that causes distension and dilation of the renal pelvis, resulting in enlargement of the kidney
   a. hydronephrosis
   b. pyelonephritis
   c. uremia
   d. polyuria

_____ 6. condition in which the bladder herniates, or protrudes, through the vaginal wall
   a. cystocele
   b. vesicocele
   c. hypercystocele
   d. both a and b

_____ 7. cystitis and urethritis are two common types of
   a. renal pelvis infections
   b. hernial conditions of the bladder
   c. urinary tract infections
   d. diseases that require renal dialysis treatment

SCORECARD: How Did You Do?

Number correct (_____), divided by 7 (_____), multiplied by 100 equals _____ (your score)

Multiple Choice: Procedures and Treatments

Directions: Choose the procedure or treatment that matches each definition. You can also complete this activity online using *EduHub*.

_____ 1. visual examination of the bladder using a very thin, flexible, tube-like instrument
   a. cystoscopy
   b. cystogram
   c. cystourethrogram
   d. intravenous pyelogram

_____ 2. radiographic procedure in which a contrast agent is injected into the body to visualize the urinary tract
   a. cystogram
   b. urethrogram
   c. catheterization
   d. intravenous pyelogram

_____ 3. test used to determine the most effective antibiotic for treating a urinary tract infection
   a. urinalysis
   b. cystoscopy
   c. culture and sensitivity test
   d. renal scan

_____ 4. nuclear medicine imaging procedure that shows the size, shape, position, and function of the kidneys
   a. renal scan
   b. intravenous pyelogram
   c. cystoscopy
   d. cystogram

5. lab analysis of urine that may be performed using a dipstick or a microscope
   a. culture and sensitivity test
   b. urinalysis
   c. urinary catheterization
   d. intravenous pyelogram

6. procedure in which a tube is inserted through the urinary meatus of the urethra and then manipulated into the bladder
   a. urinary catheterization
   b. cystoscopy
   c. intravenous pyelogram
   d. renal dialysis

7. artificial method of filtration used to remove excess waste and water from the body
   a. hemodialysis
   b. peritoneal dialysis
   c. both a and b
   d. neither a nor b

8. imaging technique in which high-frequency sound waves and a computer are used to generate images of the kidneys
   a. cystogram
   b. intravenous pyelogram
   c. renal scan
   d. renal ultrasound

SCORECARD: How Did You Do?

Number correct (_____), divided by 8 (_____), multiplied by 100 equals _____ (your score)

Assessment 12.9

Identify Abbreviations

Directions: Supply the correct abbreviation for each medical term. You can also complete this activity online using *EduHub*.

Medical Term	Abbreviation
1. urinalysis	_____
2. cystoscopy	_____
3. urinary tract infection	_____
4. intravenous pyelogram	_____
5. urinary catheterization	_____
6. culture and sensitivity (test)	_____

SCORECARD: How Did You Do?

Number correct (_____), divided by 6 (_____), multiplied by 100 equals _____ (your score)

Analyzing the Intern Experience

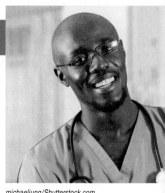

michaeljung/Shutterstock.com

In the Intern Experience described at the beginning of this chapter, we met Thomas, an intern who was assigned to assist Dr. Nefron, a general practitioner with the Middletown Clinic. Thomas listened and observed as Dr. Nefron met with Shara, a college student who came to the clinic because of symptoms that included fatigue, general bodily discomfort, lower back pain, urinary frequency, and a burning sensation upon urination.

Dr. Nefron obtained Shara's personal and family health history, performed a physical examination, and ordered a urinalysis. He then made a diagnosis and formulated a treatment plan for Shara. Later, he made a dictated recording of the patient's health information, which was subsequently transcribed into a chart note.

We will now learn more about Shara's condition from a clinical perspective, interpreting the medical terms in her chart note as we analyze the scenario presented in the Intern Experience.

Audio Activity: Shara Brown's Chart Note

Directions: Access your *EduHub* subscription and listen to the recording of the physician reading Shara Brown's chart note. Read along with the physician and pay attention to the pronunciation of each medical term.

CHART NOTE

Patient Name: Brown, Shara
ID Number: 89736
Examination Date: October 1, 20xx

SUBJECTIVE
Shara presents with **frequency**, urgency, fever, and burning upon urination for 3–5 days accompanied by malaise, **flank** pain, **hematuria**, and **renal colic**. She delayed care until completion of final exams. Patient has a history of multiple bladder infections.

OBJECTIVE
BP (blood pressure) 120/80, pulse 76, respirations 22/min. Dipstick **urinalysis** showed yellow urine, cloudy with 80–100 WBCs (white blood cells), and many bacteria.

ASSESSMENT
UTI and **cystitis**.

TREATMENT PLAN
Cephalexin 500 mg p.o. t.i.d. x 10 days (take one 500-mg tablet of the antibiotic cephalexin by mouth 3 times a day for 10 days). Recommend follow-up with **urologist**. Chronic cystitis vs. **pyelonephritis**.

Interpret Shara Brown's Chart Note

Directions: Access your *EduHub* subscription and listen to the recording of the physician reading Shara Brown's chart note. After listening to the recording, supply the medical term that matches each definition.

Example: inflammation of the kidney   *Answer:* nephritis

1. specialist in the study and treatment of diseases and disorders of the urinary tract _____

2. urinating often _____

3. painful spasms in the lower back _____

4. inflammation of the bladder _____

5. chemical analysis of the urine _____

6. infection in the urinary tract _____

7. lower back _____

8. condition of blood in the urine _____

9. inflammation of the kidney and renal pelvis _____

SCORECARD: How Did You Do?

Number correct (_____), divided by 9 (_____), multiplied by 100 equals _____ (your score)

Working with Medical Records

In this activity, you will interpret the medical records (chart notes) of patients with health conditions related to the urinary system. These examples illustrate typical medical records prepared in a real-world healthcare environment. To interpret these chart notes, you will apply your knowledge of word elements (prefixes, combining forms, and suffixes), diseases and disorders, and procedures and treatments related to the urinary system.

Audio Activity: Elizabeth Townsend's Chart Note

Directions: Access your *EduHub* subscription and listen to the recording of the physician reading Elizabeth Townsend's chart note. Read along with the physician and pay attention to the pronunciation of each medical term.

CHART NOTE

Patient Name: Townsend, Elizabeth
ID Number: 12333
Examination Date: February 23, 20xx

SUBJECTIVE
This 14-year-old female presents with urinary **frequency** and **incontinence** for the past 2 days. She has had pain on urination for the past 3–5 days; no **hematuria** noted. No **flank** pain. Patient did complain that her stomach hurt. Fever of 101° for the past 24 hours. No vomiting. Patient has a history of a urinary tract infection several months ago; however, no repeat **urinalysis** was performed. She has not had an **intravenous pyelogram** or **renal ultrasound**. Family history is significant; paternal grandmother had a **nephrectomy**.

OBJECTIVE
Alert and in no distress. Abdomen is soft with no masses, tenderness, or hepatosplenomegaly (enlargement of the liver and spleen). No guarding (a reflexive response to protect an area of pain).

LABORATORY
Urinalysis shows 60–80 WBCs (white blood cells) and 80–100 RBCs (red blood cells) and positive nitrates.

ASSESSMENT
Recurrent **UTI**.

TREATMENT PLAN
Ciprofloxacin 500 mg b.i.d. x 10 days (take 500 mg of ciprofloxacin twice a day for 10 days). Obtain urine **C&S**. Repeat urinalysis and urine culture 2 days after completion of antibiotics. Follow up with renal ultrasound.

Assessment 12.11

Interpret Elizabeth Townsend's Chart Note

Directions: Access your *EduHub* subscription and listen to the recording of the physician reading Elizabeth Townsend's chart note. After listening to the recording, supply the medical term that matches each definition.

Example: suture of the kidney   *Answer:* nephrorrhaphy

1. excision of the kidney   _____

2. lower back   _____

3. procedure in which high-frequency sound waves are used to study the kidneys   _____

4. urinary tract infection   _____

5. lab test used to determine the most effective antibiotic for treating a urinary tract infection   _____

6. chemical analysis of the urine   _____

7. urinating often   _____

8. loss of bladder control

    _____

9. condition of blood in the urine

    _____

10. radiographic procedure used to visualize
    the urinary tract

    _____

Audio Activity: Brian Simmons's Chart Note

Directions: Access your *EduHub* subscription and listen to the recording of the physician reading Brian Simmons's chart note. Read along with the physician and pay attention to the pronunciation of each medical term.

CHART NOTE

Patient Name: Simmons, Brian
ID Number: 53589
Examination Date: March 13, 20xx

HISTORY OF PRESENT ILLNESS
Patient had onset 2 hours ago of **colicky**, right **flank** pain that radiates around to the right lower quadrant and into the **urethra**. Patient states urine seems to have blood in it along with the **dysuria**. Pain becomes more severe for 1–10 minutes and then eases off. When pain is severe, he rates it at 8 on a scale of 1–10. Patient denies fever, chills, nausea, vomiting, or diarrhea.

PAST MEDICAL HISTORY
Denies history of **nephrolithiasis** or **cholelithiasis**. Denies prior, similar episodes. No drug allergies.

EXAMINATION
Patient is a 52-year-old male, appearing intermittently uncomfortable. There is mild tenderness noted to the lower portion of the right kidney upon palpation (examination using the hands or fingers). Lungs are clear. Abdomen is soft and nontender. No suprapubic (above the pubic bone) tenderness. Extremities have good pulses without edema.

LABORATORY
Clean-catch urinalysis showed **hematuria** and **pyuria**.

DIAGNOSIS
Right **ureterolithiasis**.

TREATMENT PLAN
Pain subsided. However, shortly after examination, severe pain returned in right flank and right lower quadrant. Patient was given ketorolac tromethamine 60 mg and sent for an **IVP**.

Interpret Brian Simmons's Chart Note

Directions: Access your *EduHub* subscription and listen to the recording of the physician reading Brian Simmons's chart note. After listening to the recording, supply the medical term that matches each definition. You may encounter definitions and terms introduced in previous chapters.

Example: excision of the kidney   *Answer:* nephrectomy

1. condition of blood in the urine

2. tube that carries urine to the outside of the body

3. abnormal condition of a stone in the kidney

4. lower back

5. characterized by painful spasms

6. painful or difficult urination

7. abnormal condition of a stone in the ureter

8. intravenous pyelogram; radiographic procedure used to visualize the urinary tract

9. condition of pus in the urine

10. abnormal condition of a stone in the gallbladder

SCORECARD: How Did You Do?

Number correct (_____), divided by 10 (_____), multiplied by 100 equals _____ (your score)

Chapter Review

Word Elements Summary

Prefixes

Prefix	Meaning
a-	not; without
an-	not; without
dys-	painful; difficult
intra-	inside; within
peri-	around
poly-	many; much

Combining Forms

Root Word/Combining Vowel	Meaning
cyst/o	bladder; sac containing fluid
glyc/o	sugar; glucose
glycos/o	sugar; glucose
hem/o, hemat/o	blood
hydr/o	water
lith/o	stone
meat/o	opening
nephr/o	kidney
noct/o	night
olig/o	scanty; few
py/o	pus
pyel/o	renal pelvis
ren/o	kidney
son/o	sound
sten/o	narrow; constricted
ur/o	urine; urinary tract
ureter/o	ureter
urethr/o	urethra
urin/o	urine
vesic/o	bladder

Suffixes

Suffix	Meaning
-al	pertaining to
-algia	pain
-cele	hernia; swelling; protrusion
-dipsia	thirst
-ectomy	surgical removal; excision
-emia	blood condition
-gram	record; image
-ia	condition
-iasis	abnormal condition
-itis	inflammation
-logist	specialist in the study and treatment of
-logy	study of
-lysis	destruction
-megaly	large; enlargement
-oma	tumor; mass
-osis	abnormal condition
-pexy	surgical fixation
-plasty	surgical repair
-ptosis	drooping; downward displacement
-rrhaphy	suture
-scope	instrument used to observe
-scopy	process of observing
-stomy	new opening
-tomy	incision; cut into
-tripsy	process of crushing

More Practice: Activities and Games

The following activities will help you reinforce your skills and check your mastery of the medical terminology you learned in this chapter. Access your *EduHub* subscription to complete more activities and vocabulary games for mastering the word parts and terms you have learned.

Medical Term Identification

Directions: Complete each statement using the correct medical term.

1. Laboratory analysis of the urine: _____.

2. Condition that causes distension and dilation of the renal pelvis, resulting in enlargement of the kidney: _____.

3. Condition associated with renal failure in which the kidneys do not remove urea and other waste products from the blood: _____.

4. Inflammation of the urinary bladder: _____.

5. Inflammation of the urethra: _____.

6. Artificial method of filtration for removing waste products and excess water from the body when the kidneys fail to perform this function:

   _____.

7. Procedure that involves placing a tube through the urinary meatus into the urethra: _____.

8. Nephrolithiasis is the formation of stones in the _____.

9. When a person has had a nephrectomy, his or her _____ has been surgically removed.

10. The urinary tract is composed of the kidneys, ureters, bladder, and

    _____.

11. At the end of the urethra is an opening called the

    _____, which expels urine to the outside of the body.

12. A physician who specializes in the study, diagnosis, and treatment of urinary tract diseases and disorders is called a _____.

True or False

Directions: Indicate whether each statement is true or false.

True or False?

_____ 1. The prefix **dys-** means "painful" or "difficult."

_____ 2. The root word **nephr** means "night."

_____ 3. The root words **glyc** and **glycos** both mean "sugar."

_____ 4. The root word **ureter** means "urethra."

_____ 5. The suffix **-lysis** means "destruction."

_____ 6. The suffix **-iasis** means "normal condition."

_____ 7. The suffix **-dipsia** means "thirst."

_____ 8. The term *hydronephrosis* contains a prefix, a root word, and a suffix.

_____ 9. The term *ureterostenosis* contains two root words and one suffix.

True or False?

_____ 10. We have close to one million nephrons in each kidney.

_____ 11. The act of excreting urine is called *micturition*.

_____ 12. Frequency is urinating often and usually in large amounts.

_____ 13. A dipstick is a chemical stick used in urinalysis.

_____ 14. Cystitis is an inflammation of the kidney and renal pelvis.

_____ 15. Urinary retention is the voluntary holding of urine.

_____ 16. An intravenous pyelogram is a radiographic procedure in which a contrast agent is injected into the body to visualize the urinary tract.

Break It Down

Directions: Dissect each medical term into its word parts (prefix, root word, combining vowel, and suffix) using one or more slashes. Then define each term.

Example:

Medical Term: pyuria

Dissection: py/ur/ia

Definition: condition of pus in the urine

Medical Term	Dissection
1. hematocele	h e m a t o c e l e

Definition: _____

_____

| 2. urogram | u r o g r a m |

Definition: _____

_____

| 3. perirenal | p e r i r e n a l |

Definition: _____

_____

| 4. meatorrhaphy | m e a t o r r h a p h y |

Definition: _____

_____

Medical Term	Dissection
5. hydrocele	h y d r o c e l e

Definition: _____

_____

6. lithotomy   l i t h o t o m y

Definition: _____

_____

7. meatoscope   m e a t o s c o p e

Definition: _____

_____

8. urolithiasis   u r o l i t h i a s i s

Definition: _____

_____

9. renogram   r e n o g r a m

Definition: _____

_____

10. intrarenal   i n t r a r e n a l

Definition: _____

_____

11. cystopyelonephritis   c y s t o p y e l o n e p h r i t i s

Definition: _____

_____

12. uronephrosis   u r o n e p h r o s i s

Definition: _____

_____

Audio Activity: Mara Rodriguez's Chart Note

Directions: Access your *EduHub* subscription and listen to the recording of the physician reading Mara Rodriguez's chart note. Read along with the physician and pay attention to the pronunciation of each medical term.

CHART NOTE

Patient Name: Rodriguez, Mara
ID Number: 65588
Examination Date: August 29, 20xx

SUBJECTIVE

This 43-year-old female presents with **subcostal** pain and episodes of gross (visible to the naked eye) **hematuria**. She was seen in the ER approximately 3 weeks ago for similar symptoms. At that time, a **renal ultrasound** was performed. It showed no evidence of **hydronephrosis** or renal mass. Today patient complains of some nausea and vomiting. She denies fever, chills, **dysuria**, or **frequency**. There is no previous history of urinary tract infections, **calculus** formation, or genitourinary (reproductive and urinary system) surgery.

OBJECTIVE

On physical examination, the abdomen appears relatively soft but diffusely tender (not limited to one location), particularly in the left upper and left lower quadrants. Some guarding was noted with no clearly elicited rebound tenderness. (When the areas were palpated, no rebound tenderness occurred when the physician's palpating hand was withdrawn.) **Urinalysis** today shows 6–10 erythrocytes (red blood cells) per high power field. There is no suggestion of infection with leukocytes or bacteria.

ASSESSMENT

The **etiology** of the pain remains unclear, although possibilities include a calculus, cholecystitis (inflammation of the gallbladder), or ovarian cyst. With absence of obstruction on the renal ultrasound, the cause of pain is not suggestive of a stone. Negative urinalysis also mitigates against **pyelonephritis**, and the pain is clearly abdominal. The etiology of the gross hematuria remains unclear.

TREATMENT PLAN

A surgical consultation for further evaluation of the abdomen is advised.

Interpret Mara Rodriguez's Chart Note

Directions: Access your *EduHub* subscription and listen to the recording of the physician reading Mara Rodriguez's chart note. After listening to the recording, supply the medical term that matches each definition. You may encounter definitions and terms introduced in previous chapters.

Example: inflammation of the bladder   *Answer:* cystitis

1. condition of blood in the urine

2. abnormal condition of water in the kidney

3. a stone composed of mineral salts, which can block passage of urine through the ureters

4. cause

5. procedure that uses high-frequency sound waves to study the kidneys

6. chemical analysis of the urine

7. painful or difficult urination

8. below the ribs

9. urinating often

10. inflammation of the renal pelvis and kidney

Spelling

Directions: For each medical term that is misspelled, provide the correct spelling.

1. cistoplasty

2. hydranephrosis

3. haematuria

4. nocturea

5. cistytis

6. periurrethral

7. nephrolithiosis

8. polydipsea

9. urethrascope

10. lythotripsy

11. cystosele

12. urrologist

13. oligurea

14. pyalonephritis

15. nerphoma

Cumulative Review

Chapters 11–12: Endocrine System and Urinary System

Directions: Check your mastery of word elements used in medical terminology related to the endocrine system and urinary system by defining the following prefixes, combining forms, and suffixes.

Prefixes

a-　　　　　_____

an-　　　　_____

dys-　　　 _____

endo-　　 _____

hyper-　　_____

hypo-　　 _____

intra-　　 _____

para-　　 _____

poly-　　 _____

Combining Forms

acr/o　　　　　　　_____

aden/o　　　　　　 _____

adren/o, adrenal/o　_____

carcin/o　　　　　 _____

crin/o　　　　　　 _____

cyst/o　　　　　　 _____

dips/o　　　　　　 _____

gluc/o　　　　　　 _____

glyc/o　　　　　　 _____

glycos/o　　　　　 _____

hem/o, hemat/o _____

hydr/o _____

lith/o _____

meat/o _____

nephr/o _____

noct/o _____

olig/o _____

py/o _____

pyel/o _____

ren/o _____

son/o _____

sten/o _____

thym/o _____

thyr/o, thyroid/o _____

ur/o _____

ureter/o _____

urethr/o _____

urin/o _____

vesic/o _____

Suffixes

-al _____

-algia _____

-cele _____

-dipsia _____

-e _____

-ectomy _____

-emia _____

-gram _____

-ia _____

-iasis _____

-ic _____

-ism _____

-itis _____

-logist _____

-logy _____

-lysis _____

-megaly _____

-oid _____

-oma _____

-osis _____

-pathy _____

-pexy _____

-phagia _____

-plasty _____

-ptosis _____

-rrhaphy _____

-scope _____

-scopy _____

-stomy _____

-tomy _____

-tripsy _____

Appendix A

Medical Word Elements

Prefixes

Prefix	Meaning
a-	not; without
ad-	toward
an-	not; without
anti-	against
auto-	self
brady-	slow
dia-	through; complete
dys-	painful; difficult
endo-	within
epi-	upon; above
extra-	outside
hemi-	half
hyper-	above; above normal
hypo-	below; below normal
inter-	between

Prefix	Meaning
intra-	inside; within
meta-	change; beyond
pan-	all; everything
para-	near; beside
per-	through
peri-	around
poly-	many; much
quadri-	four
retro-	back; behind
sub-	beneath; below
supra-	above
sym-, syn-	together; with
tachy-	fast
trans-	across

Combining Forms

Root Word/Combining Vowel	Meaning
acr/o	extremity
aden/o	gland
adenoid/o	adenoids
adren/o, adrenal/o	adrenal gland
angi/o	vessel
anter/o	front
arteri/o	artery
arthr/o	joint
articul/o	joint
ather/o	fatty substance
audi/o	hearing
blephar/o	eyelid
bronch/o, bronchi/o	bronchial tube; bronchus
burs/a, burs/o	bursa; sac
carcin/o	cancerous; cancer
card/o, cardi/o	heart
carp/o	carpals (wrist bones)
celi/o	abdomen
cephal/o	head
cerebell/o	cerebellum
cerebr/o	cerebrum
cervic/o	cervix; neck
chol/e	bile; gall
cholecyst/o	gallbladder
chondr/o	cartilage
clavicul/o	clavicle (collarbone)
coccyg/o	coccyx (tailbone)
col/o, colon/o	colon; large intestine
colp/o	vagina

Root Word/Combining Vowel	Meaning
contus/o	bruising
coron/o	heart
cost/o	rib
cran/o, crani/o	skull; cranium
crin/o	to secrete
cry/o	cold
cutane/o	skin
cyan/o	blue
cyst/o	sac containing fluid; bladder
cyt/o	cell
derma/a, derm/o, dermat/o	skin
dips/o	thirst
dist/o	away from the point of origin
diverticul/o	diverticulum
dors/o	along the back (of the body)
duoden/o	duodenum
ecchym/o	blood in the tissues
electr/o	electrical activity
embol/o	plug; embolus
encephal/o	brain
enter/o	intestines
erythemat/o	redness
erythr/o	red
esophag/o	esophagus
femor/o	femur (thigh bone)
fibul/o	fibula
gastr/o	stomach

(Continued)

Root Word/ Combining Vowel	Meaning
gingiv/o	gums
gloss/o	tongue
gluc/o	glucose; sugar
glyc/o	glucose; sugar
glycos/o	glucose; sugar
gynec/o	woman; female
hem/o	blood
hemat/o	blood
hepat/o	liver
herni/o	hernia; rupture; protrusion
humer/o	humerus (upper arm bone)
hydr/o	water
hyster/o	uterus
ile/o	ileum
ili/o	ilium
immune/o	protection
infer/o	below; beneath
ir/o	iris
irid/o	iris
isch/o	to keep back
ischi/o	ischium (part of the hip bone)
jejun/o	jejunum
kerat/o	cornea
kines/o, kinesi/o	movement
kyph/o	hump
lapar/o	abdomen
later/o	side
leuk/o	white
lip/o	fat

Root Word/ Combining Vowel	Meaning
lith/o	stone
lob/o	lobe (a defined portion of an organ or structure)
lord/o	curve
lymph/o	lymph
malign/o	causing harm, cancer
mamm/o	breast
mast/o	breast
meat/o	opening
medi/o	middle
melan/o	black
men/o	menstruation
mening/o, meningi/o	meninges (membranes covering the brain and spinal cord)
metacarp/o	metacarpals (bones of the hand)
metatars/o	metatarsals (bones of the foot)
metr/o, metri/o	uterus
muscul/o	muscle
my/o	muscle
myc/o	fungus
myel/o	bone marrow; spinal cord
myring/o	tympanic membrane; eardrum
necr/o	death
nephr/o	kidney
neur/o	nerve
noct/o	night
ocul/o	eye
olig/o	scanty; few
onych/o	nail

(Continued)

Root Word/ Combining Vowel	Meaning
oophor/o	ovary
ophthalm/o	eye
opt/o	eye; vision
optic/o	eye; vision
or/o	mouth
orchid/o	testes
organ/o	organ
orth/o	straight
oste/o	bone
ot/o	ear
ox/o	oxygen
pancreat/o	pancreas
patell/a, patell/o	patella (kneecap)
path/o	disease
peps/o	digestion
phag/o	eat; swallow; engulf
phalang/o	phalanges (bones of fingers or toes)
pharyng/o	pharynx; throat
phleb/o	vein
pleg/o	paralysis
pleur/o	pleura
pneum/o, pneumon/o	lung; air
polyp/o	polyp; small growth
por/o	pore; duct; small opening
poster/o	back of the body
presby/o	old age
proct/o	anus and rectum
prostat/o	prostate gland
proxim/o	nearest the point of origin

Root Word/ Combining Vowel	Meaning
prurit/o	itching
psych/o	mind
pub/o	pubis (part of the hip bone)
pulmon/o	lung
py/o	pus
pyel/o	renal pelvis
radi/o	radius (bone of the forearm); X-ray
radicul/o	nerve root
rect/o	rectum
ren/o	kidney
retin/o	retina
rhin/o	nose
sacr/o	sacrum (bone at base of the spine)
salping/o	uterine tube; fallopian tube
scapul/o	scapula (shoulder blade)
schiz/o	split
scler/o	sclera (white of the eye)
scoli/o	crooked; bent
scrot/o	scrotum
seb/o	oil; sebum
sial/o	saliva
sigmoid/o	sigmoid colon
son/o	sound
spin/o	spine; backbone
spir/o	breathe; breathing
splen/o	spleen
spondyl/o	vertebra; spine
squam/o	scale-like

(Continued)

Root Word/ Combining Vowel	Meaning
sten/o	narrow; constricted
stern/o	sternum (breastbone)
tars/o	ankle bones
ten/o	tendon
tendin/o, tendon/o	tendon
tens/o	pressure; tension
testicul/o	testes
thorac/o	chest
thromb/o	clot
thym/o	thymus gland
thyr/o, thyroid/o	thyroid gland
tibi/o	tibia (shin bone)
tonsil/o	tonsils
topic/o	place
trache/o	trachea; windpipe

Root Word/ Combining Vowel	Meaning
trich/o	hair
tympan/o	tympanic membrane; eardrum
uln/o	ulna (bone of the forearm)
ur/o	urine; urinary tract
ureter/o	ureter
urethr/o	urethra
urin/o	urine
vagin/o	vagina
vas/o	vessel; duct
vascul/o	blood vessel
ven/o, ven/i	vein
vertebr/o	vertebra; spine
vesic/o	bladder
xer/o	dry

Suffixes

Suffix	Meaning
-ac	pertaining to
-al	pertaining to
-algia	pain
-ancy	state of
-ar	pertaining to
-ary	pertaining to
-asthenia	weakness
-atic	pertaining to
-ation	process; condition; state of being or having
-cele	hernia; swelling; protrusion
-centesis	surgical puncture to remove fluid
-clasia	surgical breaking
-cyte	cell
-desis	to bind or tie together surgically
-dipsia	thirst
-dynia	pain
-e	noun suffix with no meaning
-eal	pertaining to
-ectasis	dilatation; dilation; expansion
-ectomy	surgical removal; excision
-edema	swelling
-ema	condition
-emesis	vomiting
-emia	blood condition
-esthesia	sensation; feeling
-gen	producing; originating; causing
-gram	record; image

Suffix	Meaning
-graph	instrument used to record an image
-graphy	process of recording an image
-ia	condition
-iasis	abnormal condition
-ic	pertaining to
-ical	pertaining to
-ion	condition; process
-ior	pertaining to
-ism	condition; process
-itis	inflammation
-kinesia	movement
-kinesis	movement
-logist	specialist in the study and treatment of
-logy	study of
-lysis	breakdown; loosening; dissolving
-malacia	softening
-megaly	large; enlargement
-meter	instrument used to measure
-metry	process of measuring; measurement
-oid	like; resembling
-oma	tumor; mass
-opia	vision
-osis	abnormal condition
-ous	pertaining to
-pathy	disease
-penia	deficiency; abnormal reduction
-pexy	surgical fixation

(Continued)

Suffix	Meaning
-phagia	condition of eating or swallowing
-pharynx	pharynx; throat
-phasia	speech
-plasty	surgical repair
-pnea	breathing
-ptosis	drooping; downward displacement
-rrhage	bursting forth (of blood)
-rrhagia	bursting forth (of blood)
-rrhaphy	suture
-rrhea	flow; discharge
-rrhexis	rupture
-sclerosis	hardening
-scope	instrument used to observe

Suffix	Meaning
-scopy	process of observing
-spasm	involuntary muscle contraction
-stasis	stop; stand still
-stomy	new opening
-thorax	chest; pleural cavity
-tic	pertaining to
-tome	instrument used to cut
-tomy	incision; cut into
-tripsy	crushing
-trophy	development
-us	structure; thing
-y	condition; process

Appendix B

Medical Abbreviations and Acronyms

acquired immunodeficiency syndrome	AIDS	implantable cardioverter defibrillator	ICD
anterior cruciate ligament	ACL	incision and drainage	I&D
antidiuretic hormone	ADH	inflammatory bowel disease	IBD
arterial blood gas	ABG	insulin-dependent diabetes mellitus	IDDM
autoimmune hemolytic anemia	AIHA	intravenous pyelogram	IVP
automated external defibrillator	AED	lateral collateral ligament	LCL
benign prostatic hypertrophy	BPH	lower gastrointestinal	LGI
biopsy	Bx	lumbar puncture	LP
cardiopulmonary resuscitation	CPR	magnetic resonance angiogram	MRA
cerebral palsy	CP	magnetic resonance imaging	MRI
cerebral vascular attack	CVA	medial collateral ligament	MCL
cerebrospinal fluid	CSF	mononucleosis	mono
chest X-ray	CXR	multiple sclerosis	MS
chronic obstructive pulmonary disease	COPD	myocardial infarction	MI
computerized tomography	CT	non-insulin-dependent diabetes mellitus	NIDDM
congestive heart failure	CHF	nuclear medicine imaging	NMI
continuous positive airway pressure	CPAP	pelvic inflammatory disease	PID
coronary artery disease	CAD	physical therapy	PT
culture and sensitivity test	C&S	premenstrual syndrome	PMS
cystoscopy	cysto	pulmonary function test	PFT
diabetes insipidus	DI	rest, ice, compression, and elevation	RICE
diabetes mellitus	DM	rheumatoid arthritis	RA
dilation and curettage	D&C	sexually transmitted infection	STI
Duchenne muscular dystrophy	DMD	systemic lupus erythematosus	SLE
electrocardiogram	ECG	thyroid-stimulating hormone	TSH
electroencephalogram	EEG	transient ischemic attack	TIA
electromyogram	EMG	transurethral resection of the prostate	TURP
enzyme-linked immunosorbent assay	ELISA	traumatic brain injury	TBI
esophagogastroduodenoscopy	EGD	ultraviolet light	UV
fasting blood sugar	FBS	upper gastrointestinal	UGI
gastroesophageal reflux disease	GERD	upper respiratory infection	URI
glucose tolerance test	GTT	urinalysis	UA
head, eyes, ears, nose, and throat	HEENT	urinary catheterization	cath
herpes simplex virus 1	HSV-1	urinary tract infection	UTI
human immunodeficiency virus	HIV	ventilation/perfusion scan	VPS

Index

A

abdominal cavity, 32
abdominopelvic cavity, 32, 33–34
    definition, 32
    quadrants, 33–34
    regions, 34
ACL injuries. *See* knee injuries,
    163–164
acne, 69, 75
acquired immunodeficiency
    syndrome (AIDS), 215
acromegaly, 454, 456
acute bronchitis, 383
Addison disease. *See* Addison's
    disease
Addison's disease, 466
adenocarcinoma, 454, 456
adenoid, 196, 198, 454, 456
adenoidectomy, 205, 208
adenoiditis, 205, 208
adenoma, 454, 456
adenomegaly, 454, 456
adhesions, 344
adrenal, 454, 456
adrenal gland, 447
adrenalectomy, 454, 456
adrenalopathy, 454, 456
adult-onset diabetes, 464
AED. *See* automated external
    defibrillator (AED)
age-related hearing loss. *See*
    presbycusis
AIDS. *See* acquired
    immunodeficiency syndrome
    (AIDS)
AIHA. *See* autoimmune hemolytic
    anemia (AIHA)
alcoholism. *See* liver disease
alimentary canal, 90–91, 93
allergens, 215–217, 382
    allergic reactions, 216
    definition, 215
allergy, 215
alopecia, 75
alopecia areata, 69
alveoli, 367
Alzheimer's disease, 298
amenorrhea, 333, 335
anaphylaxis, 216
anatomical planes, 25–26
anatomical position, 24–25
    anatomical planes, 25–26
    definition, 24

planes, directions, and locations,
    24–34
terms of position and direction,
    27–31
androgenetic alopecia, 69
anesthesia, 289, 291
aneurysm, 420
angina pectoris, 420
angioplasty, 412, 414
anorexia nervosa, 113
anoxia, 374, 376
anterior, 2, 147, 151
anterior (ventral), 24
anterior cruciate ligament, 163
anteroinferior, 147, 151
anteroposterior, 27
antibody, 198
antigen, 198
anuria, 493, 497
aphagia, 100, 103
aphasia, 289, 291
apnea, 374, 376
arrhythmia, 425, 426
arterial blood gas (ABG) test, 386
arteries, 404
arteriosclerosis, 24, 412, 414, 420
arthralgia, 147, 151
arthritis, 147, 151
arthrocentesis, 147, 151
arthrochondritis, 147, 151
arthrodesis, 147, 151
arthrogram, 147, 151
arthroscope, 147, 151
arthroscopy, 147, 151
arthrotome, 147, 151
ascending colon, 92
ascending urinary tract infection, 506
asthma, 217, 382
astigmatic vision, 259
astigmatism, 259
atherosclerosis, 412, 414, 420
atrophy, 147, 151
audiogram, 248, 252
audiologist, 248, 252
audiology, 248, 252
audiometer, 248, 252, 266
audiometry, 248, 252, 266–267
auditory bones, 263
aura, 299
autoimmune, 205, 208
autoimmune disorders, 197, 198,
    217–218
autoimmune hemolytic anemia
    (AIHA), 217

automated external defibrillator
    (AED), 424

B

Babinski reflex, 300–301
Babinski's sign, 300
bacterial cystitis, 504
ball-and-socket joint, 167
barium enema, 114
barium swallow, 117
barking cough. *See* croup
bedwetting. *See* enuresis
benign, 71
benign prostatic hypertrophy (BPH),
    342, 350
biopsy (Bx), 47, 48, 73, 75
bladder. *See* urinary bladder
blepharitis, 248, 252
blepharoplasty, 248, 252, 264
blepharoplegia, 248, 252
blepharoptosis, 248, 252
blepharospasm, 248, 252
blood glucose levels. *See* diabetes
    mellitus
body cavities, 32–33
body systems, 35–38
body tissues, excessive fluid. *See*
    edema
bone infection. *See* osteomyelitis
bone scan, 168
bone tissue, thinning. *See*
    osteoporosis
bone, break in the. *See* fracture
BPH. *See* benign prostatic
    hypertrophy (BPH)
bradycardia, 16, 412, 414, 426
bradykinesia, 147, 151
bradypnea, 374, 376
brain attack. *See* cerebral vascular
    attack (CVA)
brain stem, 281–282
breast cancer, 342
breasts, 324, 326
bronchi, 367
bronchiectasis, 374, 376
bronchioles, 367
bronchitis, 374, 376, 383
bronchogram, 374, 376
bronchopneumonia, 374, 376
bronchoscope, 376
bronchus. *See* bronchi
bulbourethral gland, 324, 326
bulimia nervosa, 113

burns, 70–71
   first-degree, 70
   full-thickness, 71
   second-degree, 70
   third-degree, 71
bursae, 162
bursectomy, 147, 151
bursitis, 147, 151, 162
bursotomy, 147, 151

C

CAD. *See* coronary artery disease (CAD)
calculus, 485, 486
cancer, 71
cannula, 221
capillaries, 404
carcinogen, 85
carcinogenic, 85
carcinoma, 100, 103
cardiac, 412, 414
cardiac arrhythmia, 426
cardiac catheterization, 424
cardiac hypertrophy, 422
cardiologist, 16, 405, 412, 414
cardiology, 405, 412, 414
cardiomegaly, 412, 414, 431
cardiomyopathy, 412, 414
cardiopulmonary, 412, 414
cardiopulmonary resuscitation (CPR), 387, 424
cardiorrhaphy, 148, 151
cardiorrhexis, 148, 151
cardiovascular, 404
cardiovascular system, 37, 402–439
   anatomical diagram, 404, 406
   anatomy and physiology vocabulary, 405
   breaking down and building terms, 412–413
   diseases and disorders, 420–423
   overview, 404
   procedures and treatments, 423–426
   word elements, 407
   working with medical records, 430
carpal, 148, 151
cartilage, 139
cataract, 260
cath lab, 424
cath. *See* catheterization
catheterization lab, 424
caudal, 27
celiectomy, 100, 103
central nervous system (CNS), 280, 282
cephalalgia, 289, 291
cephalic, 27, 289, 291
cerebellum, 281–282
cerebral, 289, 291

cerebral aneurysm, 296
cerebral angiography, 301
cerebral embolism, 296
cerebral palsy (CP), 297
cerebral vascular attack (CVA), 297
cerebrospinal, 289, 291
cerebrospinal fluid (CSF), 299, 303
cerebrovascular, 289, 291
cerebrum, 280, 282
cervical, 333, 335
cervicitis. 344
chancres. *See* syphilis
chest X-ray (CXR), 387
chlamydia, 343
cholecystitis, 100, 103
cholelithiasis, 100, 103
chondrocostal, 148, 151
chondrogenic, 148, 151
chondromalacia, 148, 151
chronic bronchitis, 383–385
chronic obstructive pulmonary disease (COPD), 384–385
circulatory system, 196, 404, 405
circumcision, 347
cirrhosis, 112
closed fracture. *See* fracture
CNS. *See* central nervous system (CNS)
coccygeal, 148, 151
cold sores, 72
colitis, 100, 103
collapsed lung. *See* pneumothorax
colon, 91
colonoscopy, 100, 103, 116
colostomy, 100, 103, 115
colposcope, 347
colposcopy, 333, 335, 347–348
combining forms, 10–11, 15, 18, 51–52, 95, 141–142, 202–203, 244, 285–286, 329–330, 370–371, 408, 450–451, 489–490
combining vowel, 11
comedo, 69
compound or open fracture. *See* fracture
computed tomography. *See* computerized tomography
computerized tomography (CT), 169, 299, 301
computerized tomography (CT) scan, 167
concussion, 297–298
congenital hypothyroidism, 463
congestive heart failure (CHF), 421–422
contact dermatitis, 71–72, 74
continuous positive airway pressure (CPAP), 387
contrast agent, 169. *Also see* intravenous pyelogram

contusion, 55, 58
COPD. *See* chronic obstructive pulmonary disease (COPD)
cornea, 238, 240
coronal plane, 25
coronary, 412, 414
coronary artery disease (CAD), 422
CPAP. *See* continuous positive airway pressure (CPAP)
CPR. *See* cardiopulmonary resuscitation (CPR)
cranial, 148, 151, 289, 291
cranial cavity, 32
craniotomy, 148, 151, 289, 291
cranium, 281
cretinism, 463
Crohn's disease, 110
croup, 385
cryosurgery, 74, 75
CT scanning. *See* computerized tomography
culture and sensitivity (C&S) test, 388, 507–508
culture test, 388, 507
Cushing syndrome. *See* Cushing's syndrome
Cushing's syndrome, 464
cutaneous, 46, 48
CVA. *See* cerebral vascular attack (CVA)
CXR. *See* chest X-ray (CXR)
cyanodermal, 55, 58
cyanosis, 55, 58
cyanotic, 86
cystectomy, 84, 493, 497
cystic, 55, 58
cystitis, 493, 497, 504
cysto, 508
cystocele, 493, 497, 506–507
cystolithiasis, 493, 497, 505
cystolithotomy, 493, 497
cystoplasty, 493, 497
cystoscope, 494, 497
cystoscopy, 494, 497, 508
cystotomy, 497

D

D&C. *See* dilation and curettage
debridement, 74, 75
defibrillation, 424
dementia, 298
dermal, 46, 48, 55, 58
dermatitis, 55, 58
dermatologic, 85
dermatologist, 47, 48, 55, 58
dermatology, 17, 47, 48, 55, 58
dermatopathology, 86
dermis, 47, 48
descending colon, 92
diabetes insipidus (DI), 466

diabetes mellitus (DM), 464–465
major types, 464–465
physiological overview, 464
diabetes, complications affecting
vision. See diabetic
retinopathy
diabetic retinopathy, 261
dialyzer, 510
diarrhea, 100, 103
diencephalon, 281–282
digestive system, 37, 88–131
anatomical diagram, 90, 92
anatomy and physiology
vocabulary, 91
breaking down and building
terms, 100–102
diseases and disorders, 110
main functions, 90–91
major organs, 90, 92
overview, 90
procedures and treatments,
114–117
word elements, 94
working with medical records, 121
digestive tract, 90, 91, 93
digital rectal exam, 348
dilatation, 420
dilation, 420, 505
dilation and curettage (D&C), 348
dipstick. See urinalysis
distal, 27
distension, 505
diverticula, 115
diverticulitis, 100, 103, 115
diverticulosis, 100, 103
dizziness or sensation of spinning.
See vertigo
DMD. See Duchenne muscular
dystrophy (DMD)
Doppler sonography, 425
dorsal, 27, 148, 151
dorsal cavity, 32
Duchenne muscular dystrophy
(DMD), 165
ductus deferens, 324
duodenal, 101, 103
duodenum, 91, 93
dwarfism. See acromegaly
dye. See contrast agent
dysentery, 101, 103
dyskinesia, 148, 151
dysmenorrhea, 333, 335
dyspepsia, 101, 103. Also see ulcers
dysphagia, 101, 103
dysphasia, 289, 291
dyspnea, 374, 376, 421. Also see
congestive heart failure
dystrophy, 148, 151
dysuria, 494, 497

E

ear, 262–263, 266–267
audiometry, 266–267
major structures of, 242
Ménière's disease, 262
myringotomy, 267
otitis media, 263
pain in middle ear. See otalgia
presbycusis, 263
ringing. See tinnitus
eating disorders, 112–113
ecchymosis, 55, 58, 148, 151
ecchymotic, 85
ECG. See electrocardiogram (ECG)
edema, 72, 75, 423. Also see
congestive heart failure
edematous. See varicose veins
EGD. See
sophagogastroduodenoscopy
EEG. See electroencephalogram
(EEG)
effusion. See myringotomy
electrocardiogram (ECG), 412, 414,
425
electrodes, 302
electroencephalogram (EEG), 299,
302
electromyogram (EMG), 148, 151,
170
ELISA test. See enzyme-linked
immunosorbent assay
(ELISA)
embolism, 296
EMG. See electromyogram (EMG)
encephalitis, 289, 291, 298–299
encephalomyelopathy, 289, 291
endocarditis, 17
endocrine system, 36, 444–481
anatomical diagram, 446, 448
breaking down and building
terms, 453–456
definition, 446
diseases and disorders, 462–466
major functions, 446
overview, 446–448
tests and procedures, 466–469
vocabulary, 447
word elements, 450–453
working with medical records, 473
endocrinologist, 446, 447, 454, 456
endocrinology, 446, 447, 454, 456
endocrinopathy, 454, 456
endometriosis, 333, 335, 344
endometrium, 344
endoscope, 116
endoscopy, 116
enteritis, 101, 103
enuresis, 504

enzyme-linked immunosorbent assay
(ELISA), 220
epidermal, 55, 58
epidermis, 46, 48, 55, 58
epididymis, 324, 326
epigastric, 16, 101, 103
epigastric region, 34
epilepsy, 299
epinephrine auto-injector. See
allergens
epithelial tissue, 46
eponym, 4
Epstein-Barr virus. See
mononucleosis
erythema, 70
erythematosus, 217
erythematous, 55, 58
erythematous skin. See psoriasis
erythrodermal, 56, 58
Escherichia coli, 504
esophageal, 101, 103
esophagogastroduodenoscopy, 101,
103, 116
esophagoscope, 116
esophagoscopy, 116
esophagus, 90–91, 93
estrogen, 324
etiology, 47, 48
exchange of gases, 366
exophthalmos. See Graves' disease
expiration, 366
external auditory meatus, 239, 240
external ear, 239
extraocular, 248, 252
exudate. See pneumonia
eye, 259–266
astigmatism, 259
blepharoplasty, 264
cataract, 260
clouding of the eye lens. See
cataract
diabetic retinopathy, 261
fluorescein angiography, 264
glaucoma, 261
LASIK, 265
macular degeneration, 261
major structures of, 241
presbyopia, 262
Snellen chart, 264
tonometry, 265–266
visual acuity test, 263–264
eye and ear, 236–277
anatomy and physiology
vocabulary, 239–243
breaking down and building
terms, 248–251
diseases and disorders, 259–263
ear, 239–240
eye, 238–239

overview of anatomy and physiology, 238
procedures and treatments, 263–267
special sensory organs, 236–277
word elements, 243
working with medical records, 271

F

fallopian tubes, 324
farsightedness, 259. *Also see* hyperopia
fasting, 467
fasting blood sugar (FBS) test, 466
female contraception, tubal ligation, 351
female-pattern baldness, 69
female reproductive system, 37
fever blisters, 72
fibula, 163
finger-to-nose test, 302
first-degree burns, 70
fixation. *See* spinal fusion
flank, 485, 486
fluorescein angiography, 264
fracture, 162
frequency, 485, 486
frontal plane, 25
full-thickness burns, 71

G

gangrene, 464
gastrectomy, 8
gastric bypass surgery, 117
gastritis, 101, 103
gastrodynia, 101, 103
gastroenterologist, 91, 93, 101, 103
gastroenterology, 7, 91, 93, 101, 103
gastroesophageal reflux disease (GERD), 110–111
gastroesophageal, 101
gastrointestinal (GI) tract, 90–91, 93
gastrology, 6
gastroscopy, 116
genital herpes, 345
GERD. *See* gastroesophageal reflux disease
gigantism. *See* acromegaly
gingivitis, 101, 103
glaucoma, 262
glossalgia, 101, 103
glucose meter, 465
glucose tolerance test (GTT), 467–468
glycemia, 454, 456
glycosuria, 494, 497
gonads, 324, 326
gonorrhea, 344

Graves' disease, 466
GTT. *See* glucose tolerance test (GTT)
gynecologist, 325, 333, 335
gynecology, 325, 333, 335

H

H. pylori, 114
hardening of the arteries. *See* arteriosclerosis
headache, recurring. *See* migraine headache
heart, 405
heart attack. *See* myocardial infarction (MI)
Helicobacter pylori (H. pylori), 113
helper T cells. *See* T lymphocytes, 197
hematemesis, 102, 103
hematoma, 56, 58
hematuria, 494, 497, 505
hemiplegia, 290, 291
hemodialysis, 510
hemorrhage, 413, 414
hemostasis, 413, 414
hemothorax, 374, 376
hepatitis, 102, 103, 112
hepatomegaly, 102, 103
herniated disk, 162–163
herpes, 72, 75
herpes simplex, 72
herpes simplex virus (HSV), 345
herpes simplex virus 1 (HSV-1), 72
herpes zoster, 72
hiatal hernia, 111
HIV infection, symptoms of, 215
HIV. *See* human immunodeficiency virus (HIV)
Hodgkin lymphoma, 218
Hodgkin's disease, 218
holter monitor, 425
homeostasis, 238, 280, 447
hormones, 446, 447
human immunodeficiency virus (HIV), 215
hydrocephalus, 290, 291
hydronephrosis, 494, 497, 505
hyperglycemia, 454, 456
hyperopia, 259
hyperpigmentation. *See* Addison's disease
hyperpnea, 374, 376
hypersecretion, 446
hypertension, 413, 414, 420
hyperthyroidism, 455, 456
hypertrophy, 148, 151, 413-414, 422
hypodermic, 56, 58
hypogastric region, 34
hypoglycemia, 455, 456
hypoliposis, 86

hypopnea, 374, 376
hyposecretion, 446
hypotension, 413, 414
hypothalamus, 281, 447
hypothyroidism, 455, 456, 466–467
hypotrichosis, 86
hysterectomy, 333, 335
hysterosalpingogram, 333, 335
hysterosalpingo-oophorectomy, 333, 335

I

ICD. *See* implantable cardioverter defibrillator (ICD)
idiopathic, 299
ileum, 91, 93
immune system, 197–198
immunization, 220
immunologist, 197, 198, 206, 208
immunology, 197, 198, 206, 208
implantable cardioverter defibrillator (ICD), 426
incision and drainage (I&D), 74
incontinence, 504
indwelling catheter. *See* urinary catheterization
infarct, 422
inferior, 27
inflammatory autoimmune disease. *See* multiple sclerosis
inflammatory bowel disease (IBD), 110
ingrown toenail, 74
inspiration, 366
insulin-dependent mellitus (IDDM), 464
integumentary, 46, 48
integumentary system, 36, 44–87
    anatomical diagram, 47, 49
    anatomy and physiology vocabulary, 48
    breaking down and building terms, 54–59
    diseases and disorders, 69–73
    main functions, 46
    major structures, 46–49
    medical records, 78–80
    overview, 46
    procedures and treatments, 73–76
    working with medical records, 78
intensity. *See* audiometry
intercostal, 148, 151
internal, 27
internal ear, 239–240
intervertebral, 148, 151
intestinal blockages, 115
intracystic, 85
intradermal, 56, 58
intragastric, 8

intraocular pressure (IOP). *See* glaucoma
intravenous pyelogram (IVP), 509
invasive, 342
involuntary muscle, 139
iridectomy, 249, 252
iridopexy, 249, 252
iridoplasty, 249, 252
iridoplegia, 249, 252
iris, 240
iritis, 249, 252
ischemia, 420

J

jejunum, 91, 93
joint, 139
joint effusion, 163
juvenile-onset diabetes, 464

K

keratometer, 249, 252
keratometry, 252
Kernig's sign, 303
kidney stones, 505 *See also* calculus
kidneys, 484, 486
kinesiology, 149, 151
kissing disease. *See* mononucleosis
knee injuries, 163–164
knee joint, injury. *See* ACL tear
kyphosis, 149, 151

L

lancet. *See* diabetes mellitus
laparoscope, 102, 103, 117, 221
laparoscopic hysterectomy, 349
laparoscopic splenectomy, 221
laparoscopy, 102, 103, 221, 333, 335
large intestine, 91, 93
laser eye surgery, 265
laser surgery, 74, 75
laser vision correction, 265
laser-assisted in situ keratomileusis (LASIK), 265
LASIK, 265
lateral, 27, 149, 151
lateral collateral ligament, 163
lateral epicondyle, 164
lateral epicondylitis, 164
lateral meniscus, 163
left hypochondriac region, 34
left iliac region, 34
left lower quadrant (LLQ), 33
left lumbar region, 34
left upper quadrant (LUQ), 33
lens, 240
leukocytes, 196
ligament, 139
lipocyte, 56, 58

lipoid, 56, 58
lipoma, 56, 58
lithotripsy, 494, 497
liver disease, 112
liver fibrosis, 112
lobule, 342
lordosis, 149, 151
lower gastrointestinal (LGI) series, 114
lumbar puncture (LP), 302
lungs, 366, 367
inflammatory disease affects. *See* sarcoidosis
lymph, 196, 198
lymphadenitis, 206, 208
lymphadenopathy, 206, 208
lymphadenosis, 206, 208
lymphangiopathy, 206, 208
lymphatic, 206, 208
lymphatic and immune systems, 194–235
anatomy and physiology vocabulary, 198–199
breaking down and building terms, 205–208
combining forms, 202–203
diseases and disorders, 215–219
overview, 196–201
word elements, 202
working with medical records, 225
lymphatic system, 37, 196, 199
anatomical diagram, 196, 200
major organs of, 200
lymphedema, 206, 208
lymph nodes, 73
lymphocyte, 196, 199, 206, 208
lymphocytoma, 206, 208
lymphoid, 206, 208
lymphoma, 206, 208
malignant. *See* Hodgkin's disease

M

macular area. *See* macular degeneration
macular degeneration, 261
magnetic resonance angiogram (MRA), 303
magnetic resonance imaging (MRI) scan, 167, 170–171, 299
male contraception, vasectomy, 350
male-pattern baldness, 69
male reproductive system, 37
malignancy, 56, 58
malignant, 71
malignant melanoma, 71, 75
mammary glands, 324
mammography, 333, 335, 343
Mantoux test, 388
mastectomy, 333, 335
McMurray test, 171

medial, 27
medial meniscus, 163
median plane, 25
medical abbreviations, anatomical terms of position, direction, location, 34–35
medical records, 78–80, 121–123, 176–178, 225–227, 271–272, 308–311, 355–357, 393–395, 430–432, 473–476, 514–517
medical terminology,
analyzing and breaking down terms, 14–17
analyzing and defining medical terms, 6–9
anatomical positions, planes, directions, and locations, 24–34
building plural forms, 21–22
introduction, 2–43
mastering, 37
medical word parts, 9–10
overview, 4–6
pronunciation, 22–23
spelling medical terms, 24
medical word parts, 9–15
combining forms, 10–11, 15, 18, 51–52, 95, 141–142, 202–203, 244, 285–286, 329–330, 370–371, 408, 450–451, 489–490
prefixes, 9–10, 15, 18, 51, 94, 140, 202, 244, 285, 329, 370, 408, 450, 489
root words. *See* combining forms
suffixes, 11–15, 18, 52, 96, 142–144, 203, 245, 286–287, 330, 371, 409, 451, 490
medulla oblongata, 281
melanin, 47, 48
melanocytes, 46–48, 56, 58
melanoma, 56, 58
Mèniére's disease, 262
meningeal, 290, 291
meninges, 281
meningitis, 290, 291, 299
meniscus, 139, 163–164
meniscus tears. *See* knee injuries
menorrhagia, 334
menorrhea, 334, 335
MI. *See* myocardial infarction (MI)
micturition, 485, 486
midbrain, 281
middle ear, 239, 240
middle ear bacterial/viral infection. *See* otitis media
midsagittal plane, 25
migraine headache, 299
mono. *See* mononucleosis
mononucleosis, 218
MS. *See* multiple sclerosis (MS)

multiple sclerosis (MS), 218
muscle degeneration. *See* muscular dystrophy
muscle tissue, three types, 137
muscular disorders. *See* muscular dystrophy
muscular dystrophy, 165
muscular system, 36, 139
musculoskeletal system, 132–193
  anatomical diagram, 134–135
  anatomy and physiology vocabulary, 135–136
  breaking down and building terms, 146
  diseases and disorders, 162–167
  major structures of muscular system, 134
  major structures of skeletal system, 135
  overview, 134
  procedures and treatments, 168–172
  word elements, 140
  working with medical records, 176
myalgia, 149, 151
myasthenia, 149, 151
mycotic, 17, 56, 58
myelogram, 290, 291
myitis, 149, 151
myocardial, 413, 414
myocardial infarction (MI), 422, 424
myocardial ischemia, 420
myopia, 259
myringectomy, 249, 252
myringitis, 249, 252
myringoplasty, 249, 252
myringotomy, 249, 252, 267
myxedema. *See* cretinism

N

nearsightedness. *See* myopia
necrogenic, 86
necrosis, 149, 151
necrotic, 56, 58
needle biopsy, 73
nephrectomy, 494, 497
nephritis, 494, 497
nephrolithiasis, 494, 497, 505
nephroma, 494, 497
nephrons, 484, 486
nephropexy, 494, 497
nephroplasty, 494, 497
nephroptosis, 495, 497
nephrorrhaphy, 495, 497
nephrostomy, 495, 497
nephrotomy, 497
nervous system, 36, 278–321
  anatomical diagram, 280, 283
  anatomy and physiology vocabulary, 282–284

  breaking down and building terms, 289–291
  definition, 280, 282
  diseases and disorders, 296–300
  functions and structures, 280–282
  major parts of brain, 284
  major structures, 283
  overview, 280
  procedures and treatments, 300–303
  word elements, 285
  working with medical records, 308
neural, 290, 291
neuralgia, 290, 291
neurologist, 282, 290, 291
neurology, 282, 290, 291
neurons, 281–282
neuropathy, 290, 291
neurotransmitters, 282
NIDDM. *See* diabetes mellitus
NMI. *See* nuclear imaging (NMI) test
nocturia, 342, 495, 497
non-insulin-dependent mellitus (NIDDM), 464
noninvasive, 342
nonspecific immunity, 197, 199
nuclear imaging (NMI) test, 168–169

O

obstructive sleep apnea, 386
ocular, 249, 252
oculomycosis, 249, 252
oliguria, 495, 497
onychectomy, 56, 58, 74, 75
onychocryptosis, 74
onychoma, 56, 58
onychomycosis, 56, 58, 74
onychosis, 56, 58
onychotomy, 56, 58
oophorectomy, 334, 335
ophthalmic, 249, 252
ophthalmologist, 250, 252
ophthalmology, 16, 250, 252
ophthalmoscope, 250, 252
optic, 250, 252
optic nerve, 239, 240
optic nerve damage. *See* glaucoma
orchidectomy, 334, 335
organomegaly, 102, 103
orology, 334
oropharynx, 102, 103
orthopedics, 139
oscilloscope, 170
ossicles, 239, 241
osteoarthritis, 149, 151
osteochondritis, 149, 151
osteomalacia, 149, 151
osteomyelitis, 149, 151, 165–166
osteonecrosis, 149, 151
osteopathy, 149, 151

osteopenia, 149, 151
osteoporosis, 149, 151, 166–167
otalgia, 250, 252, 263
otitis, 250, 252
otitis media, 263
otologist, 250, 252
otology, 250, 252
otomycosis, 250, 252
otoplasty, 250, 252
otorrhea, 250, 252
otoscope, 250, 252
otoscopy, 250, 252
ova, 324
ovaries, 324, 326, 447

P

pacemaker, 426
palpate, 348
pancreas, 447
pancreatography, 102, 103
pap smear, 349
pap test, 349
paraneural, 16
paraocular, 250, 252
parathyroid glands, 447
Parkinson's disease, 300
partial-thickness burn, 70
patellofemoral groove, 163
pathogen, 196, 199
pathogenic, 206, 208
pathologist, 47, 48, 57, 58, 206, 208
pathology, 206, 208
pelvic cavity, 32
pelvic inflammatory disease (PID), 345
penis, 324, 326
peptic ulcer. *See* ulcers
percutaneous, 57, 58
pericarditis, 413, 414
periocular, 250, 252
peripheral nervous system (PNS), 280, 282
peritoneal dialysis, 510
peritoneal membrane, 510
periurethral, 495, 497
PFT. *See* pulmonary function test (PFT)
phagocyte, 197, 199, 206, 208
phagocytic, 207, 208
pharyngitis, 375, 376. *Also see* mononucleosis
pharynx, 91, 93, 219, 366–367
phlebitis, 413, 414
physical therapy (PT), 171
PID. *See* pelvic inflammatory disease (PID)
pineal gland, 281, 447
pituitary gland, 447
plaque, 420
pleura, 367

pleural effusion, 386, 388
PMS. *See* premenstrual syndrome (PMS)
pneumonia, 375, 376, 382
pneumonocentesis, 375, 376
pneumothorax, 375, 383
PNS. *See* peripheral nervous system (PNS)
polydipsia, 455, 456, 495, 497
polyphagia, 455, 456
polyposis, 102, 103
polyps, 115
polyuria, 455, 456
pons, 281
posterior, 27, 150, 151
posterior (dorsal), 24
posterior cruciate ligament, 163
posteroanterior, 27
PPD skin test, 388
prefixes, 9–10, 15, 18, 51, 94, 140, 202, 244, 285, 329, 370, 408, 450, 489
premenstrual syndrome (PMS), 345
presbycusis, 263
presbyopia, 262
proctoplasty, 102, 103
progesterone, 324
prognosis, 47, 48
prolapsed bladder, 506
prone, 27
prostate cancer, 345–346
prostate gland, 324, 326
prostatectomy, 334, 335
prostatic, 334, 335
prostatitis, 334, 335
proximal, 27
pruritic, 57, 58
psoriasis, 72–73, 75
psychology, 290, 291
PT. *See* physical therapy
pulmonary function test (PFT), 388
pulmonary infection. *See* sensitivity test
pulmonologist, 367, 376
pulmonology, 367, 375, 376
pupil, 238, 241
pustule, 69
pyelitis, 504
pyelogram, 495, 497
pyelonephritis, 495, 497, 504, 505
pyelonephrosis, 495, 497
pyogenic, 57, 58
pyonephritis, 495, 497
pyorrhea, 57, 58
pyuria, 495, 497, 504

Q

quadriplegia, 150, 151, 290, 291
quadrants of the abdomen, 33

R

RA. *See* rheumatoid arthritis (RA)
radiculitis, 290, 291
radiopaque contrast agent, 301
rales. *See* croup
rectoscope, 102, 103
rectum, 91, 93
red rash on face. *See* erythematosus
reflex, 300
refractive errors. *See* astigmatism
renal calculi. *See* kidney stone
renal colic, 485, 486, 505
renal dialysis, 510
renal pelvis, 484, 486
renal scan, 509
renal sonogram, 510
renal ultrasound, 510
reproductive systems,
    anatomy and physiology vocabulary, 326
    breaking down and building terms, 332–334
    diseases and disorders, 342–346
    female anatomical diagram, 325, 327
    male anatomical diagram, 324, 327
    male and female, 322–363
    overview, 324–325
    procedures and treatments, 347–351
    word elements, 328
    working with medical records, 355
resectoscope, 350
respiratory system, 36, 364–401
    anatomical diagram, 366, 368
    anatomy and physiology vocabulary, 367
    breaking down and building terms, 373
    diseases and disorders, 382–386
    functions, 367
    gas exchange, 367
    overview, 366–369
    procedures and treatments, 386–389
    protection, 367
    regulation of acid-base (pH) levels, 367
    word elements, 369
    working with medical records, 393
rest, ice, compression, and elevation (RICE), 172
retina, 239, 241
retinal, 251, 252
retinitis, 251, 252
rheumatoid arthritis (RA), 217
rhinitis, 375, 376
RICE, 172

right hypochondriac region, 34
right iliac region, 34
right lower quadrant (RLQ), 33
right lumbar region, 34
right upper quadrant (RUQ), 33
Romberg sign. *See* Romberg test
Romberg test. *See* Romberg's sign
Romberg's sign, 303
root words, 10–11. *See also* combining forms
rotator cuff tear, 167

S

sagittal plane, 25
salpingitis, 334, 335
sarcoidosis, 218–219
scalp hair, acute loss. *See* alopecia
schizotrichia, 57, 58
sclera, 239, 241, 252
scleral, 251
scleritis, 251, 252
sclerotomy, 251, 252
scoliosis, 150, 151
scratch test, 220
scrotum, 324, 326
sebaceous, 46, 48
sebaceous glands. *See* acne
seborrhea, 57, 58
seborrheic, 85
sebum, 46, 48
second-degree burns, 70
seizures. *See* epilepsy
semicircular canals, 239, 241
seminal vesicles, 324, 326
sensitivity test, 388, 507
sensory ataxia, 303
sensory organs
    anatomy and physiology vocabulary, 240–241
    breaking down and building terms related to eye and ear, 248
    diseases and disorders
        ear, 262–263
        eye, 259–262
    ear, anatomical diagram, 240, 242
    eye, anatomical diagram, 239, 241
    eye and ear, 236–277
    overview, 238
    procedures and treatments
        ear, 266–267
        eye, 263–266
    word elements, 243
    working with medical records, 271
sexually transmitted infection (STI), 343
sexually transmitted infections, chlamydia, 343–344

genital herpes, 345
gonorrhea, 344
syphilis, 346
Shaken Baby Syndrome, 298
shingles, 72
sialorrhea, 102, 103
sigmoid, 91, 93
sigmoid colon, 91
sigmoidoscopy, 102, 103, 116
simple fracture. *See* fracture
skeletal system, 36, 139
skeletal system, major bones of, 138
skin cancer, 71
skin cancer. *See* malignant
    melanoma
SLE. *See* systemic lupus
    erythematosus (SLE)
sleep apnea. *See* obstructive sleep
    apnea
slipped disk, 163
slit lamp. *See* tonometry
small intestine, 91, 93
Snellen chart, 264
sound waves. *See* Doppler
    sonography
specific immunity, 199
speculum, 349
sperm, 324, 326
sphincter muscles, 484
spinal cavity, 32
spinal disks, 162
spinal fusion, 172
spinal tap. *See* lumbar puncture
spirometer, 375, 376, 388
spleen, 197, 199
splenectomy, 207, 208, 221
splenic, 207, 208
splenitis, 207, 208
splenoid, 207, 208
splenoma, 207, 208
splenomalacia, 207, 208
splenomegaly, 207, 208
splenopexy, 207, 208
splenorrhaphy, 207, 208
spondylarthritis, 150, 151
spondylodesis, 150, 151, 172
spondylolysis, 150, 151
spondylosis, 150, 151
sprain, 172
sputum, 383
sputum culture and sensitivity (C&S)
    test, 388
squamous, 57, 58
staging, 343
STI. *See* sexually transmitted
    infection (STI)
stenotic, 413, 414, 420
sternal, 150, 151
sternocostal, 150, 151
stimulus, 300

stoma. *See* colostomy
stomach, 90, 91, 93
stomach acid. *See* gastroesophageal
    reflux disease
stomach protrudes through
    abdomen. *See* hiatal hernia
strain, 172
Streptococcus, 219
striae, 464
stroke. *See* cerebral vascular attack
    (CVA)
subcostal, 150, 151
subcutaneous, 47, 48, 57
subdermal, 85
sudoriferous, 46, 48
suffixes, 11–15, 18, 52, 96, 142–144,
    203, 245, 286–287, 330, 371,
    409, 451, 490
    definition, 11
    general rules for use of, 13–14
superior, 27
supine, 27
suprapharyngeal, 16
synaptic cleft, 282
synkinesis, 150, 151
synovial compartment of joint. *See*
    joint effusion
syphilis, 346
systemic autoimmune disease. *See*
    rheumatoid arthritis,
systemic lupus erythematosus (SLE),
    217

T

T cells. *See* T lymphocytes
T lymphocytes, 197
tachycardia, 17, 413, 414
tachypnea, 375, 376
TB skin test, 388
tendinitis, 150, 151
tendon, 139
tennis elbow. *See* lateral epicondylitis
testes, 324, 326, 447
testicles, 324
testosterone, 324
thalamus, 281
third-degree burns, 71
thoracentesis, 389
thoracic cavity, 32
thrombophlebitis, 413, 414
thrombosis, 413, 414
thrombus, 296
thymectomy, 207, 208, 455, 456
thymic, 207, 208, 455, 456
thymoma, 207, 208, 455, 456
thymus, 197, 199
thymus gland, 197, 447
thyroid gland, 447
thyroid scan, 468

thyroidectomy, 455, 456
thyroiditis, 455, 456
thyroid-stimulating hormone (TSH),
    469
thyroid-stimulating hormone test,
    468–469
thyromegaly, 455, 456
thyroxine test, 469
TIA. *See* transient ischemic attack
    (TIA)
tinnitus, 262
tone. *See* audiometry
tonometry, 265–266
tonsillar, 207, 208
tonsillectomy, 207, 208, 221
tonsillitis, 207, 208, 219
tonsils, 196, 199
tonsils and throat, symptoms of
    tonsillitis, 219
tonsils, inflammation. *See* tonsillitis
topical, 57
trachea, 366–367
tracheal, 375, 376
tracheitis, 375, 376
tracheostenosis, 375, 376
tracheotomy, 375, 376
transcutaneous, 85
transdermal, 57
transient ischemic attack (TIA), 300
transport of oxygen, 366
transurethral resection of the
    prostate (TURP), 350
transverse colon, 92
transverse plane, 26
traumatic brain injury (TBI), 297
trichoid, 86
trichomycosis, 57, 58
TSH test. *See* thyroid-stimulating
    hormone test
tubal ligation, 351
tuberculin skin test, 388
TURP. *See* transurethral resection of
    the prostate
tympanectomy, 251, 252
tympanic, 251, 252
tympanic membrane, 239, 241, 267
tympanometer, 251, 252
tympanometry, 251, 252
tympanoplasty, 251, 252, 267
tympanorrhexis, 251, 252
tympanostomy, 251, 252, 267
type 1 diabetes, 464
type 1 diabetes mellitus, 464
type 2 diabetes, 465
type 2 diabetes mellitus, 465

U

UGI. *See* upper gastrointestinal
    (UGI) series

ulcers, 113–114
umbilical region, 34
underactive thyroid. *See* hypothyroidism
upper arm inflammation of lateral part. *See* lateral epicondylitis
upper gastrointestinal (UGI) series, 117
upper GI and small bowel series, 117
urea, 506
uremia, 495, 497, 506
ureter, 486
ureterolithiasis, 496, 497, 505
ureteropyelonephritis, 496, 497
ureterostenosis, 496, 497
ureterovesicostomy, 496, 497
ureters, 484
urethra, 324, 326, 484, 486
urethral, 496, 497
urethralgia, 496, 497
urethritis, 344, 594
urethrocystitis, 496, 497
urethroscope, 496, 497
urinalysis (UA), 507
urinary bladder, 484
urinary catheterization, 508
urinary incontinence, 504
urinary meatus, 484, 486
urinary retention, 342, 505
urinary system, 37, 482–527
   anatomical diagram, 485, 487
   anatomy and physiology vocabulary, 485–486
   breaking down and building terms, 493
   diseases and disorders, 504–507
   main functions, 484

   major organs and structures, 484–485
   overview, 484
   procedures and treatments, 507–510
   word elements, 488
   working with medical records, 514
urinary tract, 325, 484
urinary tract infection (UTI), 504
urination, 485, 486
urine, 486
urogram, 496, 497. *See also* intravenous pyelogram
urological, 485
urologist, 325, 334, 335, 485, 486, 496, 497
urology, 325, 335, 485, 486, 496, 497
uterine tubes, 324, 326
uterus, 324, 326
UTI. *See* urinary tract infection (UTI)
UV damage, 71
UVA rays, 71
UVB rays, 71
uvula, 219

V

V/Q scan, 389
vaccination, 220
vaccine, 220
vagina, 324, 326
vaginitis, 334, 335
varicose veins, 423
vas deferens, 324, 326
vasculitis, 150, 151
vasectomy, 334, 335, 350

veins, 404, 405
venipuncture, 467
venous, 413, 414
ventilation, 366
ventilation/perfusion scan (VPS), 389
ventral, 27
ventral cavity, 32
venules, 404
vertebrae, 162
vertebral, 150–151
vertebral cavity, 32
vertebral column, 281
vertebral disk, rupture. *See* herniated disk
vertebral disks. *See* spinal disks
vertebrectomy, 150, 151
vertigo, 262
vesicocele, 507
viral infection. *See* mononucleosis
vision blurred. *See* astigmatism
visual acuity test, 263–264
voiding, 485, 486
voluntary muscle, 139

W

weight-loss surgery. *See* gastric bypass surgery
Western blot test, 220–221
whitehead, 69
word parts. *See* medical word parts

X

xeroderma, 57, 58